Clinico Radiological Series
SINONASAL IMAGING

Clinico Radiological Series
SINONASAL IMAGING

Editors

Ashu Seith Bhalla MD MAMS FICR
Professor
Department of Radiodiagnosis
All India Institute of Medical Sciences
New Delhi, India

Manisha Jana MD DNB FRCR
Associate Professor
Department of Radiodiagnosis
All India Institute of Medical Sciences
New Delhi, India

Co-Editor

Smita Manchanda MD DNB MNAMS
Assistant Professor
Department of Radiodiagnosis
All India Institute of Medical Sciences
New Delhi, India

Surgical contents edited by
Suresh C Sharma MS
Professor and Head
Department of Otorhinolaryngology and Head & Neck Surgery
All India Institute of Medical Sciences
New Delhi, India

Foreword
Niranjan Khandelwal MD Dip NBE FICR FAMS

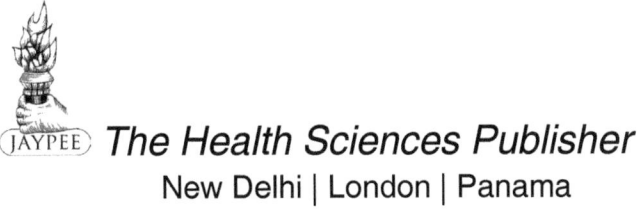

JAYPEE *The Health Sciences Publisher*
New Delhi | London | Panama

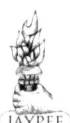
Jaypee Brothers Medical Publishers (P) Ltd

Headquarters
Jaypee Brothers Medical Publishers (P) Ltd.
4838/24, Ansari Road, Daryaganj
New Delhi 110 002, India
Phone: +91-11-43574357
Fax: +91-11-43574314
E-mail: jaypee@jaypeebrothers.com

Overseas Offices

JP Medical Ltd.
83, Victoria Street, London
SW1H 0HW (UK)
Phone: +44-20 3170 8910
Fax: +44(0)20 3008 6180
E-mail: info@jpmedpub.com

Jaypee-Highlights Medical Publishers Inc.
City of Knowledge, Bld. 235, 2nd Floor, Clayton
Panama City, Panama
Phone: +1 507-301-0496
Fax: +1 507-301-0499
E-mail: cservice@jphmedical.com

Jaypee Brothers Medical Publishers (P) Ltd.
17/1-B, Babar Road, Block-B, Shyamoli
Mohammadpur, Dhaka-1207
Bangladesh
Mobile: +08801912003485
E-mail: jaypeedhaka@gmail.com

Jaypee Brothers Medical Publishers (P) Ltd.
Bhotahity, Kathmandu, Nepal
Phone: +977-9741283608
E-mail: kathmandu@jaypeebrothers.com

Website: www.jaypeebrothers.com
Website: www.jaypeedigital.com

© 2018, Jaypee Brothers Medical Publishers

The views and opinions expressed in this book are solely those of the original contributor(s)/author(s) and do not necessarily represent those of editor(s) of the book.

All rights reserved. No part of this publication may be reproduced, stored or transmitted in any form or by any means, electronic, mechanical, photocopying, recording or otherwise, without the prior permission in writing of the publishers.

All brand names and product names used in this book are trade names, service marks, trademarks or registered trademarks of their respective owners. The publisher is not associated with any product or vendor mentioned in this book.

Medical knowledge and practice change constantly. This book is designed to provide accurate, authoritative information about the subject matter in question. However, readers are advised to check the most current information available on procedures included and check information from the manufacturer of each product to be administered, to verify the recommended dose, formula, method and duration of administration, adverse effects and contraindications. It is the responsibility of the practitioner to take all appropriate safety precautions. Neither the publisher nor the author(s)/editor(s) assume any liability for any injury and/or damage to persons or property arising from or related to use of material in this book.

This book is sold on the understanding that the publisher is not engaged in providing professional medical services. If such advice or services are required, the services of a competent medical professional should be sought.

Every effort has been made where necessary to contact holders of copyright to obtain permission to reproduce copyright material. If any have been inadvertently overlooked, the publisher will be pleased to make the necessary arrangements at the first opportunity. The **CD/DVD-ROM** (if any) provided in the sealed envelope with this book is complimentary and free of cost. **Not meant for sale.**

Inquiries for bulk sales may be solicited at: jaypee@jaypeebrothers.com

Clinico Radiological Series: Sinonasal Imaging

First Edition: **2018**

ISBN: 978-93-5270-171-1

Dedicated to

All those who motivated us to write the book—
Now read it!

Contributors

Adarsh W Barwad MD
Assistant Professor
Department of Pathology
All India Institute of Medical Sciences
New Delhi, India

Ajay Garg MD DM
Professor
Department of Neuroradiology
All India Institute of Medical Sciences
New Delhi, India

Alok Thakkar MS DNB FRCS
Professor
Department of Otorhinolaryngology and
Head & Neck Surgery
All India Institute of Medical Sciences
New Delhi, India

Ankur Goyal MD DNB MNAMS
Assistant Professor
Department of Radiodiagnosis
All India Institute of Medical Sciences
New Delhi, India

Anuj Prabhakar MD DM
Assistant Professor
Department of Neuroradiology
All India Institute of Medical Sciences
New Delhi, India

Arvind Kumar Kairo MS
Assistant Professor
Department of Otorhinolaryngology and
Head & Neck Surgery
All India Institute of Medical Sciences
New Delhi, India

Ashu Seith Bhalla MD MAMS FICR
Professor
Department of Radiodiagnosis
All India Institute of Medical Sciences
New Delhi, India

Asit R Mridha MD
Associate Professor
Department of Pathology
All India Institute of Medical Sciences
New Delhi, India

Atin Kumar MD MNAMS FICR
Professor
Department of Radiodiagnosis
All India Institute of Medical Sciences
New Delhi, India

Chandrashekhara SH MD DNB MNAMS
Associate Professor
Department of Radiodiagnosis
All India Institute of Medical Sciences
New Delhi, India

Chirom Amit Singh MS
Associate Professor
Department of Otorhinolaryngology and
Head & Neck Surgery
All India Institute of Medical Sciences
New Delhi, India

David Victor Kumar Irugu MS
Assistant Professor
Department of Otorhinolaryngology and
Head & Neck Surgery
All India Institute of Medical Sciences
New Delhi, India

Deepali Jain MD DNB FIAC
Associate Professor
Department of Pathology
All India Institute of Medical Sciences
New Delhi, India

Devasenathipathy Kandasamy
MD DNB FRCR
Associate Professor
Department of Radiodiagnosis
All India Institute of Medical Sciences
New Delhi, India

Dodul Mondal MD DNB MNAMS
Consultant Radiation Oncology
Dharamshila Narayana
Super Speciality Hospital
New Delhi, India

Hitesh Verma MD DNB MNAMS
Assistant Professor
Department of Otorhinolaryngology and
Head & Neck Surgery
All India Institute of Medical Sciences
New Delhi, India

Jyoti Kumar MD DNB MNAMS
Professor
Department of Radiology and Imaging
Maulana Azad Medical College
New Delhi, India

Kapil Sikka MD DNB MNAMS
Associate Professor
Department of Otorhinolaryngology and
Head & Neck Surgery
All India Institute of Medical Sciences
New Delhi, India

Manisha Jana MD DNB FRCR
Associate Professor
Department of Radiodiagnosis
All India Institute of Medical Sciences
New Delhi, India

Mukesh Yadav MD
Assistant Professor
Department of Radiodiagnosis
All India Institute of Medical Sciences
New Delhi, India

Prem Sagar MS DNB MNAMS
Assistant Professor
Department of Otorhinolaryngology and
Head & Neck Surgery
All India Institute of Medical Sciences
New Delhi, India

Priyanka Naranje MD DNB MNAMS
Assistant Professor
Department of Radiodiagnosis
All India Institute of Medical Sciences
New Delhi, India

Rajeev Kumar MS DNB MNAMS
Assistant Professor
Department of Otorhinolaryngology and
Head & Neck Surgery
All India Institute of Medical Sciences
New Delhi, India

Rakesh Kumar MS
Professor
Department of Otorhinolaryngology and
Head & Neck Surgery
All India Institute of Medical Sciences
New Delhi, India

Shuchita Singh MS DNB MNAMS
Assistant Professor
Department of Otorhinolaryngology and
Head & Neck Surgery
All India Institute of Medical Sciences
New Delhi, India

Smita Manchanda MD DNB MNAMS
Assistant Professor
Department of Radiodiagnosis
All India Institute of Medical Sciences
New Delhi, India

Surabhi Vyas MD DNB MNAMS
Associate Professor
Department of Radiodiagnosis
All India Institute of Medical Sciences
New Delhi, India

Suresh C Sharma MS
Professor and Head
Department of Otorhinolaryngology and
Head & Neck Surgery
All India Institute of Medical Sciences
New Delhi, India

Foreword

Nose and Paranasal sinuses constitute one of the fundamental aspects of radiology of the Head and Neck, holding great importance for both practicing radiologists and surgeons due to the diverse clinical implications and behavior of lesions in this region. In addition, from a surgical point of view, this region has wide variation in anatomy, knowledge of which is essential prior to exploration in this area to avoid complications and therapeutic failure. Multiplanar imaging has revolutionized evaluation of this region and allows us far deeper understanding than was previously possible.

It is not unusual to find chronic complaints among patients with seemingly straightforward diagnosis, and this book addresses multiple such imaging dilemma, while giving a perspective on prognostication and management of described lesions, the so called 'way forward'.

This book has combined input from an expert team of dedicated radiologists from the All India Institute of Medical Sciences, along with Head and Neck surgeons and pathologists to give a truly multidisciplinary overview of the subject.

Lucid illustrations covering anatomical details complemented by succinct bulleted text make it immensely user-friendly and readable. Detailed description of pathology with a wide range of illustrative cases make it a comprehensive guide useful to all. In addition, a structured reporting format has been provided which is a must for the current generation due to the advent of functional endoscopic sinus surgery (FESS).

This book will serve as the 'one-stop' for residents and postgraduates of Radiology as well as Otorhinolaryngology, with its unique format and extensive coverage. In addition, it promises to benefit both practicing radiologists and clinicians, providing an overview of all aspects of sinus disease.

Niranjan Khandelwal MD Dip NBE FICR FAMS
Professor and Head
Department of Radiodiagnosis and Imaging
Postgraduate Institute of Medical Education and Research
Chandigarh, India

Preface

In clinical practice, it is not uncommon to find 'sinus' equated to 'sinusitis', an omniscient complaint responsible for much chronic morbidity among its victims. The paranasal sinuses are a group of complex structures with challenging anatomy, further showing diverse anatomical variation. A thorough knowledge of these variations and pathology affecting this region is therefore necessary, as subtle findings may sometimes confound even a trained eye.

All diseases of the paranasal sinuses are not sinusitis, and differentiation between what is benign vs more sinister disease is essential for optimal management and protection of adjacent critical structures—orbit and skull base.

Otorhinolaryngology and Head & Neck surgery is a rapidly expanding specialty which relies heavily on imaging. Therefore, radiologists practicing Head and Neck radiology need to adopt a systematic approach in reporting in order to provide a structured and comprehensive report to the surgeon. Likewise, especially in the era of endoscopic surgery, attention to detail is a must for surgeons in order to successfully negotiate the complex labyrinths of bony anatomy. For this purpose, this book contains a separate dedicated chapter on Functional Endoscopic Sinus Surgery (FESS) imaging.

This book is not intended to be a detailed text on sinus imaging but we hope that it will help the busy radiologists and surgeons in interpreting images of the paranasal sinuses. The variety of illustrative cases and proposed structured reporting format are aimed at this.

We welcome any feedback on enhancing the content of the book, which can be incorporated in the subsequent editions.

Ashu Seith Bhalla
Manisha Jana

Acknowledgments

We wish to thank all the contributors for their efforts in compiling this text. We sincerely thank Prof Suresh C Sharma for guiding us in this new endeavor. We are especially thankful to our Radiology colleagues without the help of whom this effort would not have been possible. We are also grateful to our colleagues from the Department of Otorhinolaryngology and Pathology for their contributions.

We would also like to extend our appreciation to Shri Jitendar P Vij (Group Chairman), Mr Ankit Vij (Group President), Ms Chetna Malhotra Vohra (Associate Director-Content Strategy), Mr Subrata Adhikary (Commissioning Editor), Ms Ritika Chandna (Development Editor), Mr Shakil (Proofreader) and all the staff of M/s Jaypee Brothers Medical Publishers, New Delhi, India, for their efforts and input enabling timely publication of the book.

Contents

SECTION 1: NORMAL ANATOMY AND IMAGING

1. **Imaging Modalities and Techniques**   3
   Devasenathipathy Kandasamy, Chandrashekhara SH

2. **Sinonasal Anatomy: Structure-wise**   14
   Jyoti Kumar, Ashu Seith Bhalla, Manisha Jana

3. **Sinonasal Anatomy: Section-wise**   41
   Jyoti Kumar

SECTION 2: INFLAMMATORY NASAL CONDITIONS

4. **Imaging in Rhinosinusitis (Inflammatory Diseases)**   57
   Ashu Seith Bhalla, Smita Manchanda

5. **Imaging in Polyps and Mucoceles**   77
   Smita Manchanda, Ashu Seith Bhalla

6. **Chronic Rhinosinusitis: Clinical Aspects**   94
   Arvind Kumar Kairo, Hitesh Verma

7. **Imaging in Fungal Sinusitis**   99
   Ashu Seith Bhalla, Smita Manchanda

8. **Fungal Diseases of Nose and Paranasal Sinuses: Surgical Aspects**   113
   Suresh C Sharma, Kapil Sikka

9. **Pre- and Post-Functional Endoscopic Sinus Surgery Imaging**   118
   Ankur Goyal, Ashu Seith Bhalla, Arvind Kumar Kairo

SECTION 3: TUMOR AND TUMOR-LIKE CONDITIONS

10. **Pathology of Sinonasal Lesions**   137
    Deepali Jain

11. **Pathology of Bony/Cartilaginous Sinonasal Tumors**   150
    Asit R Mridha, Adarsh W Barwad

12. **Benign Tumors of the Nose and Paranasal Sinuses: Imaging**   160
    Smita Manchanda, Ashu Seith Bhalla

13. **Benign Sinonasal Tumors: Surgical Perspective**   182
    Chirom Amit Singh, Suresh C Sharma

14. **Malignant Tumors of Sinonasal Cavities: Imaging**   188
    Mukesh Yadav, Devasenathipathy Kandasamy

15. **Malignant Tumors of Nose and Paranasal Sinuses: Surgical Perspective**   201
    Rajeev Kumar, Hitesh Verma

16. **Radiation and Chemotherapy in Management of Malignant Sinonasal Tumors**   209
    Dodul Mondal

SECTION 4: TRAUMA

17. **Imaging in Sinonasal Trauma**   219
    Manisha Jana, Ashu Seith Bhalla

18. **Imaging of Cerebrospinal Fluid Leaks**   236
    Atin Kumar, Ajay Garg

19. **Sinonasal Trauma and Cerebrospinal Fluid Rhinorrhea: Surgical Aspects**   249
    Kapil Sikka, Alok Thakkar

SECTION 5: CONGENITAL/PEDIATRIC DISEASES

20. **Pediatric Sinonasal Disorders: Imaging**   257
    Priyanka Naranje

21. **Pediatric Sinonasal Disorders: Surgical Perspective**   290
    Prem Sagar, Shuchita Singh

SECTION 6: SYSTEMIC DISORDERS/SURROUNDING STRUCTURES INVOLVING PNS

22. **Systemic Disorders Affecting Sinonasal Cavity**   301
    Surabhi Vyas, Ashu Seith Bhalla

23. **Anterior Skull Base Lesions: Imaging**   316
    Ajay Garg, Anuj Prabhakar

24. **Imaging of Dental Lesions and Sinonasal Cavity**   332
    Smita Manchanda, Ashu Seith Bhalla

25. **Imaging of Disorders Involving Sinonasal Cavity and Orbit** 348
    Ashu Seith Bhalla, Smita Manchanda

SECTION 7: CLINICO-RADIOLOGICAL APPROACH

26. **Approach to Nasal Obstruction** 361
    Rakesh Kumar, Ashu Seith Bhalla, Manisha Jana

27. **Approach to Epistaxis** 382
    David Victor Kumar Irugu, Manisha Jana, Ashu Seith Bhalla

28. **Imaging Approach to Sinus Lesions** 392
    Smita Manchanda, Ashu Seith Bhalla

Index 417

Section 1

Normal Anatomy and Imaging

1. Imaging Modalities and Techniques
2. Sinonasal Anatomy: Structure-wise
3. Sinonasal Anatomy: Section-wise

CHAPTER 1

Imaging Modalities and Techniques

Devasenathipathy Kandasamy, Chandrashekhara SH

- Introduction
- Imaging Modalities
  - Radiographs
  - CT Scan
- Multidetector Row Computed Tomography (MDCT)
- Cone Beam CT
  - MRI
  - F-18 FDG PET-CT

INTRODUCTION

- Paranasal sinuses (PNS) are air-filled structures located around the nasal cavity and formed with in the bones of the skull and face. The various functions are decreasing the weight of head, conditioning the inhaled air with moisture and heat and increasing the resonance of speech.
- There are four sets of sinuses on either sides namely, maxillary, frontal, ethmoid and sphenoid sinuses.
- Imaging of sinonasal pathology has evolved over the last three decades and advances in imaging have changed the way we look at diseases.
- The unprecedented detail in which the PNS and skull base anatomy are visualized in current generation imaging was not possible earlier.
- Parallel growth of new techniques and approaches, such as endoscopic and image guided surgeries have also increased the demand on imaging.
- Sinonasal inflammatory pathology is very common and usually secondary to infection or allergy.
- Most of them do not need imaging evaluation.
- There specific scenarios where imaging evaluation is indicated.
- American Academy of Otolaryngology-Head and Neck Surgery (AAO-HNS) published a consent statement in 2012 aiming to guide the choice of imaging in the evaluation of sinonasal diseases (Table 1.1).[1]

The consent statement also published the scenarios where imaging is not indicated:

- Uncomplicated sinusitis or upper respiratory tract infections.
- Responding to medical treatment.
- Children less than 3 years with uncomplicated acute sinusitis.

Table 1.1: Indications for imaging.	
S. No.	Indications
1.	Chronic sinusitis not responding to medical treatment
2.	Recurrent sinusitis
3.	Complication of sinusitis
4.	CSF rhinorrhea
5.	Invasive fungal sinusitis in immunocompromised individuals
6.	Tumor evaluation
7.	Preoperative planning for new or revision surgeries
8.	Complications of surgery

To prevent misuse of imaging modalities American College of Radiology (ACR) has published its ACR appropriateness criteria in 2013, which rates the usefulness of an imaging modality in a given situation.[2]

IMAGING MODALITIES

The imaging modalities which are used to evaluate sinonasal diseases are:
- Radiographs
- Computed tomography (CT)
  - Multidetector CT (MDCT)
  - Cone-beam CT (CBCT)
- Magnetic resonance imaging (MRI)
- F-18 FDG positron emission tomography (PET).

Radiographs

Plain radiographs were used to evaluate PNS before the advent of CT scans.

Techniques

- Standard four view sinus series include (Table 1.2):
  - Water's view (occipitomental) (Fig. 1.1)
  - Caldwell's view (occipitofrontal) (Fig. 1.2)
  - Lateral view (Fig. 1.3)
  - Submentovertical view.
- The above standard set of views provide good assessment of PNS (Figs. 1.4A to D). Amongst these Water's view is most frequently employed.
- Abnormalities manifest as opacification of sinuses, bone destruction, soft tissue or displacement of structures.
- However, the sensitivity and specificity of plain radiographs are poor compared to newer modalities which make it a less favored modality.
- In a properly exposed radiograph, PNS density is identical to orbital density.
- Erect or sitting position used during radiography of PNS to identify presence or absence of fluid and to differentiate fluid and thickening caused by other pathology.
- The recent AAO-HNS guidelines are also not in favor of using plain radiographs for the evaluation of sinusitis.[1]
- Currently, the utility of radiographs is very limited.

Table 1.2: Various radiographic views of paranasal sinuses (PNS).

Projection	Method/name	Technique	PNS visualized	Structures visualized
Lateral	R or L	Head in true lateral position	All paranasal sinuses	Integrity of the posterior antral bony margins Air-fluid level in the sphenoid sinus Sella turcica and nasopharynx are well seen
PA axial 15° (Occipitofrontal)	Caldwell	Radiographic baseline (OM line) is perpendicular to the bucky CR angled caudal 15°	Frontal and anterior ethmoidal sinuses	Best projection for examining the frontal and ethmoid sinuses in the frontal projection
Occipitomental	Water's Closed mouth	OM baseline or radiographic baseline 45° from horizontal CR perpendicular to IR	Maxillary sinuses	Evaluation of maxillary antra, roof of orbit, frontal sinus
Occipitomental	Water's Open mouth	OM baseline or radiographic baseline 45° from horizontal. Open mouth	Maxillary and sphenoidal sinuses	Better evaluate lower posterior sphenoid sinus
Submentovertical	Basal view	Infraorbitomeatal line is parallel to the IR and bucky	Ethmoidal and sphenoidal sinuses	Anterior and posterior walls of the frontal sinuses The lateral and medial walls of the maxillary antrum

(OM line: Orbitomeatal line; CR: Central ray; IR: Image receptor).

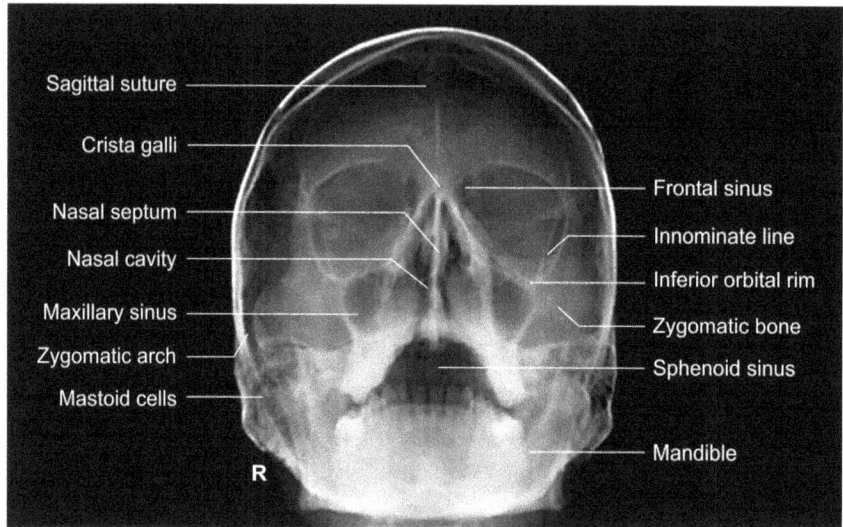

Fig. 1.1: Radiograph of paranasal sinuses (PNS)—Water's view.

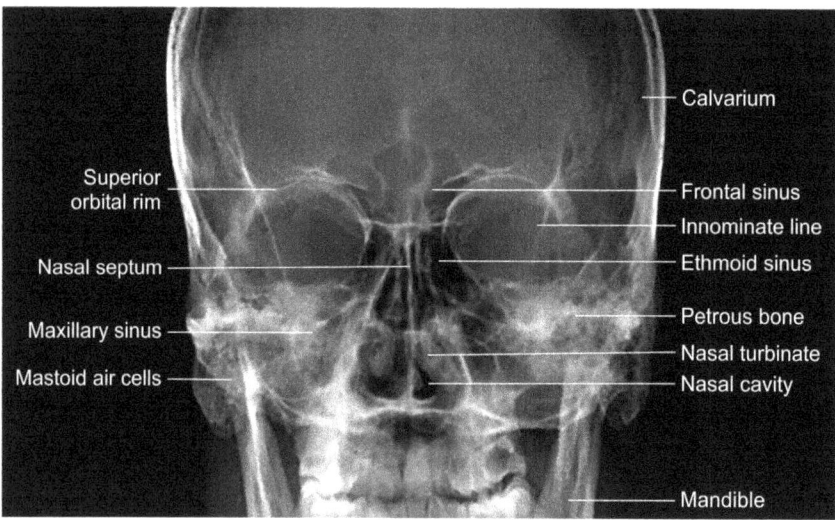

Fig. 1.2: Radiograph of paranasal sinuses (PNS)—Caldwell's view.

Chapter 1 Imaging Modalities and Techniques 7

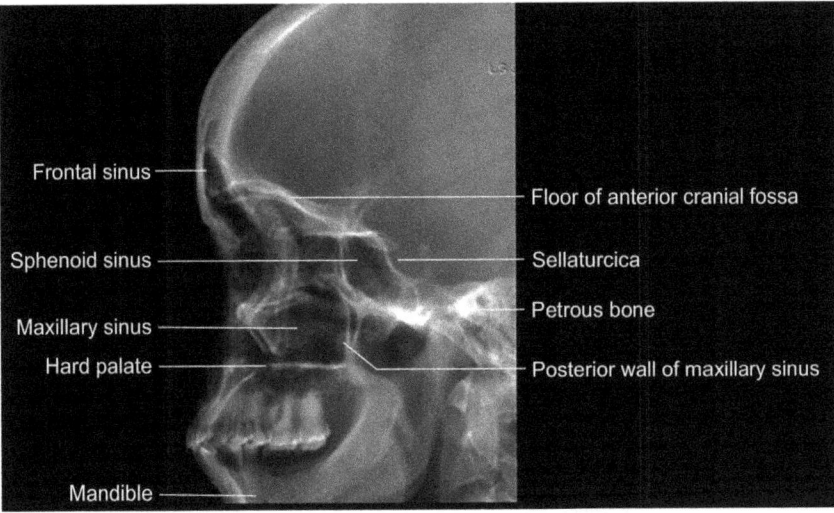

Fig. 1.3: Radiograph of paranasal sinuses (PNS)—Lateral view.

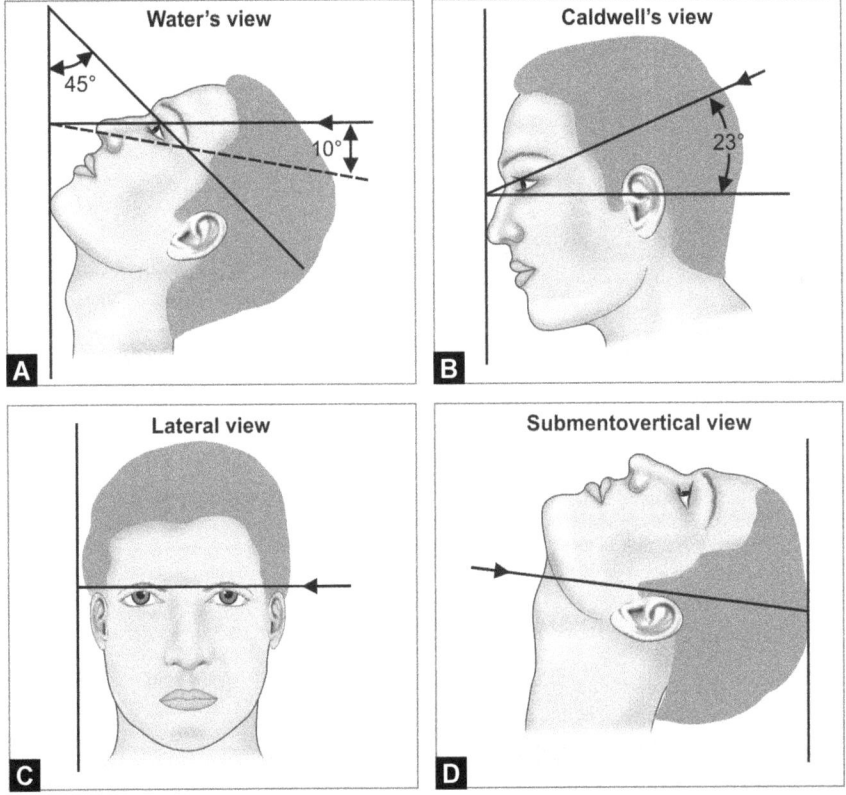

Figs. 1.4A to D: Schematic diagram of various radiographic views of paranasal sinuses (PNS).

CT Scan (Figs. 1.5A to C and Table 1.3)

- CT scan is the modality of choice and the workhorse for the evaluation of sinonasal diseases.
- The ability of CT scan to show the sinuses in much better detail coupled with good spatial resolution has practically replaced plain radiographs.
- Findings, such as sinus opacification, bone destruction, mucoperiosteal thickening and normal variations in the anatomy are not only valuable in the diagnostic point of view but also for the preoperative planning in these patients.

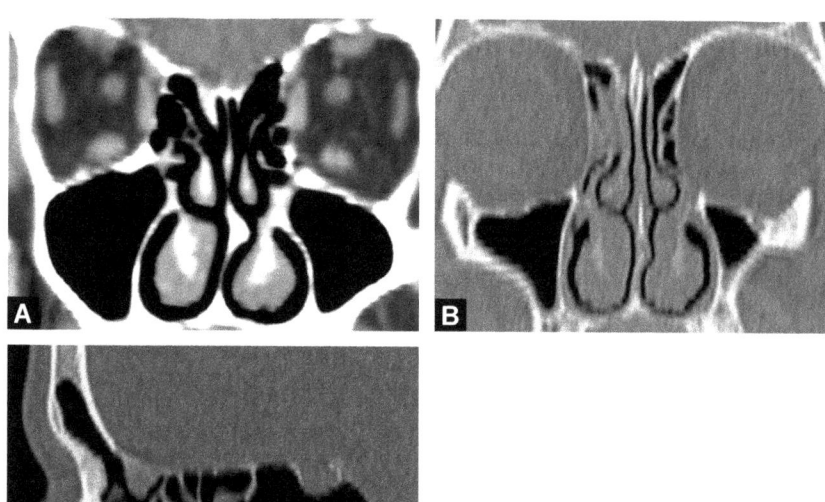

Figs. 1.5A to C: Computed tomography (CT) of paranasal sinuses (PNS). (A) Coronal soft tissue window; (B) Coronal bone window; and (C) Sagittal bone window sections used for PNS evaluation.

Table 1.3: Computed tomography (CT) techniques.
1. Axial plane: parallel to the infraorbitomeatal plane
2. Craniocaudal: Frontal sinus to hard palate
3. Tube current: 120 kVp, tube current modulation with quality reference mAs of 80
4. 0.6 mm acquisition with reconstruction of data into 1–3 mm sections in axial, coronal and sagittal planes
5. Bone windows: Width 3500, center 300
6. Soft tissue windows: Width 270, center 70
7. Sinus windows: Width 2000, center 400

Multidetector Row Computed Tomography (MDCT)

- *Role of MDCT*
  - Axial scanning avoids the extension of head
  - Lack of obscuration of important anatomy by spray artifact from dental restoration
  - Allow more refined reconstructions in other plane than the primary scan plane.
- *Role of Coronal Reconstructions*
  - Primary imaging orientation
  - Best shows osteomeatal unit
  - Relationship of ethmoid roof to brain
  - Correlate with surgical orientation.
- *Role of Sagittal Reconstructions*
  - Better visualization of frontal recess and frontal sinus, these are areas of persistent and recurrent sinus disease
  - Better show sphenoid sinus and basal lamella and agger nasi cell, contributing the safer and accurate endoscopic procedure.
- Whenever CT scan images are reviewed, it is best to visualize all three planes simultaneously and they must be linked. So that when the cursor is kept on any plane the other two planes will align accordingly to the same point of interest (Figs. 1.6A to D).

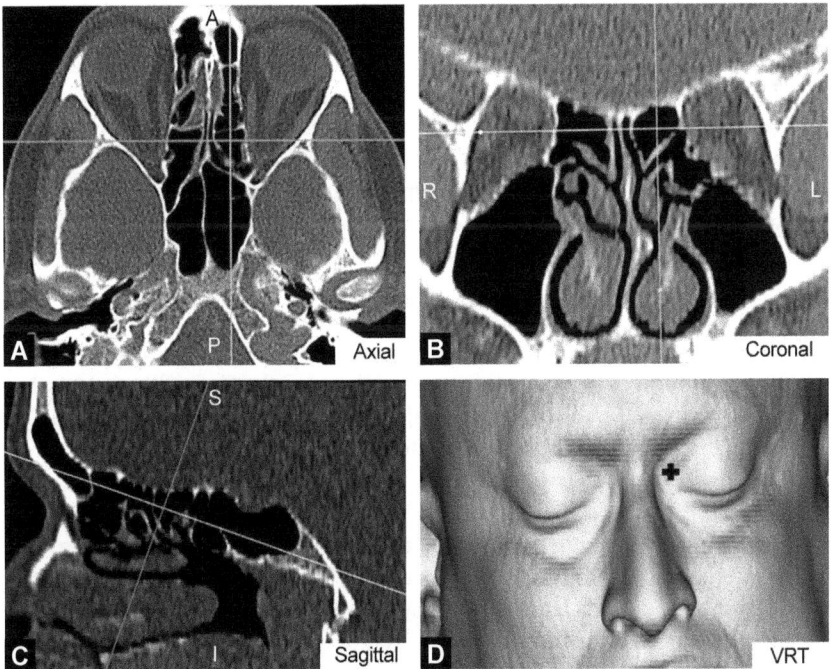

Figs. 1.6A to D: Reviewing method of CT images. Images are viewed in all three planes simultaneously and they are linked to each other. Wherever cursor or cross-hair is placed on an image the other planes align to that point automatically.

- Noncontrast CT (NCCT) is usually done for sinonasal inflammatory diseases unless there is a suspicion of extrasinus involvement. Contrast-enhanced CT (CECT) is generally recommended for the evaluation of tumors.
- Demonstration of the pathology or the normal structures in multiple planes, such as coronal (most important), axial and sometimes sagittal is crucial for the surgical point of view.
- Multiplanar reformations (MPR) were not possible in older CT scanners, hence direct acquisition of images in both axial and coronal planes were performed. The axial acquisition is done in supine position and coronal acquisition is usually done in prone position with hyperextension at neck. This doubled the radiation dose and increased artifacts due to motion (patient discomfort due to awkward positioning) and dental implants.
- With the advent of MDCT, scenario changed and with the capability of rapid thin section acquisition it is now possible to acquire the entire sinonasal region in seconds. Once the volume data is acquired images can be reformatted in any plane. This technique negates the limitations of older scans.
- The volume data can be post processed to generate various types of 3D images such as volume rendering technique (VRT), surface shaded display (SSD), etc.
- The major limitation of CT scan is the radiation dose involved in the process. Roughly a standard dose CT PNS gives four times radiation dose than a standard three set plain radiographs.[3] There are various methods available to reduce the radiation dose by maintaining the diagnostic quality. Two most important techniques which are widely used to reduce the radiation dose are—(1) tube current modulation, and (2) iterative reconstruction.
- Tube current modulation is a type of automatic exposure control in which the radiation dose is adjusted in accordance with the patient habitus, attenuation of body part and the desired image quality. The implementation of this technique varies with the vendors and it can bring down the radiation dose up to 60%.
- Iterative reconstruction is actually an older technique but the advances in computing have made it feasible only recently. Generally, it is added on to the existing filtered back projection method. It has the potential to bring down the radiation dose up to 85%.

Cone Beam CT

- CBCT is getting wide acceptance as a point of care imaging tool and it is compact, portable and cheap compared to main stream CT scanners.
- They use area detectors in contrast to multiple thin rows of detectors in conventional CT. The scanning of area of interest is completed in single rotation as compared to multiple rotations in conventional CT scanners (Table 1.4).
- Major advantages of CBCT compared to conventional CT are superior spatial resolution and lesser radiation dose.

Table 1.4: Advantages and disadvantages of cone-beam computed tomography (CBCT) compared to multidetector CT (MDCT).

Advantages	Disadvantages
• Excellent spatial resolution • Bony structures are shown in great detail • Lower radiation dose	• Poor contrast resolution due to increased scatter • Poor visualization of soft tissues • Poor temporal resolution • Limited Z-axis coverage • Lower dynamic range of the flat panel detectors • Contrast studies cannot be done

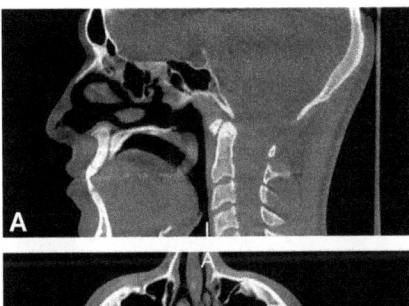
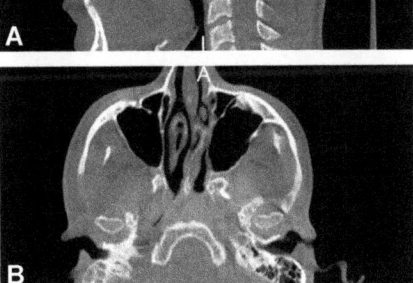
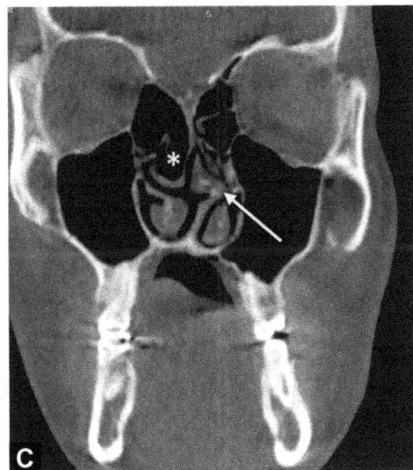

Figs. 1.7A to C: Cone-beam computed tomography (CBCT) images in all three planes (A to C) showing deviated nasal septum with bony spur (arrow) and concha bullosa (asterisk) on the right side. Note that CBCT images are good for bony structures and but soft tissues are not well-visualized.

- In spite of the above advantages it is currently not able to replace conventional CT for routine evaluation of sinonasal diseases because of various limitations.
- The contrast resolution and signal-to-noise ratio (SNR) is poor in CBCT which is because of scattering effect on area detectors. Hence, it is good in evaluating only the high contrast structures, such as bones (Figs. 1.7A to C).
- The lower dynamic range and poor temporal resolution of the flat panel detectors also pose major limitations.

MRI (Table 1.5)

- Although CT is the preferred modality in the evaluation of sinonasal diseases, MRI has its own place in many situations and it is used as a complementary modality to CT.
- The main advantages of MRI over CT are as follows:
  - Better contrast resolution and hence better characterization of soft tissues (differentiating tumor from secretions)

Table 1.5: Magnetic resonance (MR) planning.
1. Coronal, axial and sagittal images
2. Scan thickness 3–5 mm, interslice distance 1 mm
3. Routine sequence T1W and T2W
4. Contrast enhanced sequences (3D or 2D)
5. T2W/FLAIR sequence for brain
6. Fat suppressed used to evaluate complications of sinusitis or suspected neoplastic disease involve orbit and skull base

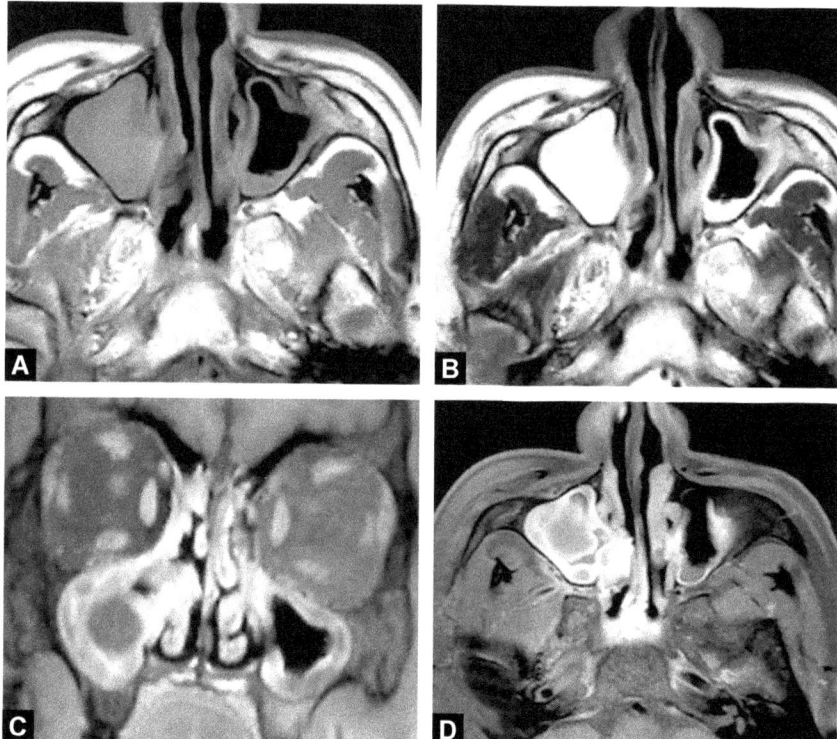

Figs. 1.8A to D: Magnetic resonance imaging (MRI) of paranasal sinuses (PNS) for sinusitis. (A and B) Axial T1W image and T2W image showing diffuse mucosal thickening in bilateral maxillary sinuses with hyperintense content. (C and D) Coronal and axial postcontrast T1W image revealing diffuse mucosal enhancement.

- Better evaluation of tumor spread outside the bony outline of sinuses
- Perineural spread of tumor is best visualized on MRI
- Spread of pathology in to orbit or cranium are also better evaluated on MRI.
- Apart from routine morphological imaging on MRI using T1 and T2 weighted sequences, there are functional imaging techniques, such as diffusion weighted imaging (DWI) and perfusion imaging which can evaluate newer paradigms (Figs. 1.8 and 1.9).

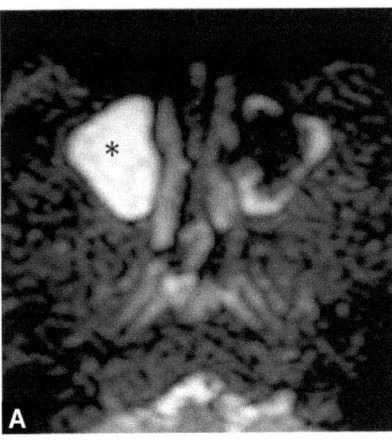 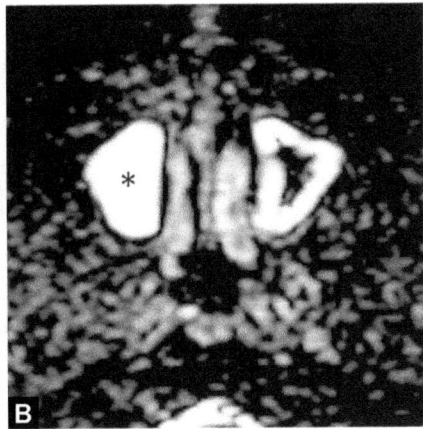

Figs. 1.9A and B: Diffusion weighted MRI in sinusitis. Diffusion weighted MRI (b value 0) image showing hyperintense bilateral maxillary sinus mucosal thickening (asterisk on A), which on corresponding ADC image showing hyperintensity (asterisk on B) suggesting facilitated diffusion.

- Although there are overlapping features on DWI and perfusion imaging to differentiate benign and malignant lesions, they can be a valuable addition nonetheless.

F-18 FDG PET-CT

- PET-CT is another complementary modality mainly reserved for patients with malignant sinonasal masses to look for metastasis.
- It is also used to look for postoperative residual or recurrent lesions in patients with malignancy.

CONCLUSION

Imaging is not indicated in vast majority of cases of inflammatory lesions of sinus. However, imaging plays a vital role in the diagnosis, preoperative evaluation and intraoperative guidance for surgeons in neoplastic, traumatic, developmental and specific situations in inflammatory conditions. CT is the workhorse in the evaluation of pathology complemented by MRI. With the ever-growing technical advancements in imaging, the value it adds to the management of patient is becoming indispensable.

REFERENCES

1. Setzen G, Ferguson BJ, Han JK, et al. Clinical consensus statement: Appropriate use of computed tomography for paranasal sinus disease. Otolaryngol-Head Neck Surg. 2012;147(5):808-16.
2. Cornelius RS, Martin J, Wippold FJ, et al. ACR Appropriateness Criteria Sinonasal Disease. J Am Coll Radiol. 2013;10(4):241-6.
3. Abul-Kasim K, Strömbeck A, Sahlstrand-Johnson P. Low-dose computed tomography of the paranasal sinuses: radiation doses and reliability analysis. Am J Otolaryngol. 2011;32(1):47-51.

2
CHAPTER

Sinonasal Anatomy: Structure-wise

Jyoti Kumar, Ashu Seith Bhalla, Manisha Jana

- Introduction
- Anatomy of Nasal Cavity
- Anatomical Variants of Nasal Cavity
  - Nasal Septum
  - Nasal Turbinates
- Anatomy of Frontal and Anterior Ethmoidal Sinuses
  - Frontal Sinus
    - Frontal Sinus Ostium
    - Frontal Beak or Frontonasal Process of Maxilla
    - Frontal Recess
    - Frontal Sinus Drainage Pathway
    - Frontoethmoidal Cells
    - International Frontal Sinus Anatomy Classification
  - Ethmoid Sinuses
    - Anterior Ethmoidal Air Cells
- Other Anatomic Variants in Frontal and Ethmoidal Sinus Cells
- Anatomy of Maxillary Sinus
- Anatomical Variants of Maxillary Sinus
- Anatomy of Osteomeatal Unit (OMU)
  - Anatomy of Uncinate Process
- Anatomical Variants of Uncinate Process, Ethmoid Infundibulum and Maxillary Ostium
- Anatomy of Lamina Papyracea (LP) and Anterior Ethmoidal Artery
- Anatomical Variants of LP
- Anatomy of Olfactory Fossa and Median Anterior Skull Base (ASB)
- Anatomic Variants of ASB
- Anatomy of Posterior Ethmoid Air Cells
- Anatomic Variants of Posterior Ethmoid Cells
- Anatomy of Sphenoid Sinus and Median Central Skull Base (CSB)
- Anatomic Variants of CSB
- Relevant Orbital Anatomy

INTRODUCTION

Sinonasal cavity includes the nose, nasal cavity and paranasal sinuses including frontal, ethmoid, maxillary and sphenoid sinuses.
- *Nose* refers to the part projecting above the mouth, containing the nostrils, and used for breathing and smelling.
- *Nasal cavity* refers to is a large air filled space above and behind the *nose* in the middle of the face.

- *Paranasal sinuses* are mucosa-lined air filled spaces located within the facial/calvarial bones.
- Mucosa from the sinuses drains into the nasal cavity. Sinuses have numerous functions which include decreasing the weight of the head and humidifying and warming the air inhaled through nose. Sinuses also increase the resonance of speech.
- There are four sets of sinuses: (1) frontal, (2) ethmoid, (3) maxillary, and (4) sphenoid. Surface anatomy of the nose is depicted on 3D volume rendered image (Fig. 2.1).

ANATOMY OF NASAL CAVITY

- Its superior boundary is the cribriform plate and inferior boundary is formed by hard and soft palate (Fig. 2.2).
  - Midline nasal septum separates the nasal cavities on the two sides (Fig. 2.3). It comprises of an anterior cartilaginous and posterior bony part formed by vomer and perpendicular plate of ethmoid.
- The lateral wall bears the nasal turbinates
  - Three turbinates on the lateral wall—superior, middle, inferior (Fig. 2.4)
  - Occasionally there is a fourth/supreme turbinate
  - The middle turbinate has an anterior vertical attachment to skull base lateral to medial lamella of cribriform plate; and then a more posterior oblique attachment (also called basal lamella) to lamina papyracea and further posterior horizontal attachment to medial wall of maxillary sinuses (Figs. 2.5A to C)
- Meati refers to passages of the nasal cavity
  - There are three meati—superior, middle and inferior, each beneath the corresponding turbinate
  - A fourth supreme meatus may be there beneath the supreme turbinate, if present
  - Sphenoid and posterior ethmoid air cells drain into superior meatus

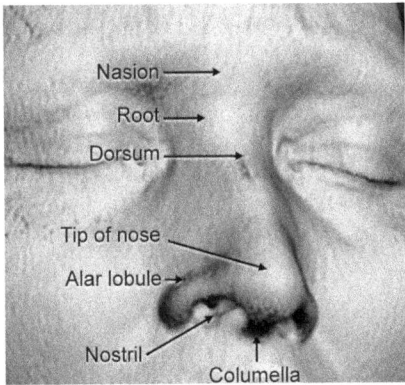

Fig. 2.1: Volume rendered image of the nose.

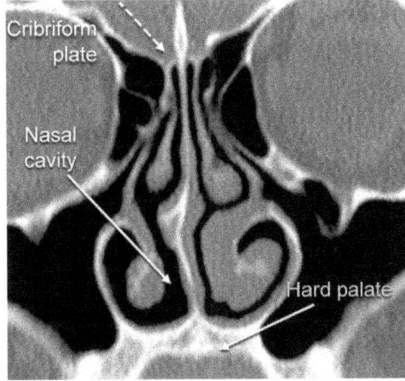

Fig. 2.2: Nasal cavity boundaries—superior cribriform plate and inferior hard palate.

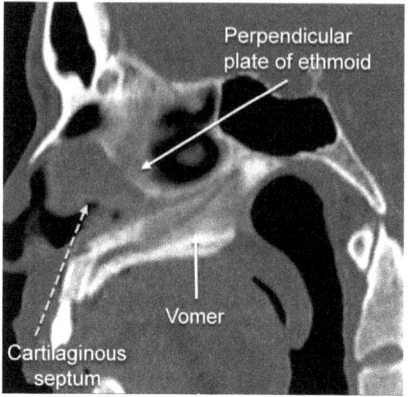

Fig. 2.3: Nasal septum parts—anteriorly cartilaginous part and posteriorly bony part (perpendicular plate of ethmoid and Vomer).

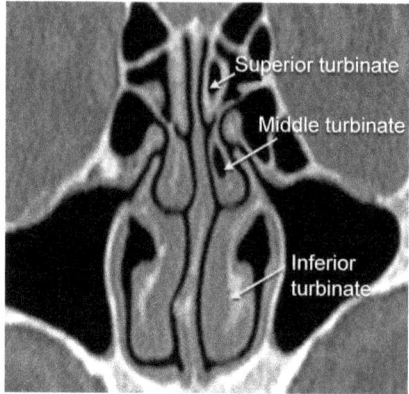

Fig. 2.4: Lateral wall of nasal cavity. Meati are beneath the corresponding turbinates.

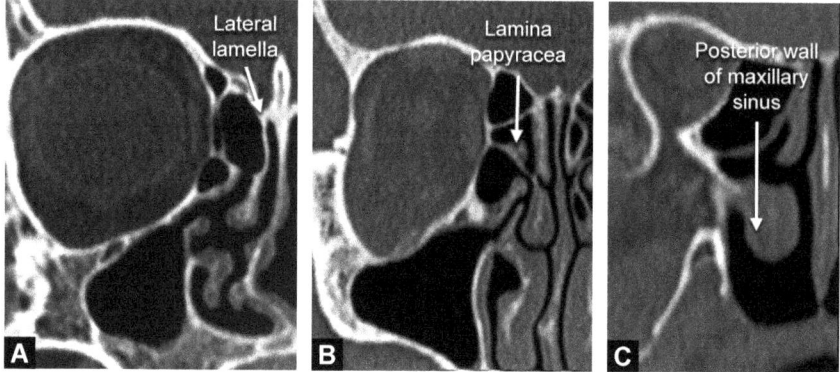

Figs. 2.5A to C: Middle turbinate attachments. (A) Anteriorly to lateral lamella superiorly; (B) Then obliquely to lamina papyracea; and (C) posteriorly to medial wall of maxillary sinus.

- Frontal, maxillary and anterior ethmoidal cells drain into middle meatus
- Nasolacrimal duct drains into inferior meatus.

ANATOMICAL VARIANTS OF NASAL CAVITY

Nasal Septum
- *Septal Deviation (Figs. 2.6A and B)*
  - Most common at chondrovomeral junction
  - Can narrow middle meatus and impair access to the meatus during functional endoscopic sinus surgery (FESS)
  - Septal deviation can be either S-shaped deviation to either side of midline, or septal spur

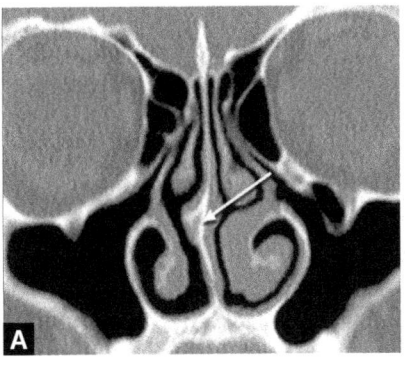 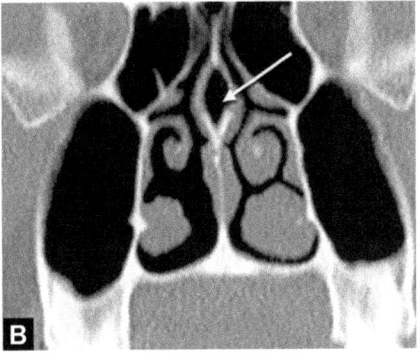

Figs. 2.6A and B: (A) **Nasal septal deviation with spur** (arrow); (B) **Posterior septal pneumatization** (arrow).

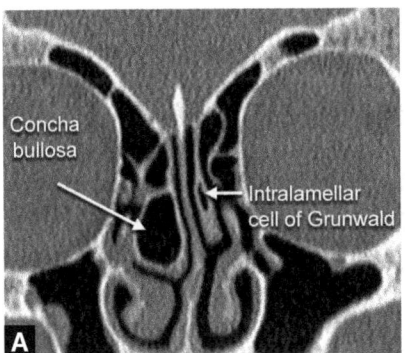 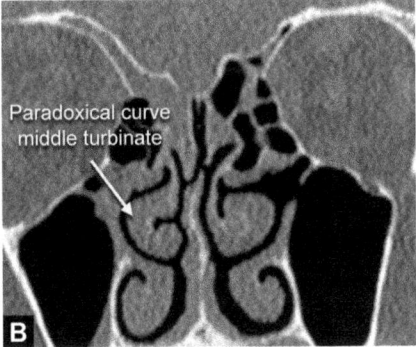

Figs. 2.7A and B: (A) Right sided **concha bullosa** and left sided **intralamellar cell of Grunwald**. (B) **Paradoxical curvature** of right sided middle turbinate.

- *Septal spurs* (Figs. 2.6A and B) are often seen with septal deviation. It can narrow middle meatus and ethmoid infundibulum
- *Septal Pneumatization (Figs. 2.6A and B)*
  - Anteriorly (from crista galli) or posteriorly (from sphenoid sinus)
  - Posteriorly pneumatized septum can impair access to sphenoid ostium during FESS.

Nasal Turbinates

- Superior and inferior turbinates do not show any functionally significant variant.
- Middle turbinate variants are commonly significant. These include:
  - Concha bullosa (Fig. 2.7A): It is pneumatization of bulbous portion of middle turbinate. It is often bilateral, associated with septal deviation; and can obstruct the infundibulum if large
  - Intralamellar cell of Grunwald/conchal neck air cell/lamellar bulla (Fig. 2.7A): It refers to pneumatization above level of OMU involving vertical lamella; and does not have any impact on sinonasal physiology.

- Paradoxical curvature (Fig. 2.7B) refers to turbinate with lateral convexity which can impede access to OMU, if significant sized
- Turbinate sinus is deep invagination produced by sharp folding of middle turbinate on itself
- Pneumatized basal lamella is significant as it can be confused as an ethmoid air cell.

ANATOMY OF FRONTAL AND ANTERIOR ETHMOIDAL SINUSES

Frontal Sinus

- Frontal sinuses (FS) are located in the frontal bone superomedial to the orbit.
- These are formed by upward migration of the ethmoid cells after the age of 2 years. These are last sinuses to be pneumatized.
- Frontal sinuses are paired structures separated by a septum.
- FS has a thicker anterior wall, and a thinner posterior wall which abuts the anterior cranial fossa.
- On CT, Frontal sinuses have scalloped margins with internal septae typically (Figs. 2.8A and B).
- Each frontal sinus is funnel shaped with an ostium located in its inferior which drains through the frontal sinus drainage pathway (FSDP) into the middle meatus.
- Underdeveloped frontal sinus can result in intracranial penetration during intervention (Fig. 2.9).
- FSDP is surrounded by several frontoethmoidal and anterior ethmoidal air cells.
- The terminology used in the description of FSDP and the associated air cells is confusing and has been classified/modified by several authors

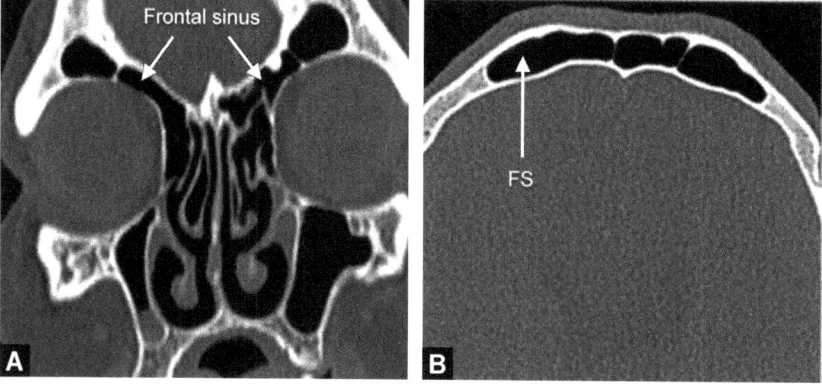

Figs. 2.8A and B: Frontal sinus with typical scalloped margins and internal septae.

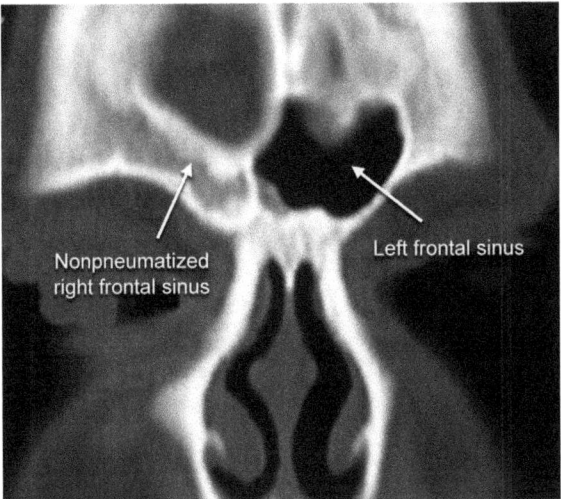

Fig. 2.9: Nonpneumatized frontal sinus.

(Aleya, Kuhn, Wormald).[1-3] A recent classification has been proposed by Wormald et al. as an international consensus statement.[3] In this chapter we attempt to amalgamate some of this content.

Frontal Sinus Ostium
- Transition zone between the frontal sinus and frontal recess.
- It is the narrowest part located at the level of the frontal beak.

Frontal Beak or Frontonasal Process of Maxilla
- It corresponds to level of frontal ostium (Fig. 2.10)
  - Thicker the frontal beak, narrower is the ostium
  - Above the frontal beak is the frontal sinus and below it is the FSDP.

Frontal Recess
- Frontal recess is below the ostium, and is the space into which the FS drains.

Frontal Sinus Drainage Pathway
- Frontal sinus drainage pathway (FSDP) can be evaluated in coronal images but is best evaluated in parasagittal images.
- It is inverted funnel shaped with apex at frontal ostium.
- FSDP has superior and inferior compartments.
- The superior compartment communicates with the frontal ostium above and inferior compartment below. It is located at the junction

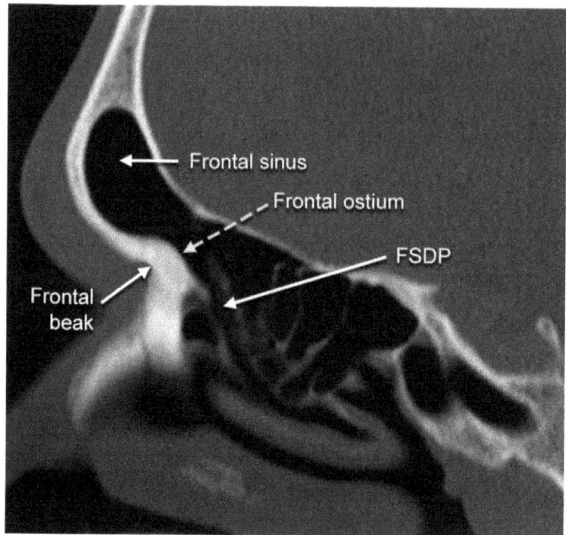

Fig. 2.10: Frontal beak at the level of frontal ostium. Above the frontal beak is the frontal sinus and below is the frontal sinus drainage pathway (FSDP).

of air spaces of the frontal and ethmoidal bones and is bordered by the *"frontoethmoidal air cells"*. The variable anatomy of these air cells governs the shape and size of FSDP.
- The inferior compartment is a narrow passage formed by the ethmoid infundibulum or the middle meatus, depending on the attachment of the uncinate process.
- Variants of inferior compartment are discussed later in the chapter.
- Anterior to FSDP is agger nasi air cell, posteriorly lies the ethmoidal bulla, laterally is lamina papyracea and medially the lateral wall of olfactory fossa and middle turbinate, superiorly lies the fovea ethmoidalis (Figs. 2.11A and B).

Frontoethmoidal Cells
- Also known as Kuhn cells after the name of the researcher who first described them. These have variable anatomy and are clinically important as they have an impact on FSDP.
- Frontoethmoidal cells (FES) lie superior to agger nasi cell (ANC).
- Several classification systems are described.
- A recent modification of International Frontal Sinus Anatomy Classification 2016 is described in Table 2.1.

International Frontal Sinus Anatomy Classification[3]
- Wormald modified classification is also used frequently and classified FES into the following types (Figs. 2.13A to F):
  - Type 1: Single cell above ANC and below frontal beak

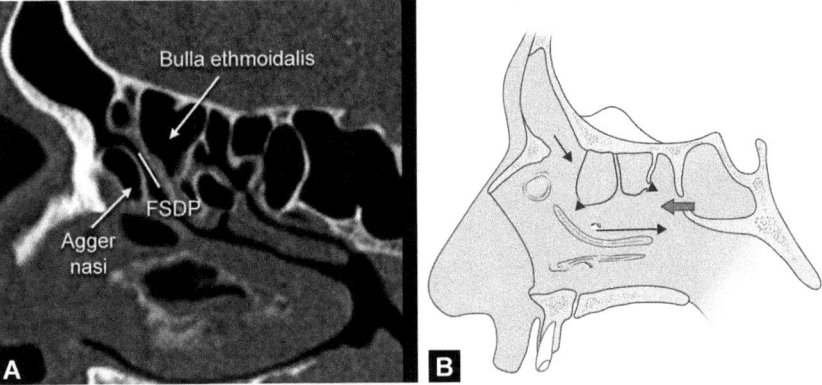

Figs. 2.11A and B: Frontal sinus drainage pathway (FSDP). (A) Agger nasi cell anterior to FSDP and bulla ethmoidalis posterior to FSDP. (B) Diagrammatic representation of drainage pathways of frontal sinus (arrow), maxillary ostium (long arrow), anterior ethmoidal (arrowheads) and sphenoid sinuses (block arrow). *Courtesy:* Dr Arvind K Kairo.

Table 2.1: The International Frontal Sinus Anatomy Classification (IFAC) modified classification of frontoethmoidal cells (FES).[3]	
Anterior cells (push FSDP posteriorly, medially or posteromedially)	• Agger nasi cell (Figs. 2.12A and B) • Supra agger cell • Supra agger frontal cell
Posterior cells (push FSDP anteriorly)	• Suprabulla cell • Suprabullar frontal cell • Supraorbital ethmoidal cell
Medial cells (push FSDP laterally)	• Frontal septal cell

(FSDP: Frontal sinus drainage pathway).

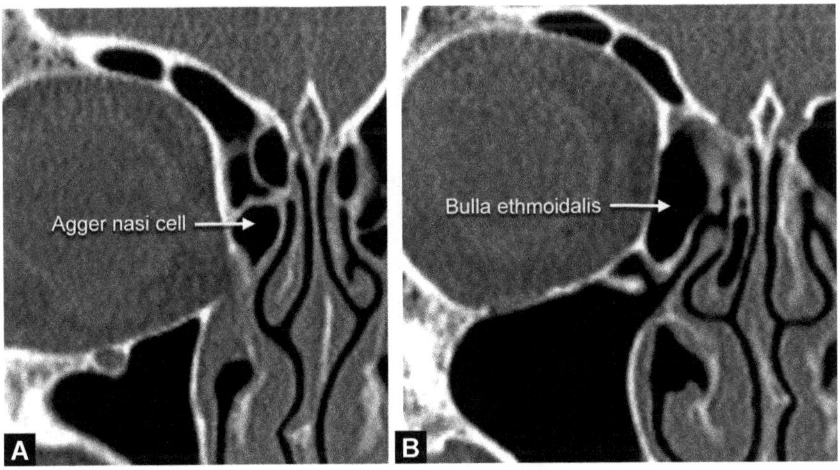

Figs. 2.12A and B: Agger nasi cell. It is the anterior most anterior ethmoidal air cell and anteroinferior to FSDP. Bulla ethmoidalis is the largest cell of the anterior ethmoidal cells and is posterior to FSDP.

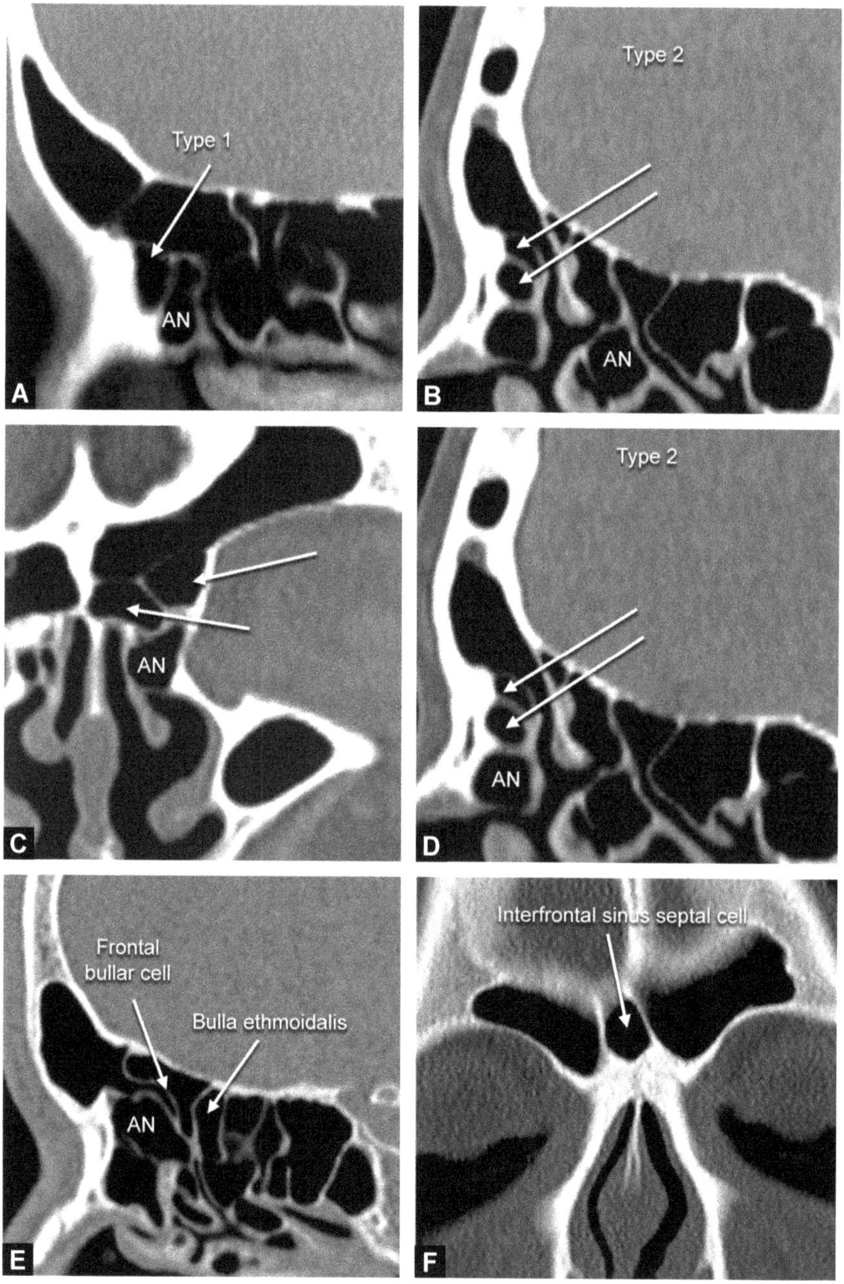

Figs. 2.13A to F: Types of frontoethmoidal cells. (A) Type 1 FES; (B and C) Type 2 FES. (D) Type 3 FES; (E and F) Types of frontoethmoidal air cells—frontal bullar cell and interfrontal sinus septal cell. This is seen in between frontal sinuses. (AN: Agger nasi cell).

- Type 2: Two or more cells above ANC and below frontal beak
- Type 3: Single cell above ANC and extending into frontal sinus not exceeding 50% height of frontal sinus

- Type 4: Single cell above ANC and extending into frontal sinus exceeding 50% of vertical height of frontal sinus or completely contained within frontal sinus
- Frontal bullar cell—single cell above bulla ethmoidalis along the undersurface of skull base and anteriorly extending into frontal sinus
- Interfrontal sinus septal cell—cell within the septum and may compromise the frontal ostium.

Ethmoid Sinuses

- Ethmoid sinuses (ES) are composed of numerous air cells located in the lateral mass of the ethmoid bone, between the two orbits.
- At birth, these cells are fluid filled and pneumatize over time, up to the age of 12 years.
- ES are bordered by the medial orbital wall (lamina papyracea) laterally, and the middle turbinate medially.
- Superiorly ES abuts the anterior skull base (ASB). The roof of ES is formed by the sphenoid bone and orbital process of the frontal bone. ASB is discussed subsequently in this chapter.
- The ES, however, has variable number and size of cells (from 3 to 18 in number) separated by thin bony septae. ES may extend above the orbits and frontal sinuses, posteriorly these can go posterior and lateral to sphenoid sinus, and inferolaterally into the roof of the maxillary sinuses.
- Broadly these are divided into anterior and posterior air cells, being divided by the basal lamella (attachment of the middle portion of middle turbinate to the lamina papyracea).
- The anterior group of cells drains into the middle meatus, while the posterior cells drain into the superior meatus.
- As the anterior cells abut the FS and the FSDP, these are considered together in the "frontoethmoidal anatomy". Located anterior to basal or ground lamella which demarcates anterior from posterior ethmoidal air cells.
- The anterior ethmoid cells drain via the bulla, ethmoid infundibulum, then hiatus semilunaris and into the middle meatus.
- There are several named AE cells that surround/form part of FSDP, and the ostiomeatal complex.

Anterior Ethmoidal Air Cells

- Largest cell in this group is bulla ethmoidalis which is a key surgical landmark (*see* Figs. 2.12A and B).
- Hiatus semilunaris is the gap between uncinate process and anterior wall of bulla ethmoidalis and opens into ethmoidal infundibulum.
- Agger nasi air cell is the most anterior extramural ethmoidal air cell and is located anteroinferior to FSDP (*see* Figs. 2.12A and B). Access to ANC needs to be carried out prior to FSDP surgery
  - If ANC small, then frontal beak is thicker with narrow ostium

- If ANC large, then frontal beak is small with wider ostium but large ANC can still obstruct FSDP albeit more inferiorly
- ANC also is closely related to nasolacrimal duct, can result in spread of infection from one structure to another.

OTHER ANATOMIC VARIANTS IN FRONTAL AND ETHMOIDAL SINUS CELLS[3,4]

- Suprabullar recess between superior wall of bulla ethmoidalis and roof of ethmoid sinus. Can form supraorbital cells laterally (Figs. 2.14A and B)
  - May displace anterior ethmoidal artery bony canal posteriorly
- Retrobullar recess
  - Between bulla ethmoidalis and basal lamella, if bulla does not reach the basal lamella posteriorly.
- Haller cells (Fig. 2.15).
  - Anterior ethmoidal cells along floor of orbits lateral to the plane of lamina papyracea
  - Can narrow maxillary ostium.

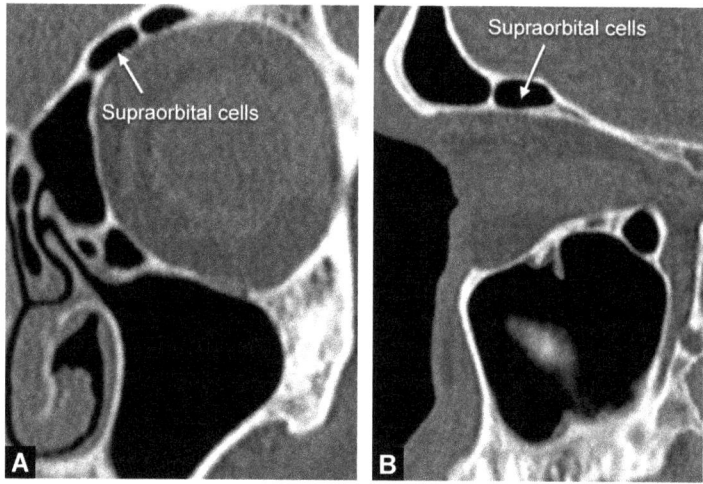

Figs. 2.14A and B: Supraorbital cells. Anterior ethmoidal cells seen to extend into the orbital plate of frontal bone.

ANATOMY OF MAXILLARY SINUS

- Located in the maxillary bone, this is the largest paranasal sinus and is first to pneumatize.
- Being fluid filled at birth, pneumatization in the horizontal posterolateral direction occurs up to 3 years of age, and then expansion inferiorly occurs from 6 years to 12 years.

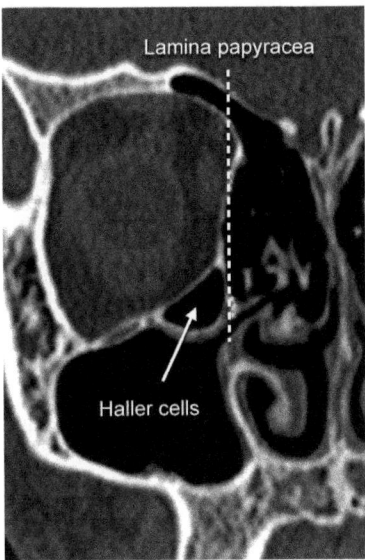

Fig. 2.15: Haller cells. Anterior ethmoidal cells along the floor of orbit lateral to plane of lamina papyracea (dotted line).

- MS is in the shape of a pyramid with the apex directed laterally, and base along the lateral nasal wall.
- It extends from orbital floor superiorly to alveolar process of maxilla inferiorly..
- Inferior orbital nerve (branch of maxillary division of trigeminal nerve) runs along the roof of the maxillary sinus (Fig. 2.16).
- Inferior orbital nerve exits through the anterior MS wall into the cheek. Anterior wall is thinnest in the region of canine fossa, providing an entry point for intervention.
- Critical structures are located posterior to the MS. Pterygopalatine fossa is located behind the posteromedial wall, while the infratemporal fossa is behind the posterolateral wall.

ANATOMICAL VARIANTS OF MAXILLARY SINUS

- Sinus hypoplasia: Risk of orbital penetration during FESS.
- Septae (Fig. 2.17) can be fibrous/bony. These often extend from infraorbital nerve canal to lateral wall and can impede drainage of sinus.
- Dehiscent bony canal of infraorbital nerve may put this nerve at risk of involvement in cases of sinus disease (Fig. 2.18).

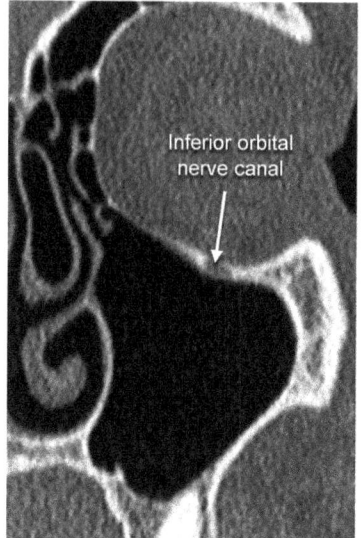

Fig. 2.16: Inferior orbital nerve canal. This runs along the superior wall of maxillary sinus.

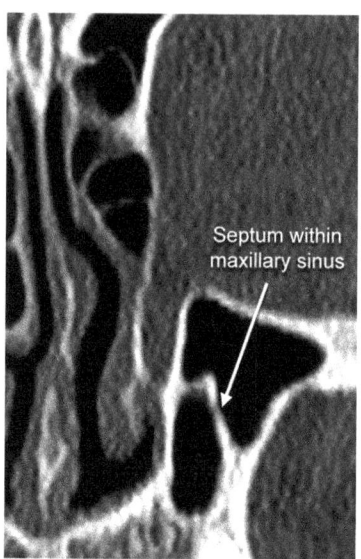

Fig. 2.17: Bony septum within left maxillary sinus.

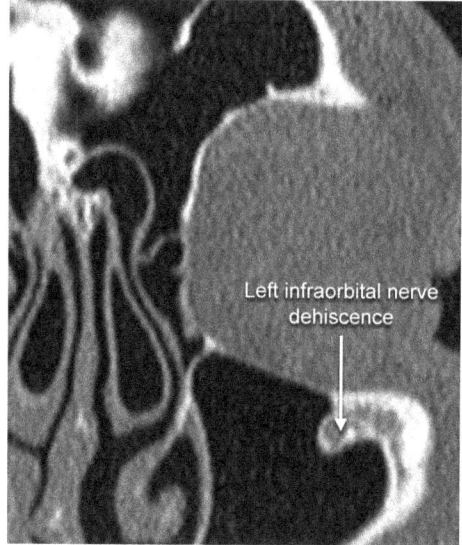

Fig. 2.18: Dehiscent infraorbital canal. Inferior orbital nerve canal projecting into the left maxillary sinus.

ANATOMY OF OSTEOMEATAL UNIT (OMU)

- It is a three dimensional space which is the drainage unit of frontal, anterior ethmoidal and maxillary sinuses.
- Comprises of maxillary ostium, ethmoidal infundibulum, middle meatus, bulla ethmoidalis, uncinate process and hiatus semilunaris (Figs. 2.19A and B)

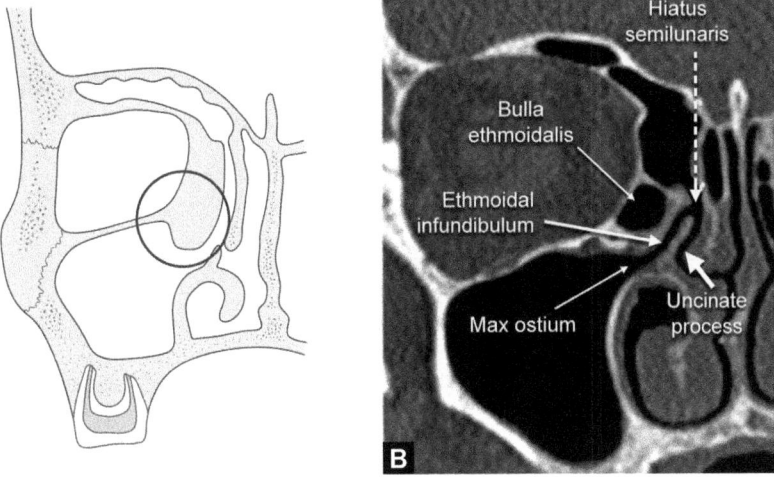

Figs. 2.19A and B: Osteomeatal complex. (A) Diagrammatic representation (*Courtesy:* Dr Arvind K Kairo); (B) NCCT coronal section.

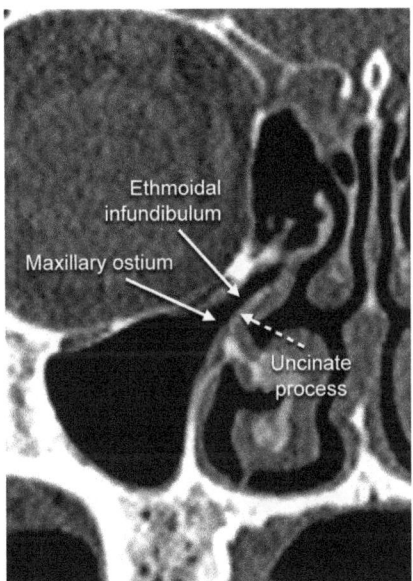

Fig. 2.20: Maxillary ostium. Maxillary ostium seen draining into ethmoidal infundibulum that lies between uncinate process and lamina papyracea.

- Lamina papyracea forms its lateral border, middle turbinate the medial border, while frontal recess and maxillary ostium mark its superior and inferior extent.
- Maxillary sinus ostium (3–10 mm) is located along the superomedial wall of the sinus; drains into ethmoidal infundibulum, which is the space between the uncinate process and lamina papyracea on coronal scan (Fig. 2.20).

Anatomy of Uncinate Process[5]

- Uncinate process is a part of the ethmoid bone.
  - It is a saber shaped bone running in sagittal plane and is a key surgical landmark before opening maxillary sinus ostium
  - It lies lateral to the middle turbinate.
- Attachments (Figs. 2.21A to D)
  - Anterior attachment to lacrimal bone
  - Posterior free concave margin

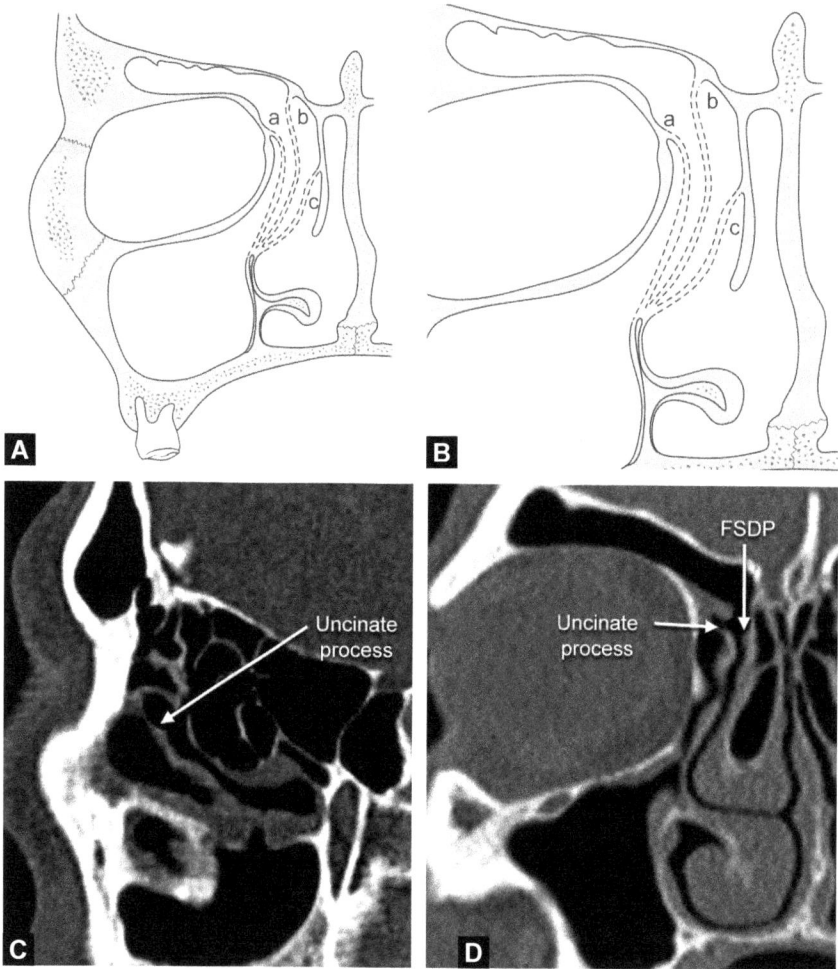

Figs. 2.21A to D: (A) Diagrammatic representation of **uncinate process** (*Courtesy:* Dr Arvind K Kairo). (B) Magnified image of variable attachments of uncinate process (diagrammatic). (C) Uncinate process—as seen on sagittal oblique image. (D) Superior attachment of uncinate process to lamina papyracea on coronal image with frontal sinus drainage pathway (FSDP) seen medial to it.

- Inferior attachment to inferior turbinate and perpendicular process of palatine bone
- Variable superior attachment to lamina papyracea (a in Figs. 2.21A and B), anterior skull base (b in Figs. 2.21A and B) or middle turbinate (c in Figs. 2.21A and B) or with multiple superior attachments.

ANATOMICAL VARIANTS OF UNCINATE PROCESS, ETHMOID INFUNDIBULUM AND MAXILLARY OSTIUM

- The site of superior attachment of the UP governs the location of the ethmoid infundibulum and hence the drainage pathway of the frontal sinus.
- *Superior attachment to lamina papyracea (Fig. 2.21A)*
  - Frontal sinus drainage pathway becomes medial to the UP and drains into middle meatus (Figs. 2.21A to D)
  - Laterally, a blind recess forms called recessus terminalis.
- *Superior attachment to anterior skull base or to the middle turbinate (Figs. 2.21B and C)*
  - FSDP is now lateral to uncinate and opens into ethmoidal infundibulum
  - Predisposes to spread of infection from ethmoid to frontal cell.

Other variants of UP
- Atelectatic uncinate process
  - UP is opposed/fused to inferomedial wall of orbit
  - Associated with hypoplastic/silent maxillary sinus
  - More prone to orbit injury during surgery.
- Hooked/pneumatized uncinate process
  - Can narrow ethmoidal infundibulum
- Absent uncinate process
- Everted uncinate process
  - Can be misinterpreted as double middle turbinate at FESS.
- *Accessory ostia/posterior fontanelle (Figs. 2.22A and B)*
  - Posterior to natural ostia
  - Can cause recurrent sinusitis
  - Surgical combination of two ostia done to prevent complications.

ANATOMY OF LAMINA PAPYRACEA (LP) AND ANTERIOR ETHMOIDAL ARTERY

- Lamina papyracea—medial wall of orbit
  - Sagittal plane drawn through lamina should pass through sagittal plane of maxillary ostium on coronal CT images (Fig. 2.23)
  - Small defects in LP are common and seen in up to 10% population.
- Anterior ethmoidal artery passes through a bony canal on upper one third of LP (Fig. 2.24)
  - Has notched appearance behind the bulla ethmoidalis.

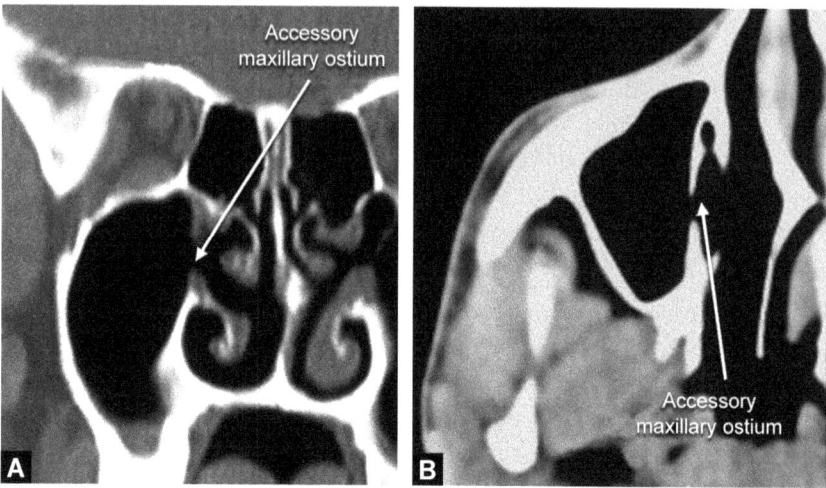

Figs. 2.22A and B: Accessory maxillary ostium. This lies behind the plane of the maxillary ostium.

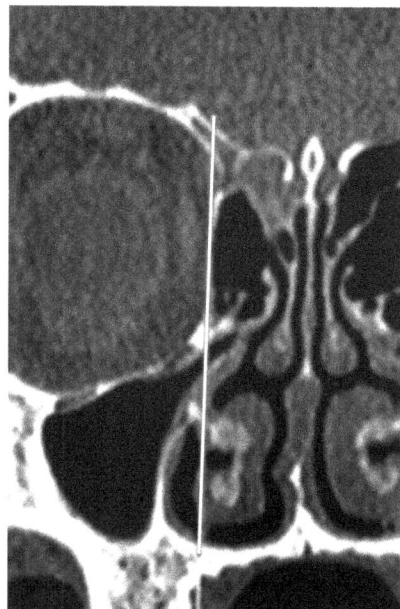

Fig. 2.23: Plane of maxillary ostium—passes through the level of lamina papyracea.

ANATOMICAL VARIANTS OF LP

- Large defects in lamina papyracea: These can predispose to orbital injury
    - Dehiscent canal of anterior ethmoidal artery: Artery can then prolapse into ethmoidal air cells on a mesentery and be predisposed to injury during surgery.

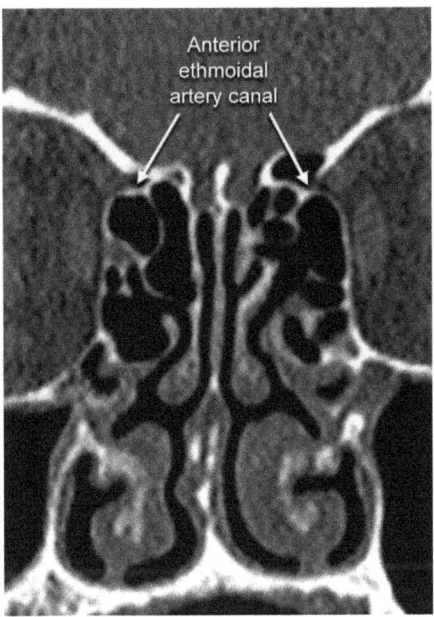

Fig. 2.24: Anterior ethmoidal artery canal seen as a notch in the upper medial wall of orbit.

ANATOMY OF OLFACTORY FOSSA AND MEDIAN ANTERIOR SKULL BASE (ASB)

- *Anterior skull base:* Constituted by parts of frontal bone (orbital plates), ethmoid bone (cribriform plate), and sphenoid bone (lesser wing).
- Orbital plates of frontal bone form the posterior wall of frontal sinus and fovea ethmoidalis (or ethmoid skull base/roof of ethmoid sinus); then continue posteriorly as planum sphenoidale.
- Cribriform plate forms the roof of nasal cavity. It is also referred to as lamina cribrosa and the olfactory nerves traverse through its perforations. The cribriform plate is joined laterally by the lateral lamella (LL) to the fovea ethmoidalis. LL has a vertical orientation.
  - Olfactory fossa—houses the olfactory bulb. It is a depression in the cribriform plate and bound by crista galli medially, medial lamella of cribriform plate inferiorly and lateral lamella of cribriform plate laterally (Fig. 2.25). Olfactory bulb is best seen on T2W coronal MR images (Fig. 2.26.)
  - Asymmetry in level of olfactory fossa can be seen in up to one-third of the population.
- Keros classification[6] of depth of olfactory fossa (Figs. 2.27A and B): Depth of the olfactory fossa depends on the height of the LL
  - Type 1 lateral lamella 1–3 mm
  - Type 2 lateral lamella 4–7 mm
  - Type 3 lateral lamella 8–16 mm.

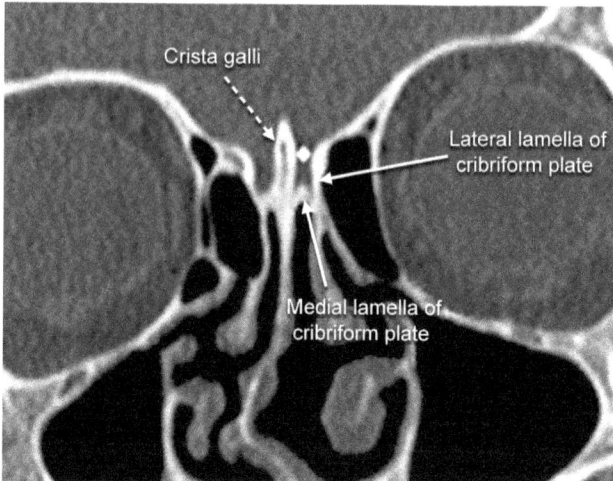

Fig. 2.25: Olfactory fossa boundaries. Olfactory fossa (dot) bounded by crista galli medially, lateral lamella of cribriform plate laterally and medial lamella of cribriform plate inferiorly.

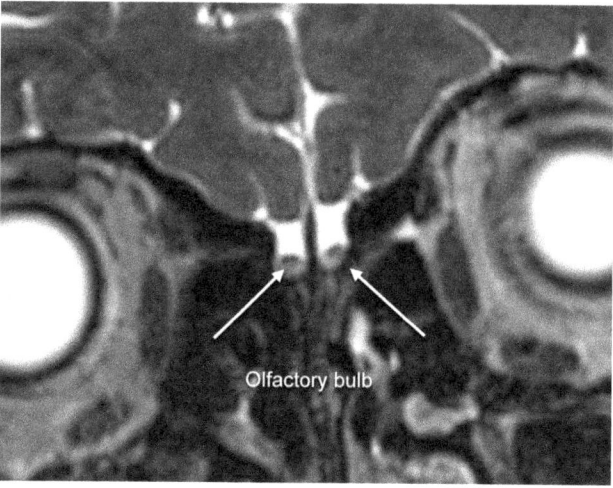

Fig. 2.26: Olfactory bulb (arrows). As seen within olfactory fossa on MRI T2W coronal image.

- Type 1 is the shallowest olfactory fossa while type 3 is the deepest.
- The anterior ethmoid artery (AEA) is a branch of the ophthalmic artery (branch of internal carotid artery). It passes through the anterior ethmoidal canal/foramen (seen as a notch on the superomedial orbital wall) to the ethmoidal labyrinth and then to the anterior skull base.
- It is identified on the lateral wall of the olfactory fossae as horizontal lucencies (anterior ethmoid sulcus).

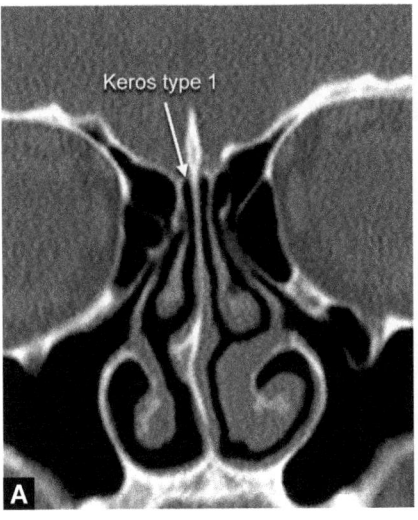 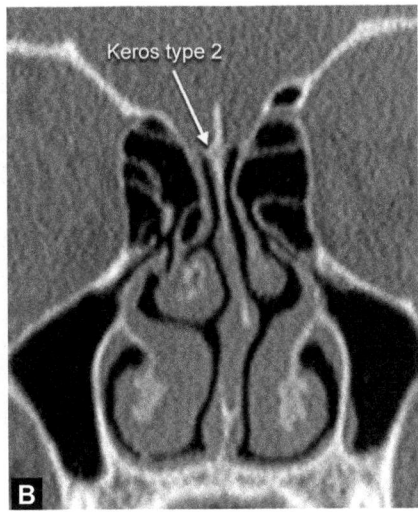

Figs. 2.27A and B: Types of olfactory fossa.

- Lateral lamella is thinnest bone in anterior skull base, hence predisposed to injury during surgery
  - Middle turbinate attaches to lateral lamella of cribriform plate anteriorly, can be injured during turbinate handling
  - Anterior ethmoidal artery also traverses the lateral lamella.
- Fovea ethmoidalis—orbital plate of frontal bone that joins lateral lamella of cribriform plate medially to lamina papyracea laterally.
- Rudmik and Smith[7] assessment of height of anterior ethmoid skull base (ESB)—vertical distance between plane of ESB and mid orbital plane as seen on coronal section showing anterior ethmoidal artery is measured (Fig. 2.28)
  - High ESB—vertical distance >7 mm
  - Moderate ESB—vertical height 4–7 mm
  - Low ESB—vertical height < 4 mm.

ANATOMIC VARIANTS OF ASB

- Type 2 olfactory fossa is the most common and least prone to injury while type 3, the least common, is most prone to injury
  - Angle between medial and lateral lamella can vary. Greater the angle, more the risk for injury during surgery.
- Lower ESB, greater the chance of injury during surgery
  - Anterior ethmoidal artery can hang within a bony mesentery and is then prone to injury
  - Aerated crista galli can attenuate frontal ostium (Fig. 2.29).

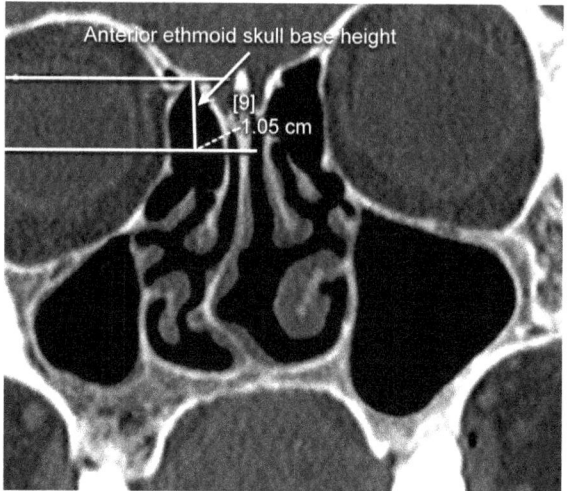

Fig. 2.28: Anterior ethmoid skull base height. Measured as vertical distance between fovea ethmoidalis and mid orbital plane (1.05 cm here). Keros type 3 and Rudmick & Smith high type ASB.

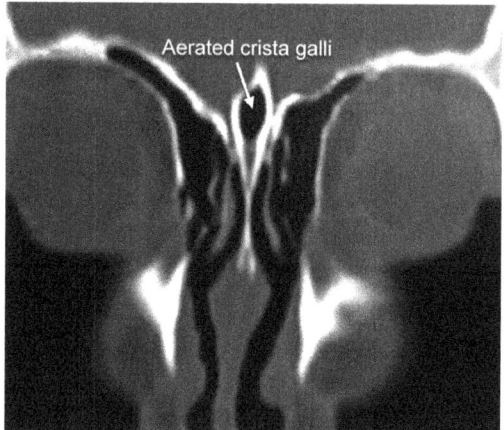

Fig. 2.29: Aerated crista galli. Coronal image shows aerated crista galli.

ANATOMY OF POSTERIOR ETHMOID AIR CELLS

- Ethmoid bone is a midline bone separating nasal cavity from the brain. It has four parts:
  - The cribriform plate (horizontal part): olfactory nerve fibers pass through it and olfactory bulb lies on it
  - Crista galli: Thick midline triangular structure on which falx cerebri attaches
  - Vertical plate (forms part of nasal septum)
  - Lateral masses or labyrinths on each side.

The posterior ethmoidal air cells are located posterior to basal lamella and anterior to sphenoid sinus (Figs. 2.30A and B)

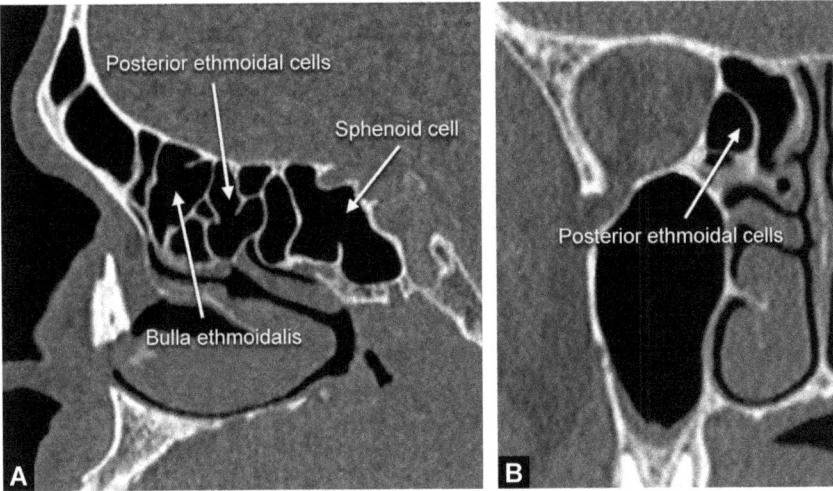

Figs. 2.30A and B: Posterior ethmoid cells. Sandwiched between bulla ethmoidalis and sphenoid sinus.

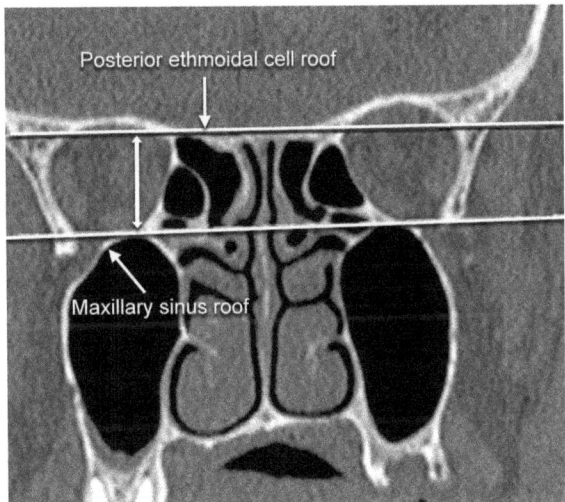

Fig. 2.31: Posterior ethmoid skull base height. Distance between roof of posterior ethmoidal cells and roof of maxillary sinus.

- Medial to lamina papyracea and lateral to superior turbinate
- These are fewer as compared to anterior ethmoid air cells
- These air cells drain via their separate ostia into the superior meatus
- Height of posterior ethmoid sinus can be measured as the distance between roofs of maxillary sinus and posterior ethmoid sinus as seen on coronal images (Fig. 2.31).

ANATOMIC VARIANTS OF POSTERIOR ETHMOID CELLS

- Onodi cell/sphenoethmoidal air cell
  - These are posterior ethmoid cells that extend superolateral to sphenoid sinus
  - An oblique or horizontal septum, if seen within sphenoid sinus is suggestive of their presence (Fig. 2.32A)
  - A cruciform septation within sphenoid air cell suggests bilateral onodi cells (Fig. 2.32B)
  - Onodi cells have a close relationship with the optic nerve and internal carotid artery, and can predispose these structures to injury during FESS.
- Low lying posterior ethmoid cells can predispose to skull base penetration during FESS.

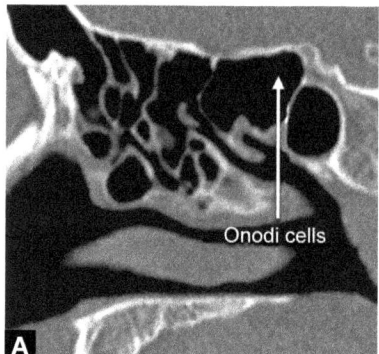
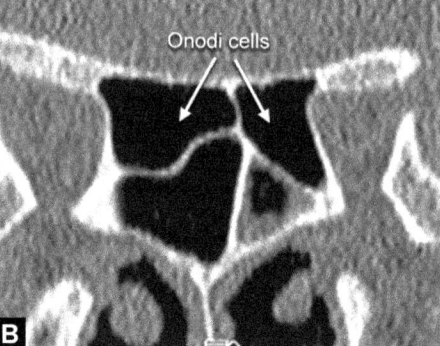

Figs. 2.32A and B: Onodi cells. Posterior ethmoidal cells lying superolateral to sphenoid sinus giving *cribriform sign* on coronal image.

ANATOMY OF SPHENOID SINUS AND MEDIAN CENTRAL SKULL BASE (CSB)

- Body of sphenoid bone houses the SS; laterally demarcated by petro-occipital suture.
- Sphenoid sinus usually bilateral and asymmetric with vertical septation within.
- Anteriorly the roof of the SS is bound by planum sphenoidale, and posteriorly is the sella turcica. Planum sphenoidale continues anteriorly with ethmoid bone. Anterior clinoid process marks the transition between anterior skull base (ASB) and central skull base (CSB).
- Anterior wall is connected to perpendicular plate of ethmoid and vomer in the midline, and can be displaced by an Onodi cell.
- Lateral walls are thin and can even have dehiscent areas. It is related to critical structures (optic nerve, cavernous sinus, ICA).
- Sphenoid sinus drains via its ostium and sphenoethmoidal recess into the superior meatus; it lies at the medial aspect of its anterior wall (Figs. 2.33A and B). The ostium is approximately 1.5 cm superior to the posterior choanae. In the majority, it lies just medial to the superior turbinate

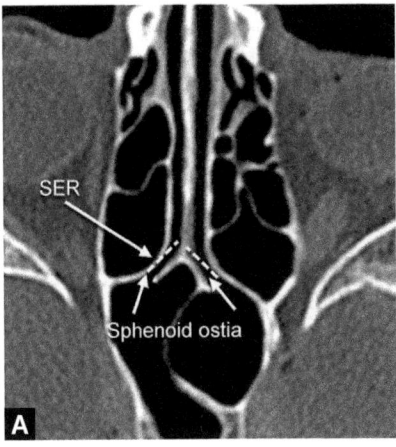
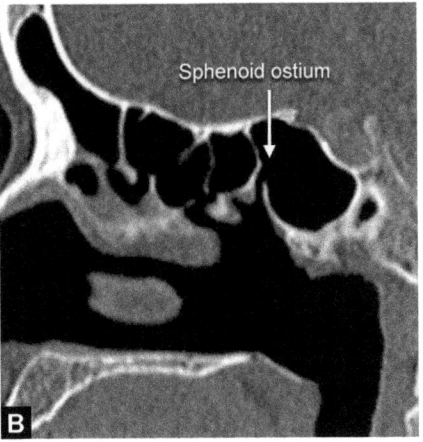

Figs. 2.33A and B: Sphenoid sinuses drain via sphenoid ostia into sphenoethmoid recess.

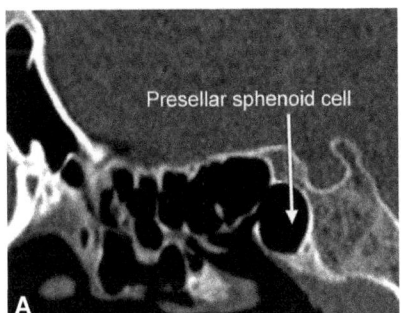
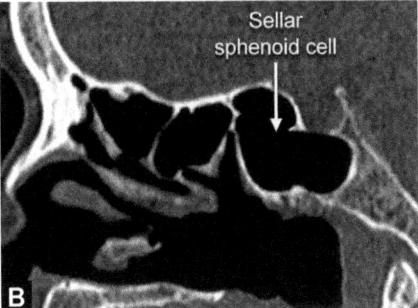

Figs. 2.34A and B: Types of sphenoid sinus based on degree of pneumatization.

- Sphenoethmoidal recess is a narrow corridor which is bound superiorly by cribriform plate, medially by nasal septum and laterally by superior turbinate. Inferiorly it leads to the superior meatus. The SS as well as posterior ethmoid cells drain into it.
- Types of sphenoid sinus based upon extent of pneumatization (Figs. 2.34A and B)
  - Nonpneumatised sphenoid sinus
  - Conchal sphenoid sinus—small air cell not reaching up to sella
  - Presellar sphenoid sinus—reaching up to anterior wall of sella
  - Sellar sphenoid sinus—reaching below sellar floor; most frequent.
- Critical structures in close relationship with sphenoid sinus (Fig. 2.35)
  - Optic nerve canal in relationship with superior wall of sphenoid sinus
  - Internal carotid artery canal in relationship with posterolateral wall of sphenoid sinus
  - Pterygoid/vidian canal along the inferior wall
  - Foramen rotundum—along the lateral wall
  - Lateral craniopharyngeal wall: Defect along lateral wall of sphenoid sinus due to fusion defect between basisphenoid and greater wing of sphenoid.

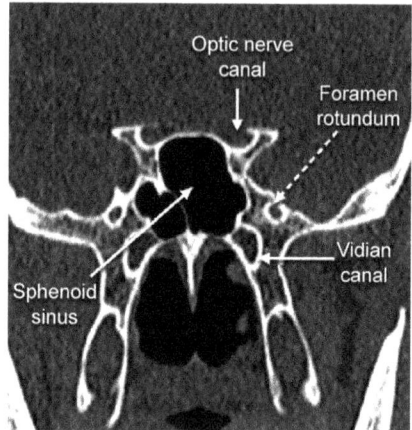

Fig. 2.35: Central skull base critical structures in close relation to sphenoid sinus.

ANATOMIC VARIANTS OF CSB

- Poor pneumatization
  - Trans-sphenoidal skull base surgery is relatively contraindicated.
- Presence of intrasinus septae
  - Variable, vertical/horizontal/oblique
  - Must be mentioned in report with attention to any attachment with critical structures especially the carotid arteries
  - Horizontal septae point to onodi cells.
- Dehiscent walls of bony walls of any of these critical structures should be carefully looked for
- Pneumatized anterior clinoid process (Fig. 2.36)
  - Results in formation of opticocarotid recess between optic nerve canal above and carotid artery below
  - Optic nerve canal may be dehiscent in up to four-fifths of these cases.

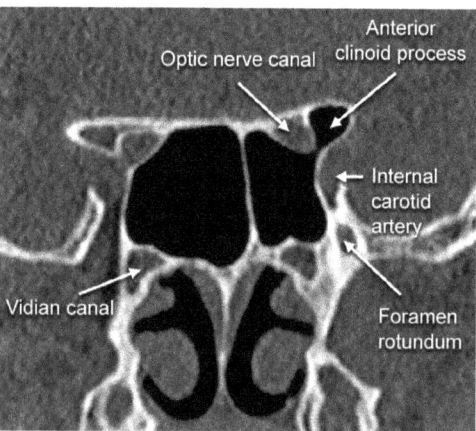

Fig. 2.36: Aerated anterior clinoid process—seen to surround the optic nerve canal on the left side.

RELEVANT ORBITAL ANATOMY (FIGS. 2.37A AND B)

The relevant orbital anatomy is given in Table 2.2.

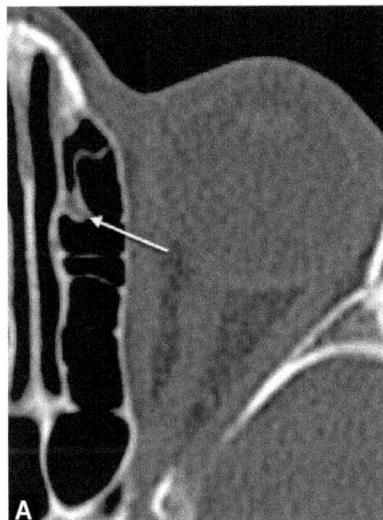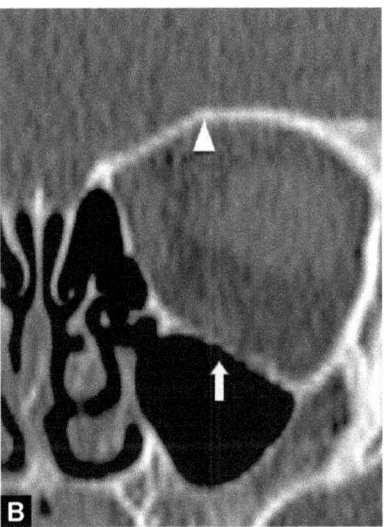

Figs. 2.37A and B: Boundaries of orbit. [Medial wall: Lamina papyracea (arrow); Roof: Frontal bone (arrowhead); Floor: Roof of MS (block arrow)].

	Table 2.2: Relevant orbital anatomy.	
Wall	Bone	Relationship to sinuses
Medial wall	Frontal bone (orbital process) Lamina papyracea (ethmoid bone) Lacrimal bone Palatine bone (orbital process)	Lateral wall of ethmoid sinuses
Lateral wall	Zygomatic bone Greater wing of sphenoid	
Floor (inferior wall)	Maxillary bone Zygomatic bone Palatine bone	Roof of MS Infraorbital nerve passes through it
Roof	Frontal bone and lesser wing of sphenoid	Floor of frontal sinuses

REFERENCES

1. van Alyea OE. Frontal cells: an anatomic study of these cells with consideration of their clinical significance. Arch Otolaryngol. 1941;34:11-23.
2. Kuhn FA. Surgery of the frontal sinus. In: Kennedy DW, Bolger WE, Zinreich SJ (Eds). Diseases of the Sinuses: Diagnosis and Management. London, UK: B.C. Decker; 2001. pp. 281-301.
3. Wormald PJ, et al. The International Frontal Sinus Anatomy Classification (IFAC) and classification of the Extent of Endoscopic Frontal Sinus Surgery (EFSS). Int Forum Allergy Rhinol. 2016;6(7):677-96.

4. Folbe AJ, Svider PF, Eloy JA. Anatomic considerations in frontal sinus surgery. Otolaryngol Clin North Am. 2016;49(4):935-43.
5. Güngör G, Okur N, Okur E. Uncinate process variations and their relationship with ostiomeatal complex: a pictorial essay of multidedector computed tomography (MDCT) findings. Pol J Radiol. 2016;81:173-80.
6. Keros P. On the practical importance of differences in the level of the cribriform plate of the ethmoid. Laryngol Otol (Stuttg). 1965;41:808-13.
7. Rudmik L, Smith TL. Evaluation of the ethmoid skull-base height prior to endoscopic sinus surgery: a preoperative computed tomography evaluation technique. Int Forum Allergy Rhinol. 2012;2(2):151-4.

CHAPTER 3

Sinonasal Anatomy: Section-wise

Jyoti Kumar

- Introduction
- Consecutive Coronal Sections
- Consecutive Axial Sections
- Consecutive Sagittal Sections

INTRODUCTION

- Coronal sections form the basic imaging plane for evaluating the paranasal sinuses and nasal cavity
- Similarly bone window is the most informative window setting
- Axial and sagittal planes delineate some structures better (see Chapters 1 and 9)
- This chapter depicts the sectional anatomy in all three planes through sequential images

CONSECUTIVE CORONAL SECTIONS

Consecutive coronal sections from anterior to posterior are depicted in Figures 3.1A to R. Coronal scans well depict the nasal turbinates and meati, nasal septum, agger nasi (AN) cell, various sinuses, components of ostiomeatal unit and adjacent skull base.

Coronal Sections (Figs. 3.1A to F)

- Most anteriorly, the nares, ala and cartilaginous septum (NS) can be seen.
- On successive scans, the nasal bones (NB) are visualized which are paired bones and join together to form the root of the nose.
- Parts of frontal (FS) and maxillary sinuses (MS) begin to be seen.
- Agger nasi cell is seen as the anterior most anterior ethmoidal cell, which is anterior to the vertical attachment of middle turbinate (MT).

Key

AE cells: Anterior ethmoid cells	AN: Agger nasi cells
FS: Frontal sinus	IT: Inferior turbinate
MS: Maxillary sinus	MT: Middle turbinate
NLD: Nasolacrimal duct	NB: Nasal bone
NS: Nasal septum	

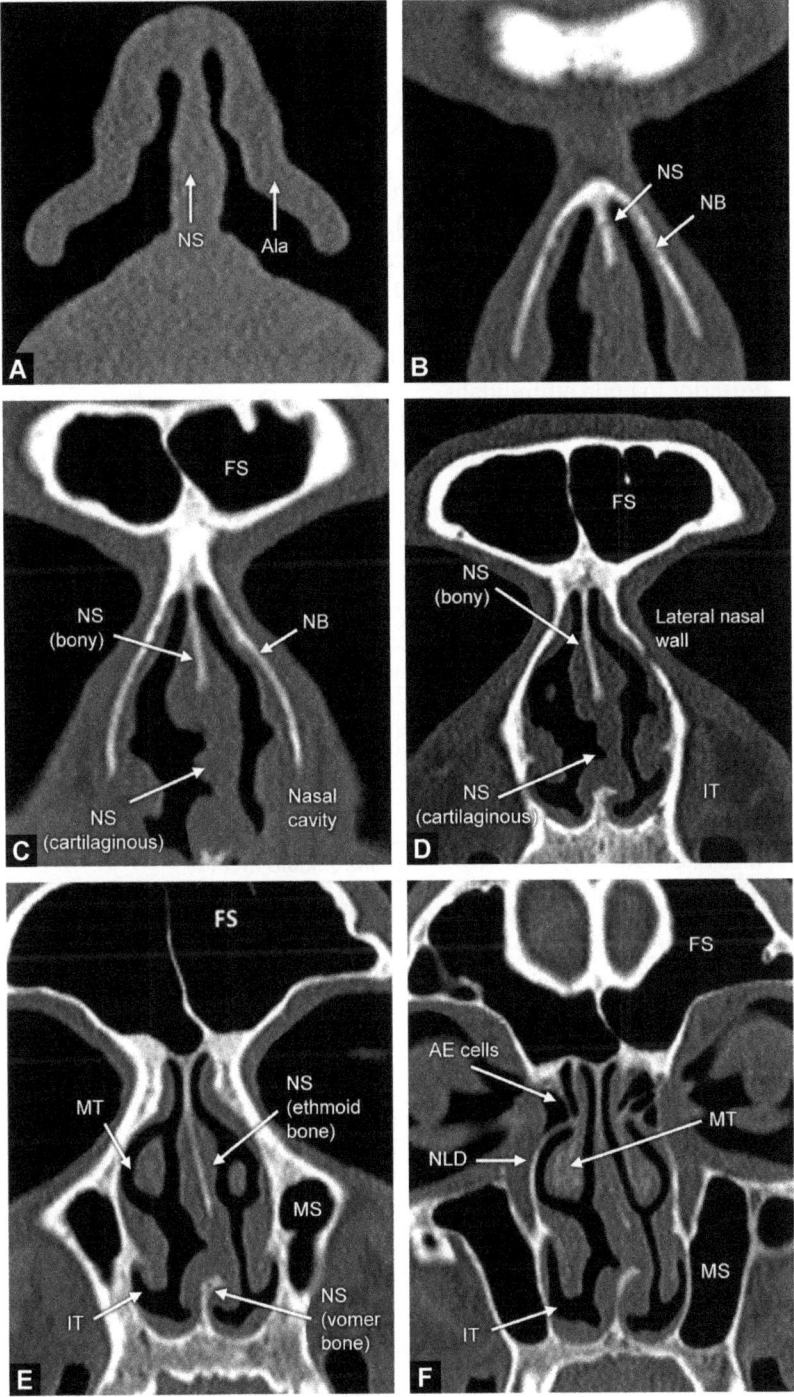

Figs. 3.1A to F: Consecutive coronal sections from anterior to posterior.

Coronal Sections (Figs. 3.1G to L)

- Frontal sinus drainage pathway (FSDP) can then be seen just posterior to the agger nasi cell.
- Canal for inferior orbital nerve (ION) is seen running along the roof of the maxillary sinus.
- Components of osteomeatal unit (Fig. 3.1K) are then well visualized namely—maxillary ostium (MO), ethmoidal infundibulum, uncinate process, hiatus semilunaris and bulla ethmoidalis (BE).
- Crista galli (CG) and medial (ML) and lateral lamella (LL) of cribriform plate are seen as boundaries of olfactory fossa.
- Oblique attachment of middle turbinate or basal lamella is seen just posterior to bulla ethmoidalis.
- Vertical attachment of middle turbinate (MT) can be seen to the anterior skull base at the junction of medial (ML) and lateral lamella (LL) of cribriform plate.

Key

AN: Agger nasi	BE: Bullae ethmoidalis
CG: Crista galli	FS: Frontal sinus
FSDP: Frontal sinus drainage pathway	IM: Inferior meatus
ION: Inferior orbital nerve canal	IT: Inferior turbinate
LL: Lateral lamella	LP: Lamina papyracea
ML: Medial lamella	MM: Middle meatus
MO: Maxillary ostium	MT: Middle turbinate
OF: Olfactory fossa	NS: Nasal septum

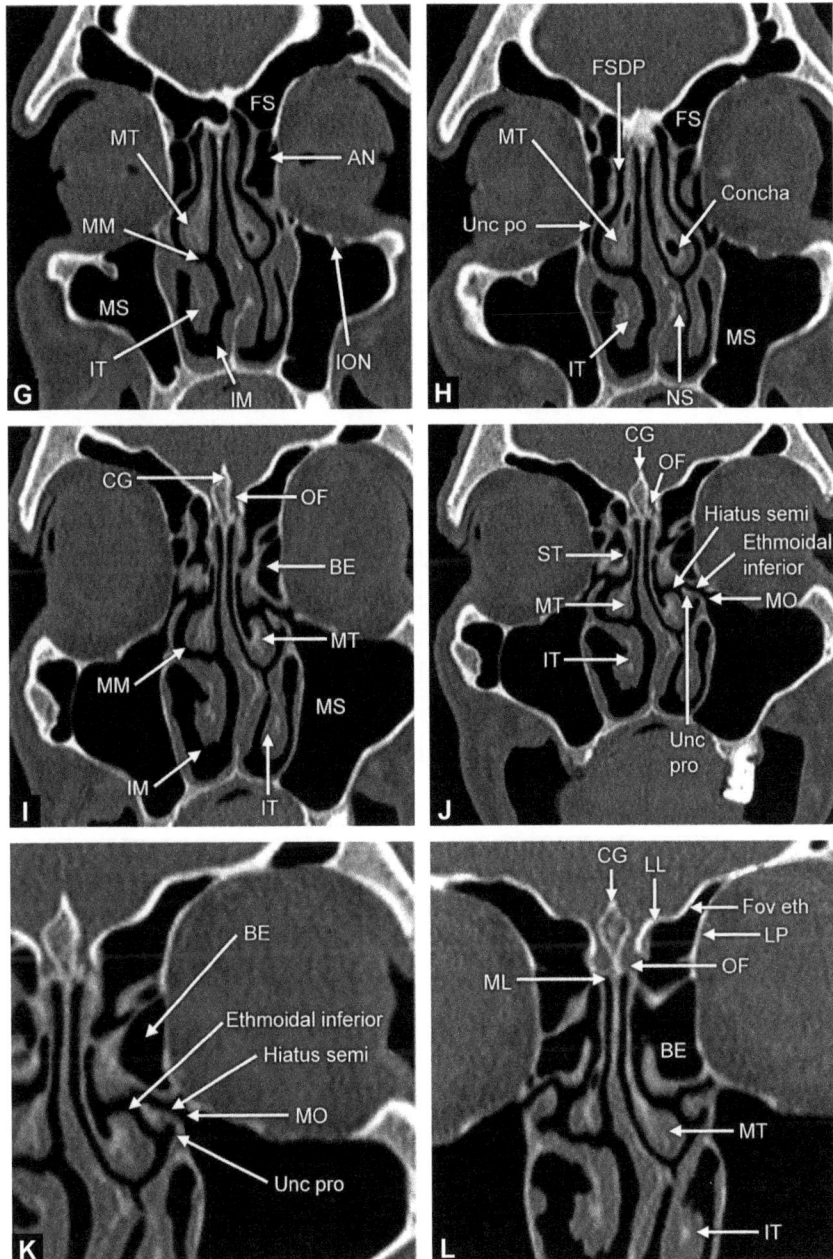

Figs. 3.1G to L: Consecutive coronal sections from anterior to posterior.

Coronal Sections (Figs. 3.1M to R)

- Canal for anterior ethmoidal artery is also seen as a notch in the lamina papyracea (LP) just behind bulla ethmoidalis.
- Behind the basal lamella lie the posterior ethmoidal cells (PE).
- These can extend posterosuperior to the sphenoid cell and are called onodi cells.
- The choana are the posterior nasal openings of the nasal cavity into the nasopharynx separated by the nasal septum (vomer) and bounded laterally by the medial pterygoid plate.

Key

CC: Carotid canal	FR: Foramen rotundum
HP: Hard palate	IM: Inferior meatus
IT: Inferior turbinate	LL: Lateral lamella
LP: Lamina papyracea	ML: Medial lamella
MM: Middle meatus	MO: Maxillary ostium
MT: Middle turbinate	NS: Nasal septum
OA: Orbital apex	OC: Optic canal
OF: Olfactory fossa	PP: Pterygoid plate
SP: Soft palate	SS: Sphenoid sinus
ST: Superior turbinate	VC: Vidian canal

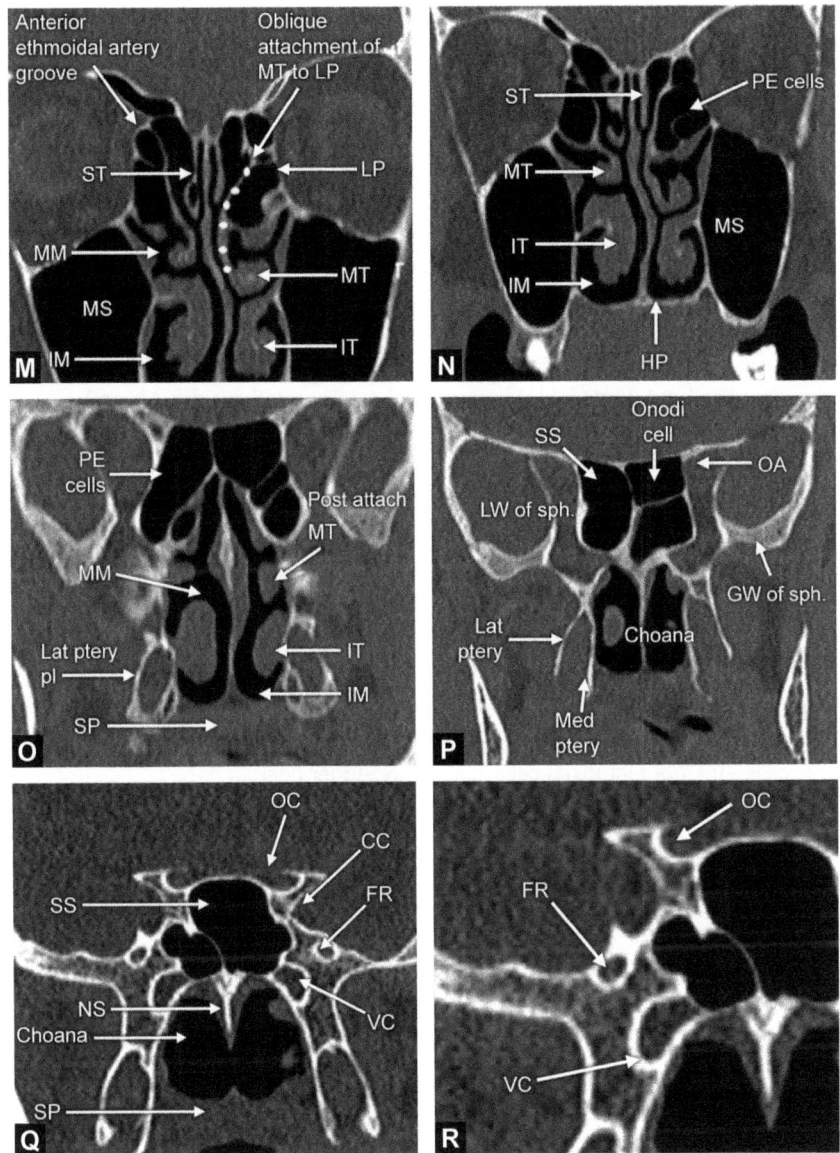

Figs. 3.1M to R: Consecutive coronal sections from anterior to posterior.

CONSECUTIVE AXIAL SECTIONS

Consecutive axial sections of paranasal sinuses from superior to inferior are depicted in Figures 3.2A to L.

Axial Sections (Figs. 3.2A to F)

- On the superior most scans, frontal sinuses (FS) can be seen, thereafter followed by crista galli (CG) and anterior skull base structures.
- Agger nasi is the most anterior ethmoidal cell seen just anterior to frontal sinus drainage pathway which is better seen on sagittal images.
- Nasolacrimal duct (NLD) is seen in close association with AN cell.
- Bulla ethmoidalis (BE) is the largest ethmoidal air cell the posterior boundary of which is the basal lamella (BL).
- Behind the basal lamella (BL), lie the posterior ethmoidal (PE) air cells.
- Piriform aperture is pear-shaped anterior bony opening of the nasal cavity bounded superiorly by nasal bone, laterally by nasal process of maxilla and inferiorly by palatine process.

Key

AE cells: Anterior ethmoidal cells	AN: Agger nasi
BE: Bullae ethmoidalis	CG: Crista galli
FS: Frontal sinus	LP: Lamina papyracea
NB: Nasal bone	NLD: Nasolacrimal duct
NS: Nasal septum	OA: Orbital apex
PE: posterior ethmoidal cells	SOF: Superior orbital fissure

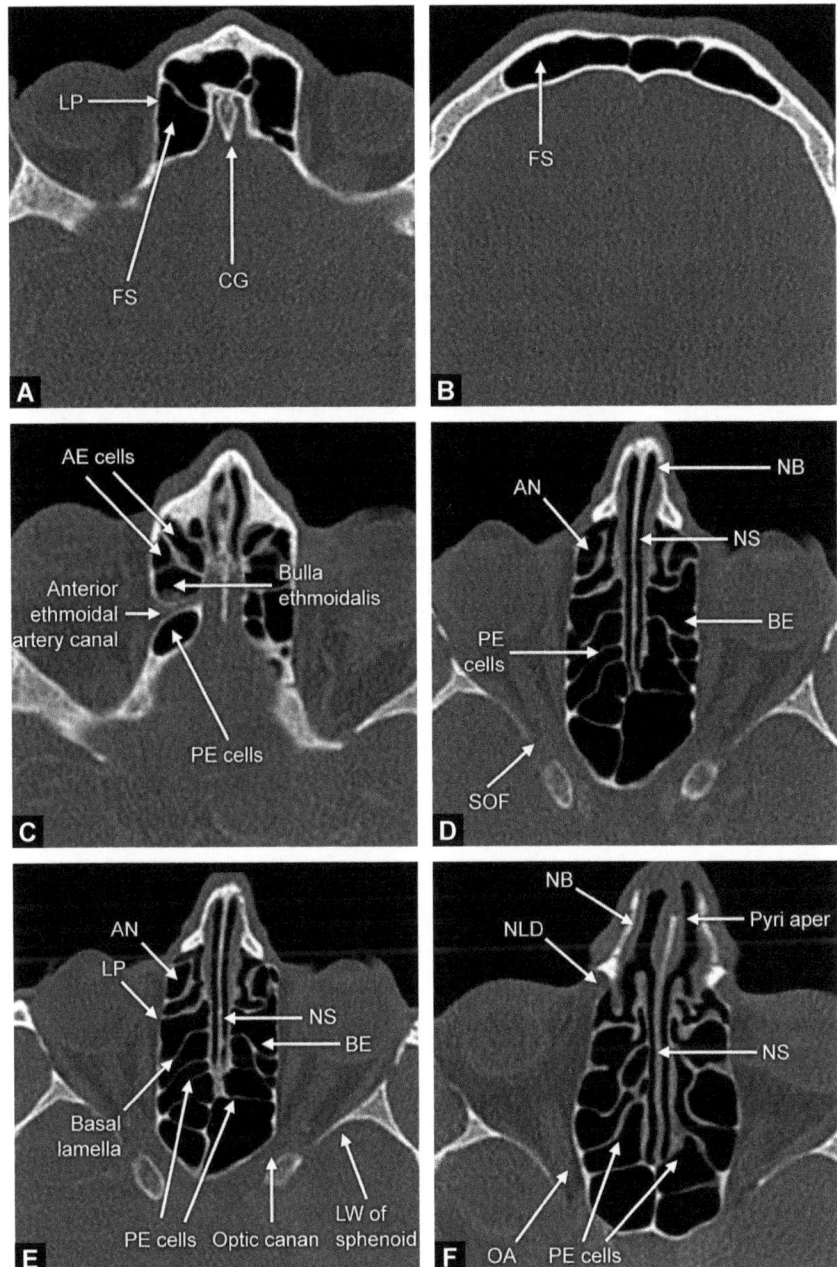

Figs. 3.2A to F: Consecutive axial sections from cranial to caudal.

Axial Sections (Figs. 3.2G to L)

- The sphenoid cells are seen behind the posterior ethmoidal cells (PE). Sphenoid ostium (SO and sphenoethmoidal recess (SER) are clearly seen on the axial scans.
- Their surrounding critical skull base structures can also be seen on axial images.
- Inferiorly, nasolacrimal duct (NLD) is seen to drain into the inferior meatus.
- The choana are the posterior nasal openings of the nasal cavity into the nasopharynx separated by the nasal septum (vomer) and bounded laterally by the medial pterygoid plate.
- Hard palate (HP) is the inferior most boundary of the nasal cavity.

Key

FR: Foramen rotundum	HP: Hard palate
IT: Inferior turbinate	MS: Maxillary sinus
MT: Middle turbinate	NB: Nasal bone
NLD: Nasolacrimal duct	NS: Nasal septum
PPF: Pterygopalatine fossa	SS: Sphenoid sinus

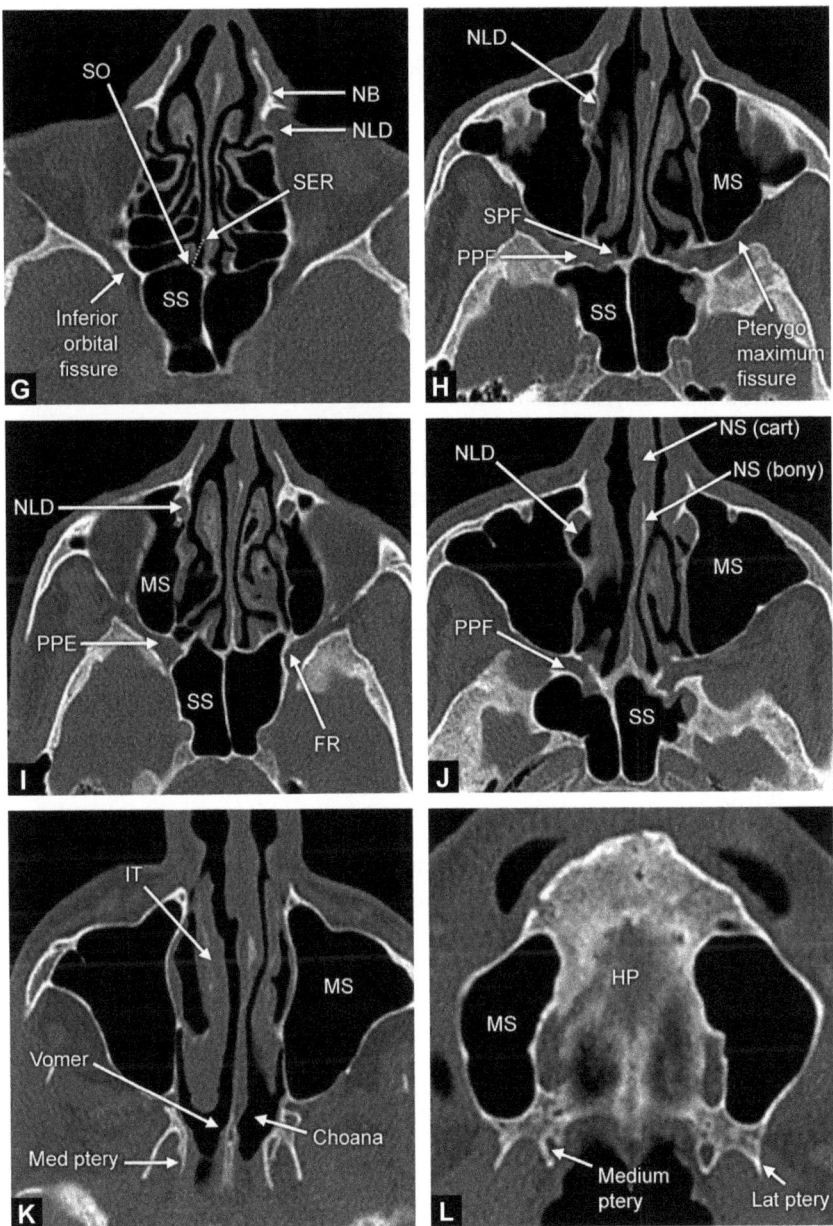

Figs. 3.2G to L: Consecutive axial sections from cranial to caudal.

CONSECUTIVE SAGITTAL SECTIONS

Consecutive sagittal sections are depicted from lateral to medial in Figures 3.3A to F. Sagittal sections well depict the drainage pathways of frontal sinus and sphenoid sinus.

Sagittal Sections (Figs. 3.3A to F)

- Laterally on these sagittal images, frontal (FS) and maxillary sinuses (MS) can be seen.
- On a more medial section through the nasal cavity, the turbinates and meati are well-visualized.
- The anterior and posterior ethmoidal cells (PE cells) are seen between the frontal and sphenoid sinuses (SS).
- Agger nasi cell is the anterior most anterior ethmoidal cell seen anterior to the frontal sinus drainage pathway.
- Bulla ethmoidalis (BE) is the largest anterior ethmoidal cell and lies behind the frontal sinus drainage pathway.
- The posterior boundary of the bulla ethmoidalis (BE) is the basal lamella (BL).
- Sphenoid ostium (SO) is the opening of the sphenoid sinus into sphenoethmoidal recess.
- Onodi cells if present can be seen projecting superior to the sphenoid sinus.
- Parts of nasal septum, both cartilaginous and bony (vomer and perpendicular plate of ethmoid) can be seen in the midline.
- Hard palate forms the inferior boundary of the nasal cavity.

Key

AN: Agger nasi cells	BE : Bullae ethmoidalis
BL: Basal lamella	FS: Frontal sinus
FSDP: Frontal sinus drainage pathway	HP: Hard palate
IM: Inferior meatus	IT: Inferior turbinate
MM: Middle meatus	MT: Middle turbinate
NB: Nasal bone	NS: Nasal septum
SO: Sphenoid ostium	SS: Sphenoid sinus

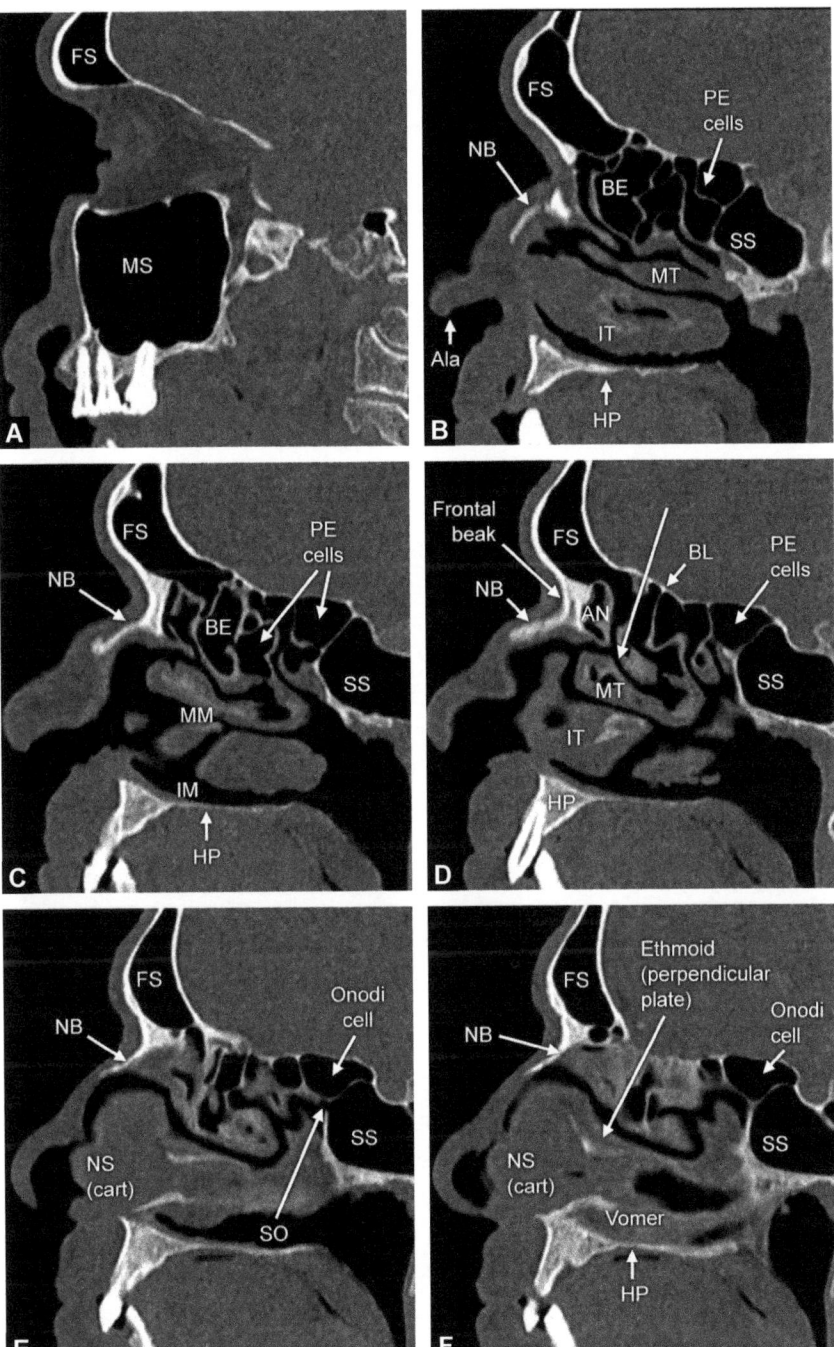

Figs. 3.3A to F: Consecutive sagittal sections.

Section 2

Inflammatory Nasal Conditions

4. Imaging in Rhinosinusitis (Inflammatory Diseases)
5. Imaging in Polyps and Mucocele
6. Chronic Rhinosinusitis: Clinical Aspects
7. Imaging in Fungal Sinusitis
8. Fungal Diseases of Nose and Paranasal Sinuses: Surgical Aspects
9. Pre- and Post-functional Endoscopic Sinus Surgery Imaging

4
CHAPTER

Imaging in Rhinosinusitis (Inflammatory Diseases)

Ashu Seith Bhalla, Smita Manchanda

- Introduction
- Classification
- Imaging Modalities
- Acute Sinusitis
  - Complications
- Chronic Rhinosinusitis
  - Imaging Findings
  - Staging
  - Patterns
  - Causes of Obstruction to Drainage Pathways
  - Chronic Complications
- Retention Cyst, Polyps, Mucocoele
- Silent Sinus Syndrome
- Atrophic Rhinitis
  - Miscellaneous Associations
- Chronic Inflammation and Cocaine Abuse
- Sinonasal Tuberculosis
- Dental Infection and Sinusitis
  - Differential Diagnosis

INTRODUCTION

- Refers to inflammation of the sinus mucosa, often accompanied by that of nasal mucosa as well.
- Incidental mucosal thickening is often detected in asymptomatic patients undergoing magnetic resonance imaging (MRI) for other indications. It is reported that up to 20-40% patients who undergo MRI may display mucosal thickening in the sinonasal (SN) cavity.[1] In asymptomatic patients this mucosal thickening may not have any clinical significance.
- *Drainage pathways*
  - Sinus lined by ciliated columnar epithelium → mucous propelled to sinus ostium by cilia → nasal cavity → pharynx
  - Any obstruction in nasociliary pathways for clearance of mucosa leads to accumulation of secretion in the sinus.

CLASSIFICATION

Various bases of classification are:
- Based on etiology: Infective (viral, bacterial or fungal), non-infective (reactive or allergic)
- Based on duration: Acute, subacute or chronic (Chapter 6)
- Based on extra-sinus or vascular infiltration: Invasive or noninvasive
- Based on extent: Various patterns are described which are detailed subsequently.

IMAGING MODALITIES

- Imaging is seldom indicated for acute sinusitis, but is performed if recurrent episodes of acute sinusitis occur, or in chronic sinusitis. Imaging is also indicated when complicated acute sinusitis is suspected.[1,2]

Plain Radiographs

- May be used in acute sinusitis or as a screening modality in those with a low clinical suspicion.
- Should be performed in sitting/standing position.
- No patient preparation is required.
- Frequently used views are Water's view (Fig. 4.1) and Caldwell's view, occasionally lateral view may be required.
- May be used for follow-up imaging.

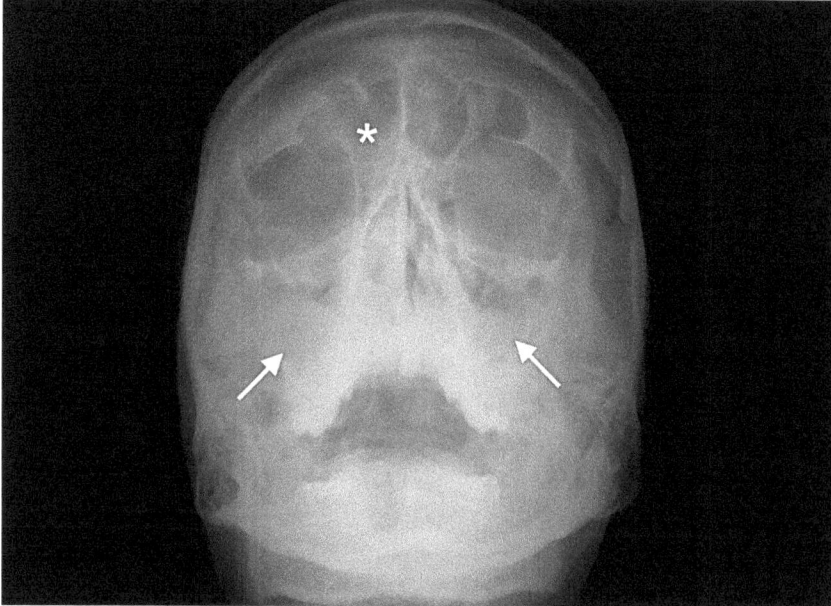

Fig. 4.1: Chronic sinusitis (Water's view). Mucosal thickening bilateral maxillary (arrows) and right frontal sinuses (asterisk).

Computed Tomography (CT) Scan

- Non-contrast computed tomography (NCCT) is the imaging modality of choice for imaging of chronic or recurrent disease.
- Low dose CT may be used, especially for follow-up imaging.
- If there is suspicion of complicated acute sinusitis clinically, then contrast administration will be required.
- NCCT should be performed only after adequate dose of antibiotics and resolution of symptoms of acute sinusitis.
- Also, it is advocated that after nasal blowing, nasal decongestants may be instilled 15 minutes prior to the scan. This is, however, not universally advocated.

Magnetic Resonance Imaging (MRI)

- Contrast enhanced MRI is the preferred modality when complications of acute sinusitis are suspected.
- However, not a preferred modality for chronic sinusitis as it can lead to underestimation of the disease. Also, calcification, air and long standing desiccated secretions all appear similar (signal voids).

ACUTE SINUSITIS

- Allergic or infective in etiology.
- Imaging is seldom indicated unless complications suspected.
- *Plain radiographs:* Sinus opacification/air fluid levels are seen.
- *CT/MRI:* Mucosal thickening with submucosal edema and/or secretions within the sinuses. Acute secretions being mucoid in nature have an attenuation similar to water (up to 25 HU). Interspersed lucencies due to air bubbles/an air fluid level (Fig. 4.2) may be seen, which is considered characteristic of acute sinusitis.
- On MRI, acute secretions appear hypointense on T_1WI and hyperintense on T_2 weighted images.
- While an air-fluid level may be seen in acute sinusitis, its presence does not necessarily imply acute sinusitis. There can be several causes for it (Table 4.1).

Complicated Acute Sinusitis (Figs. 4.3 and 4.4)

- Besides immunocompromised hosts, complications are more frequent in children.
- Complications of acute sinusitis (Table 4.2)[2] primarily result from extra-sinus spread of the inflammation.
- Complications are more severe and more frequent in immunocompromised hosts.
- Contrast enhanced MRI is required to detail the extent, when orbital or intracranial spread is suspected.

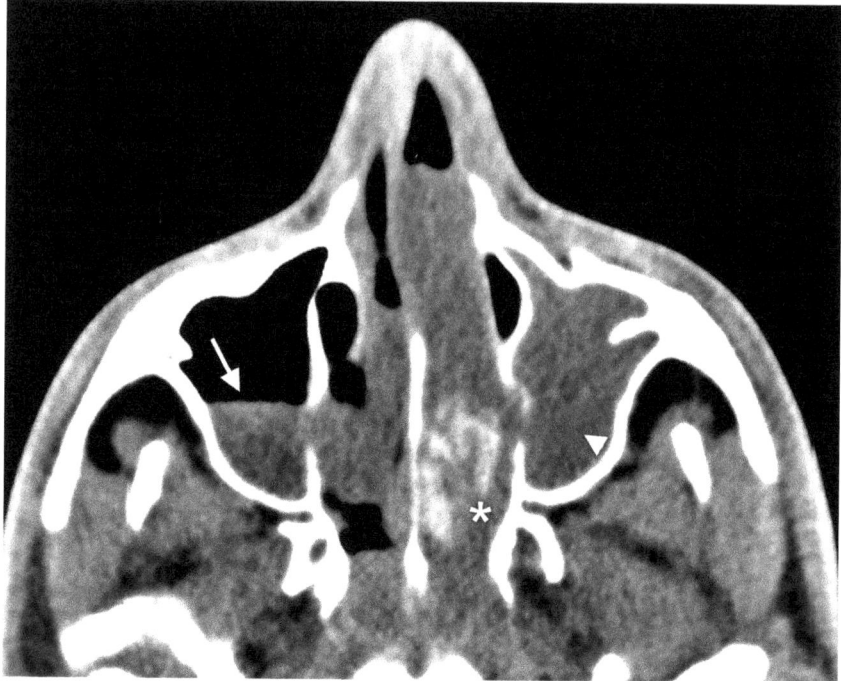

Fig. 4.2: Acute on chronic sinusitis. Air fluid level right maxillary sinus (arrow). Hypodense secretions left maxillary sinus (arrowhead) with hyperdense secretions in left posterior nasal cavity (asterisk).

Table 4.1: Causes for air-fluid level.
1. Acute sinusitis
2. Recent trauma
3. Recent surgery
4. Antral lavage or oroantral fistula
5. Hemorrhage in coagulopathies
6. Barotrauma
7. Sinonasal polyposis
8. Children who have been crying

- Fat-suppressed T_1 weighted images best delineate extent.
- *Orbital complications*
  - More frequent in children than in adults.
  - Inflammatory edema results in swelling of eyelid. As the inflammation progresses, it may result in orbital cellulitis, subperiosteal and orbital abscesses.

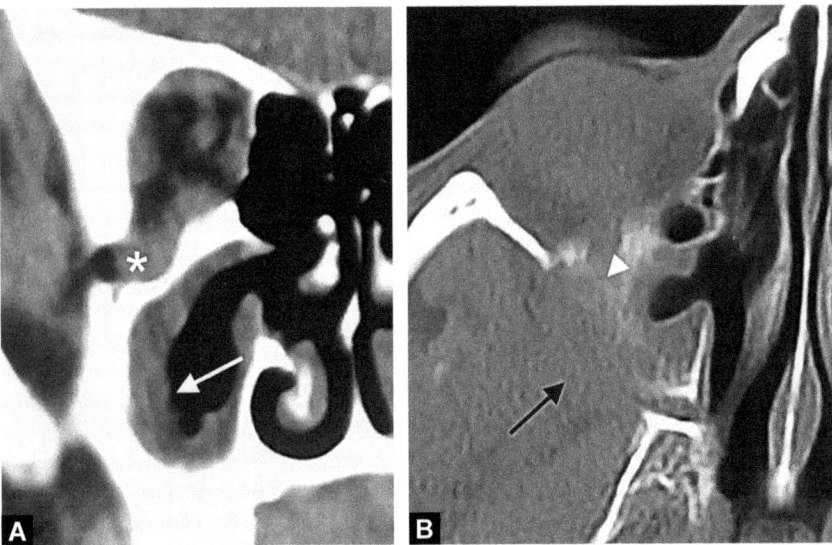

Figs. 4.3A and B: Complications of sinusitis—cellulitis and periostitis. Right maxillary mucosal disease (white arrow) with erosion of posterior wall (arrowhead). Ill-defined soft tissue in inferior orbital fissure (asterisk) and retroantral fat (black arrow).

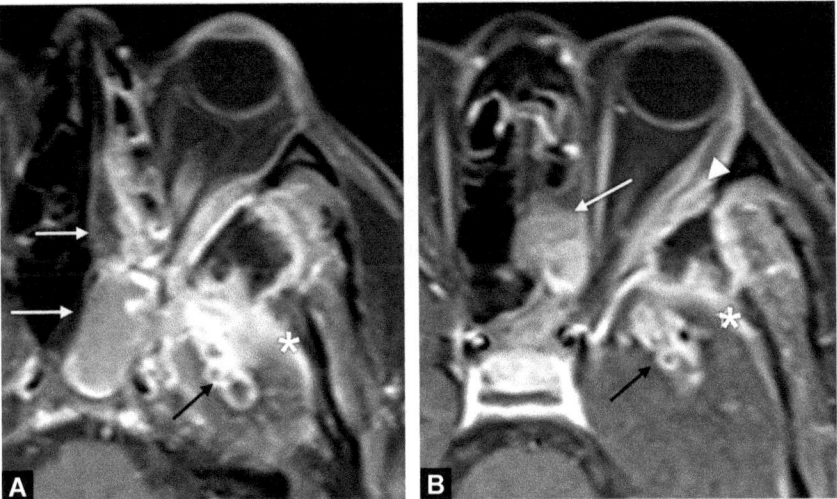

Figs. 4.4A and B: Intracranial complications of sinusitis—meningitis and cerebral abscesses. Left ethmoid and sphenoid mucosal enhancement with secretions (white arrows). Erosion of zygomatic bone with subperiosteal abscess (arrowhead). Abnormal meningeal enhancement along left temporal lobe (asterisk). Multiple small ring enhancing lesions s/o intra-axial abscesses left temporal lobe (black arrow).

- *Intracranial complications*
    - In case of frontal sinus involvement, there can be spread of infection to orbit and also intracranially through its posterior plate (when periostitis/osteomyelitis develops).

Table 4.2: Complications of acute sinusitis.	
	CECT/CEMR Findings
Orbital	
Cellulitis and periostitis (Fig. 4.3)	• Ill-defined soft tissue enhancement • Contiguous to sinus inflammation • Extra-ocular muscles may be involved • Critical structure at orbital apex
Abscess (Fig. 4.4)	• Low density collections with rim enhancement • Subperiosteal abscesses form along medial wall/roof/floor
Superior ophthalmic vein thrombosis	
Intracranial	(Less frequent than orbital complications)
	• Subdural effusion is the commonest (most common organism: *Streptococcus anginosus*)
Cavernous Sinus Thrombosis	• Enlargement with lateral convexity of unilateral/bilateral cavernous sinuses
Extra-axial abscesses	• Epidural/ subdural collections • Rim enhancing low density extra-axial collections
Cerebritis	• Edema/ill-defined enhancement of brain parenchyma • Uncommon, more often in children with frontal sinusitis
Cerebral abscess	• Walled off collections with rim enhancement • Surrounding edema

- "Pott's puffy tumor"—osteomyelitis of the frontal sinus results in edema (doughy feel) overlying the sinus. Also an accompanying subgaleal abscess contributes to the mass-like appearance.
- Rarely spread of infection from sinuses to cranium may occur through skull base defects (congenital/acquired).
- Also sphenoid sinus is a less frequent site of sinusitis (<3%), it is most common site to result in meningitis.

CHRONIC RHINOSINUSITIS

Imaging Findings

Imaging is the mainstay of diagnosis. Imaging findings include mucosal thickening, retained secretions and bony changes.
- *Mucosal thickening*[2,3]
  - Normal mucosa is not visualized on CT/MR and hence any vascularized soft tissue seen lining the air filled sinuses is labeled as "thickened".
  - However, some mucosal thickening may be seen in normal individuals (as physiologic), and the criteria vary among different sinuses (Figs. 4.5A and B).

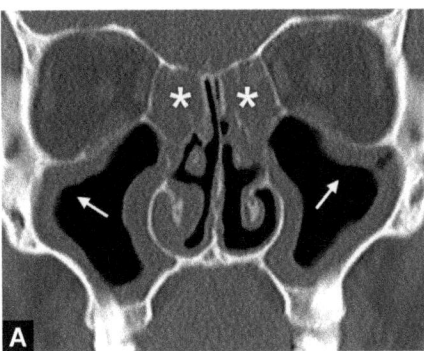
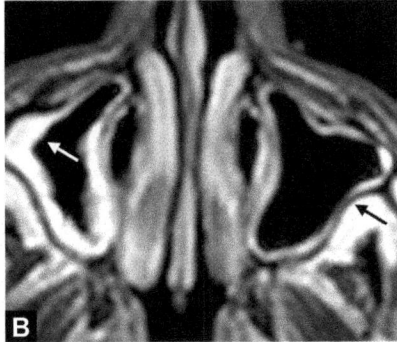

Figs. 4.5A and B: Mucosal thickening. (A) CT: Mucosal thickening of bilateral maxillary (white arrows) and ethmoid sinuses (asterisks). (B) MRI (T2WI): Right maxillary sinus: Thickened mucosa (white arrow), left maxillary sinus—normal (<3 mm) (black arrow).

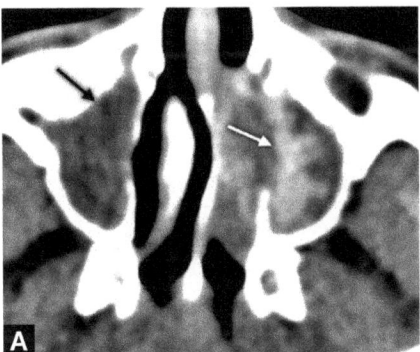
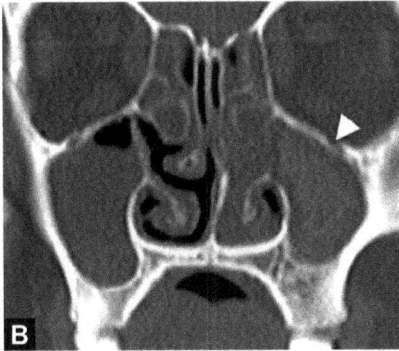

Figs. 4.6A and B: Opacification of sinuses. Right maxillary sinus: Hypodense secretions (black arrow). Left: Hyperdense inspissated secretions (white arrow) with decreased size (evolving silent sinus) (arrowhead).

- Maxillary sinuses: up to 3 mm normal, frontal sinus: any thickening is abnormal, ethmoid sinus: up to 2 mm normal.

Retained secretions[3,4]
- Accumulation of secretions leads to opacification of sinuses.
- Over a period of time, there is resorption of the fluid component and increase in the protein content of the secretions. Hence, these become thick and viscous.
- *On CT (Figs. 4.6A and B),* while acute secretions are of water density, these become increasingly more dense, and eventually long inspissated secretions appear hyperdense.
- Calcification is infrequent, has a scattered, peripheral distribution, and may give an egg-shell or round appearance. The secretions of calcific density give the appearance of an antrolith (Figs. 4.7A and B)

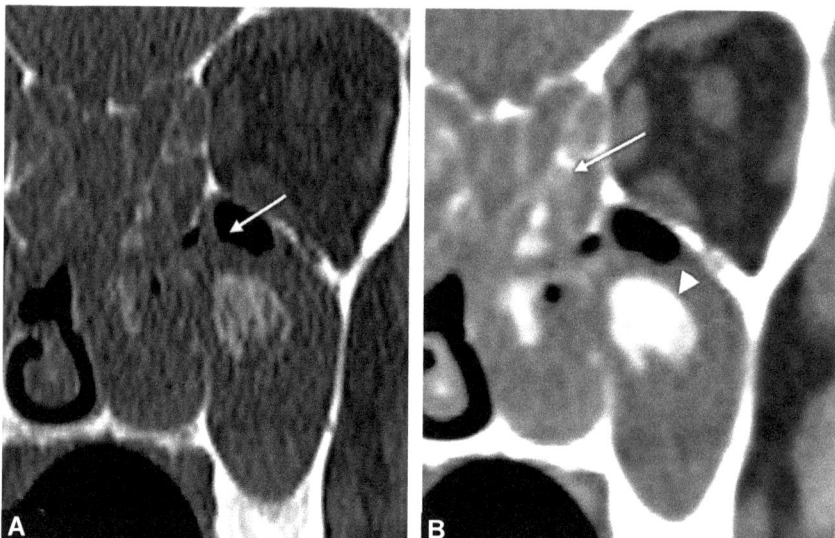

Figs. 4.7A and B: Maxillary antrolith in polyposis pattern of CRS. Opacification of left maxillary and ethmoid sinuses with widening of ostiomeatal unit (arrows). Retained secretions forming maxillary antrolith (arrowhead).

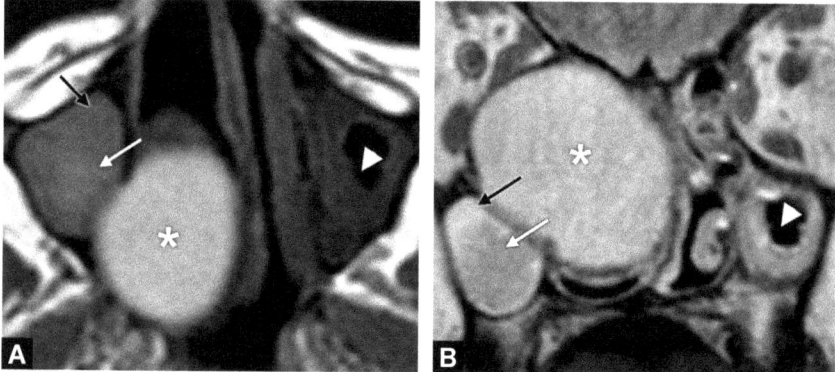

Figs. 4.8A and B: MRI appearance of secretions. (A) Axial T1WI; (B) Coronal T2WI
- Right maxillary sinus:
  – Peripheral secretions (black arrow)-T1 hypointense, T2 hyperintense
  – Central secretions (white arrow)-T1 hyperintense, T2 hypointense
- Left maxillary sinus:
  – Mucosal thickening (arrowhead)-T1 hypointense, T2 hyperintense
- Large right ethmoidal mucocoele (asterix) is seen

- Interspersed between the inspissated secretions and the bony sinus wall, the thickened mucosa and submucosal edema appears as a hypodense line.
- *On MRI (Figs. 4.8A and B), the alterations in the signal intensity of the secretions on T1 and T2 weighted images depends on the percentage of protein content and the viscosity.*[2] Different protein contents result in

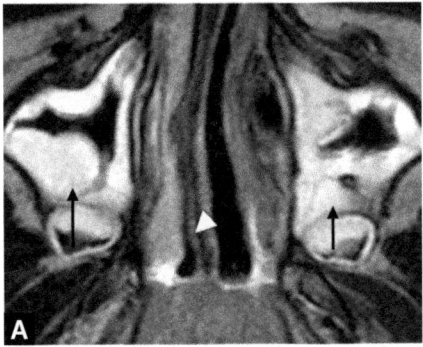 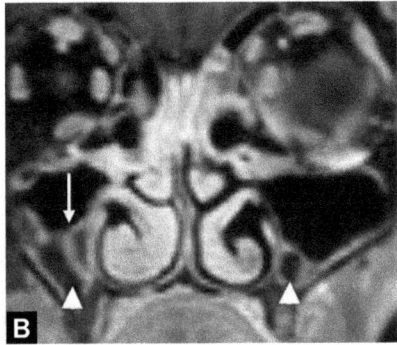

Figs. 4.9A and B: Polypoid mucosal disease with active inflammation. (A) Axial T2WI. Polypoid mucosal disease with submucosal edema in bilateral maxillary sinuses (black arrows). Both appear hyperintense. (B) Coronal postcontrast T1WI. Mucosal enhancement (white arrow) outlining nonenhancing submucosal edema (arrowheads).

different signal intensities on T1 and T2W-images with up to 5% protein content appearing hypointense on T1WI and hyperintense on T2WI. Between 5% and 25%, both the T1 and T2 signal is hyperintense whereas between 25% and 30%, the T2 signal becomes hypointense. As the protein content increases to 30–35%, both the T1 and T2 signals become hypointense. High protein content of >35% appears as signal void on T1- and T2WI mimicking an aerated sinus and hence CT correlation is necessary.

- On contrast enhanced magnetic resonance (CEMR), if active inflammation is present the mucosa enhances as a thin line, and edematous zone seen between this enhancing line and bony wall represents submucosal edema (Figs. 4.9A and B).
- In the fibrotic stage, the thickened mucosa does not enhance.

Bony changes

- Over a period of time, chronic rhinosinusitis (CRS) is accompanied by thickening and sclerosis of the sinus walls (Figs. 4.10A and B).
- Thinning or erosion is only seen in mucocele, polyps or fungal forms of the disease.

Staging

- There are various staging systems available but are not commonly used. One of these is the radiological Lund-Mackay system.
- The modified Lund-Mackay system (2) includes the following:
  - Sinus opacification (0 for normal, 1 for partial and 2 for total); OMC (0 for no obstruction, 2 for obstructed sinus) and normal variants (0 if absent and 1 for present). These variants include absent frontal sinus, paradoxic middle turbinate, concha bullosa, Haller cells, Agger nasi cell pneumatization and everted uncinate process.
- It is said that these scores correlate with the surgical treatment and its outcome.

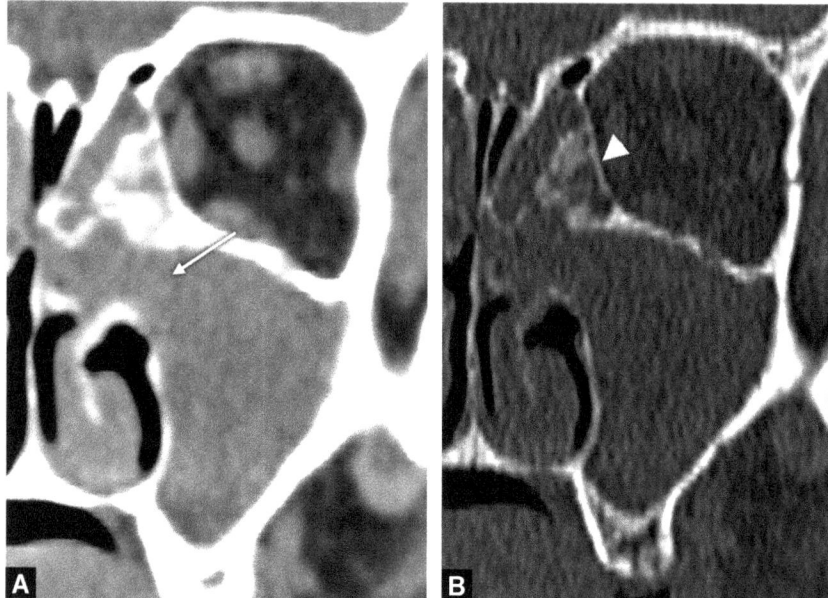

Figs. 4.10A and B: Bony changes (sclerosis) in polyposis pattern of chronic rhinosinusitis (CRS). (A) Opacification of left maxillary and ethmoid sinuses with widening of osteomeatal unit (arrow). (B) Sclerosis of ethmoid trabeculae (arrowhead).

Patterns of CRS

- Based on the distribution of the disease as seen on NCCT, CRS has been divided into five patterns (Table 4.3; Figs. 4.11 to 4.14)[5,6]
- This classification has management implications in that it covers the choice of surgical technique with patterns III and IV being labeled as complex surgical groups.

Sinonasal Polyposis

- Sinonasal polyposis is a nonobstructive form of CRS diffusely involving the sinuses and nasal cavity.
- The diffuse polyposis characteristically shows central hyperdensity on NCCT (due to inspissated secretions) with background hypodensity, which is due to secretions that are more mucoid.
- There is widening of the ostomeatal units and ethmoid infundibulum with erosion of bony ethmoidal trabeculae and nasal septum. Bulging of the bony ethmoid walls may be seen (Figs. 4.15A and B).

Causes of Obstruction of Drainage Pathways

The common cause of obstruction of drainage pathways includes mucosal inflammation (causing thickening), hypertrophied turbinates, adhesions, polyps, tumors and anatomical variants. The anatomical variants and the resultant pattern of CRS are detailed in Table 4.4.

Chapter 4 Imaging in Rhinosinusitis (Inflammatory Diseases)

Table 4.3: Patterns of chronic rhinosinusitis (CRS).

Pattern	Sinus/Sinuses involved	Site of obstruction	Surgery	Recurrence
I: Infundibular pattern (Figs. 4.11A and B)	Unilateral maxillary sinus	Ostium of • Maxillary sinus • Inferior infundibulum	Simple endoscopic procedure	Low
II: Osteomeatal Unit Pattern (Figs. 4.12A and B)	• Unilateral • Maxillary • Frontal • Anterior ethmoidal cells	• Middle meatus and • Ostiomeatal unit	More extensive surgery (vs pattern I)	Higher
Subpattern: Frontal recess pattern (Figs. 4.13A and B)	Unilateral frontal sinus	Frontal recess		
III: Sphenoethmoid recess pattern (Figs. 4.14A and B)	Sphenoid sinus ± Posterior ethmoid cells	Sphenoethmoid recess	• More complex surgery • Higher complication rate	High
IV: Sinonasal polyposis (Figs. 4.15A and B)	All sinuses and nasal cavity Diffuse involvement	Nonobstructive form	• Medical treatment • Surgery in refractory cases • Extensive difficult surgery	High
V: Sporadic pattern	• Random involvement • Not explained by drainage walls • Often single sinuses			

Note: In the presence of widening of ostium or bony erosion in the drainage pathway, polyposis or tumor should be suspected and contrast study/sampling is advised.

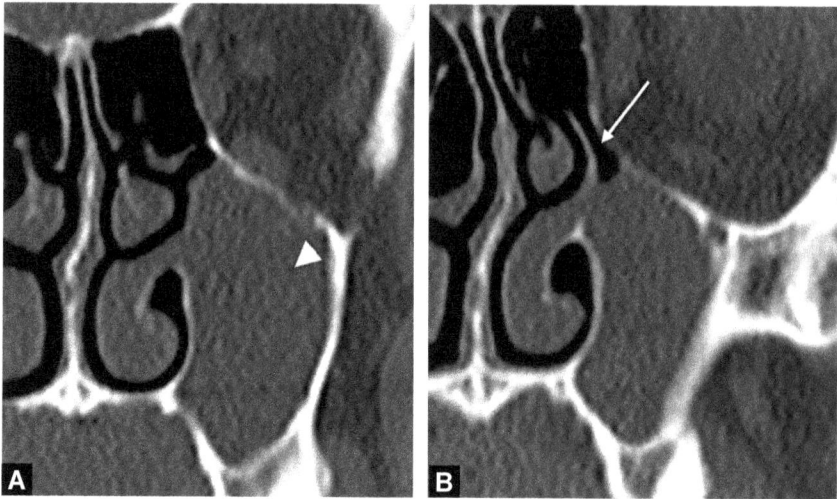

Figs. 4.11A and B: Infundibular pattern (I). (A) Opacified left maxillary sinus (arrowhead); (B) Obstruction at left infundibulum (arrow).

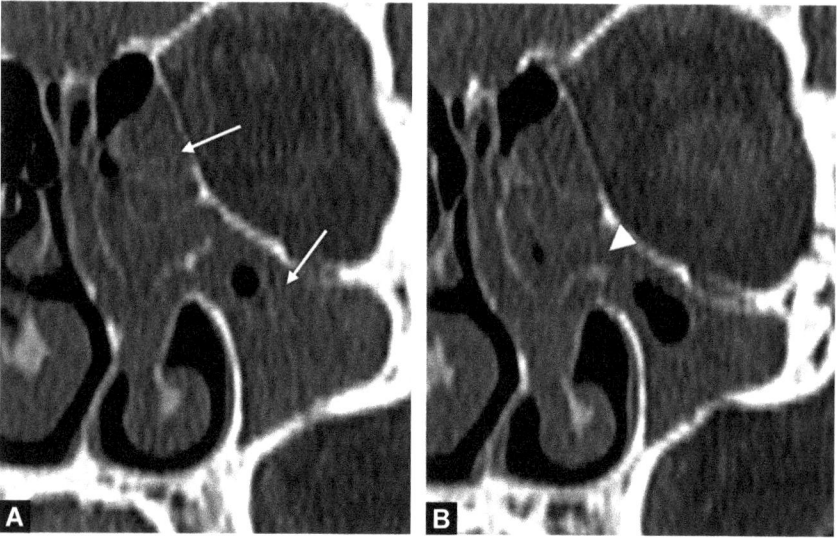

Figs. 4.12A and B: Osteomeatal unit pattern (II). (A) Opacified left anterior ethmoid air cells and maxillary sinus (arrows); (B) Obstructed osteomeatal unit (arrowhead).

Chronic Complications/Sequelae

- Chronic complications of CRS include retention cysts, polyps, mucocele, silent sinus syndrome and atrophic rhinitis. Retention cysts are detailed in Chapter 5.
- ***Silent sinus syndrome***
  - *Synonyms:* Imploding antrum syndrome, chronic maxillary sinus atelectasis

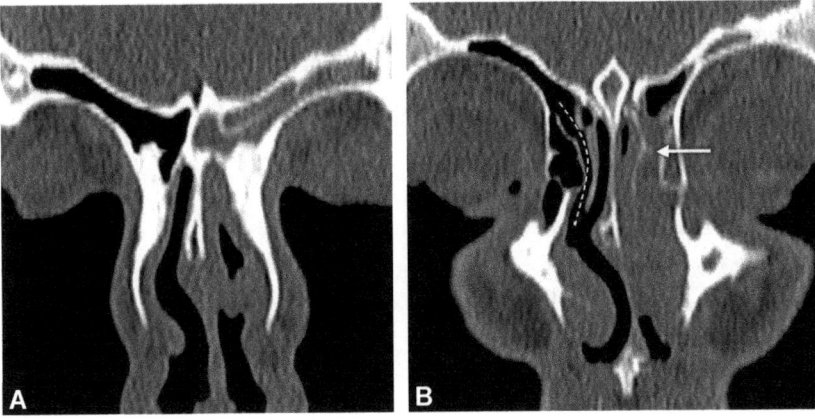

Figs. 4.13A and B: Frontal recess pattern. (A) Opacified left frontal sinus; (B) Occluded left frontonasal drainage pathway (arrow) compared with normal right side (dotted line).

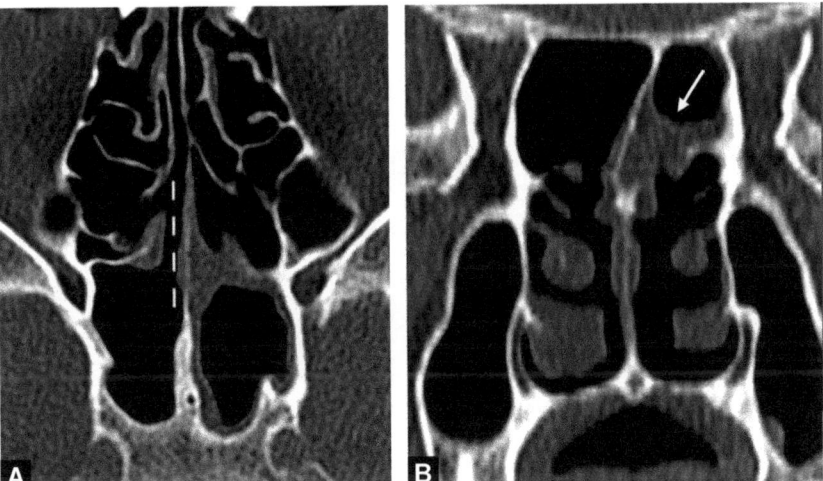

Figs. 4.14A and B: Sphenoethmoidal recess pattern (III). (A) Normal right sphenoethmoidal recess (dotted line); (B) Soft tissue thickening left sphenoid sinus (arrow) with obliteration of sphenoethmoid recess.

- Sequelae of chronic occlusion of the maxillary sinus ostium
- Leads to volume loss/shrinkage of the sinus due to negative pressure
- Clinical presentation is of gradual enophthalmos and facial asymmetry. Patient is often not symptomatic for the sinus symptoms; hence the term "silent"
- Air within the sinus is absorbed and it is filled with thick secretions (Figs. 4.17A and B)
- Seen in adults, is either the consequence of chronic sinusitis or occasionally of trauma of the lateral nasal wall.

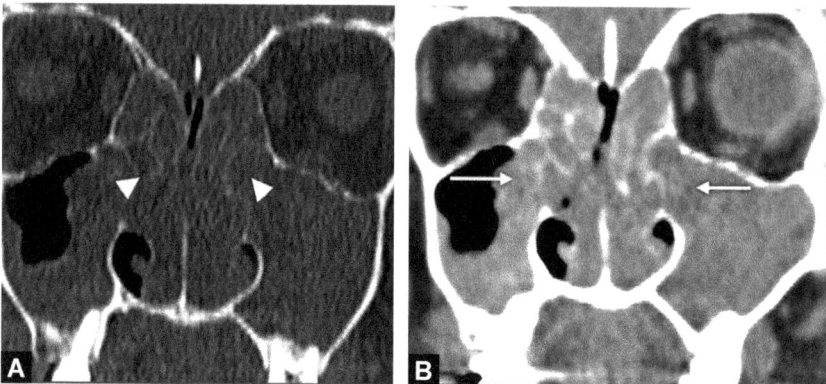

Figs. 4.15A and B: Sinonasal polyposis pattern (IV). (A) Near complete opacification of bilateral sinonasal cavities. Deossification of ethmoid trabeculae (arrowheads). (B) Widening of ostiomeatal units (arrows).

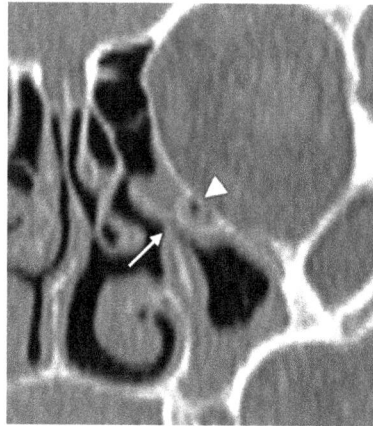

Fig. 4.16: Haller cell causing type I pattern. Left Haller cell (arrowhead) causing obstruction of left infundibulum (arrow) and maxillary sinusitis.

Table 4.4: Anatomical variants causing obstruction of sinus drainage pathways.	
Anatomical variants	Pattern of CRS
Haller cell (Fig. 4.16)	Pattern I
Pneumatized uncinate	
Enlarged ethmoidal bulla	
Hypoplastic maxillary sinuses	
Concha bullosa	Pattern II
Paradoxical middle turbinate	
Interlamellar cell of Grunwald	
Deviated nasal septum	
Agger nasi cell	Frontal recess pattern
Frontal ethmoidal cells	
Interfrontal sinus septal cell (narrow frontal ostium)	

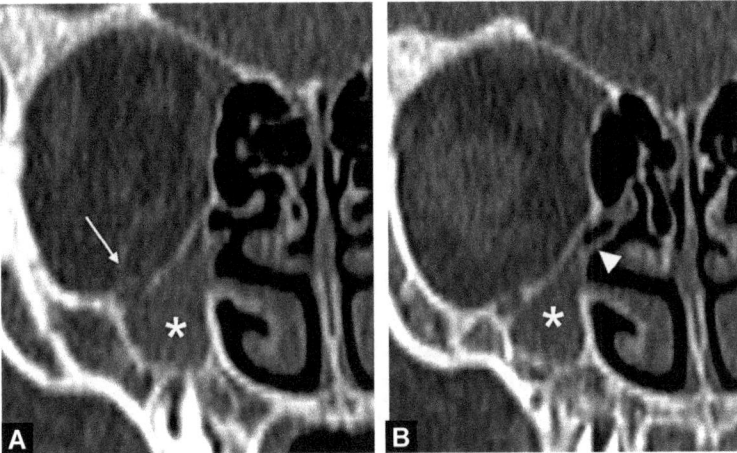

Figs. 4.17A and B: Silent sinus syndrome. Small opaque maxillary sinus with infundibular occlusion (asterisks). Enlargement of orbit with downward displacement of the floor (arrow). Lateral retraction/displacement of uncinate process (arrowhead).

- *Imaging* (Figs. 4.17A and B):
  - There is volume loss of sinus with inward bowing of sinus walls that are also thickened, sinus is opacified with dense secretions.
  - Downward displacement of the orbital floor is seen with enophthalmos. There is also increased orbital volume and even thinning of the orbital floor.
  - The osteomeatal unit/ostium is blocked.
  - There is lateral retraction of the uncinate process which rests against the inferomedial wall of the orbit. Middle meatus is thus enlarged.
  - Increase in retroantral fat pad is seen.[3]
- *Treatment:* Surgical with uncinectomy and clearance of the ostium. Additional orbital floor repair may be required.
- *Differential diagnosis:*
  - Postoperative changes: following Caldwell-Luc operation.
  - Hypoplasia: It is an important differential in the absence of history of surgery and the differentiating points are discussed in detail at the end of the chapter.
- **Atrophic rhinitis**
  - *Synonyms:* Rhinitis sicca, ozera, open-nose syndrome.
  - *Two forms:* Primary or secondary.
  - Form of CRS wherein the ciliated columnar epithelium of the sinonasal cavity is replaced by non-ciliated epithelium resulting in "roomy" space.[7]
  - *Primary:* Decreasing incidence in modern world. May still be seen in developing world in parts of India, China, Middle East and Egypt.

Multifactorial causes postulated, however, most consistent is infection by *Klebsiella ozaenae*.
- *Secondary:* More common in developed world with most common cause being postsinus surgery. Others being radiation, trauma, granulomatous disease or infections. Granulomatous diseases include granulomatosis with polyangiitis (GPA), sarcoidosis, rhinoscleroma (see Chapter 22).
- *Clinical presentation*
    ▶ Classical triad described by Dr Frenkel includes fetor (malodor), crusting and atrophy.[7]
    ▶ Females > Males, begins in puberty.
    ▶ Severity grading given by *Ssali*[8]
        - Early: Minimal crest and odor with atrophy of turbinates.
        - Advanced stage has foul odor, plenty of crusting and generalized atrophy including bony atrophy.
        - Late advanced stage is extensive with large nasal cavities and even ulcers and bleeding.
- *Pathology:*
    ▶ Endarteritis and periarteritis affecting terminal arterioles is characteristic.
- *Imaging findings:*
    ▶ Similar in primary and secondary forms. Once secondary causes reach atrophic stages, difficult to differentiate.
    ▶ Findings include (Figs. 4.18A to C):
        - Roomy enlarged nasal cavities with outward bowing of lateral walls.
        - Mucosal atrophy and resorption of bony turbinates (middle and inferior).
        - Ostiomeatal complex loses definition with resorption of uncinate process and ethmoid sella.
        - Maxillary sinuses appear hypoplastic with mucoperiosteal thickening of the sinuses.
- *Management:*
    ▶ Several modalities ranging from nasal douching to estrogen to surgical treatment.

Miscellaneous Associations

Chronic Inflammation and Cocaine Abuse

- Inhalation (snorting/sniffing) of cocaine causes multiple sinonasal complications
- Mechanism: Direct irritation/Severe vasoconstriction
- Septal perforation/synechiae
- Chronic sinusitis/bone erosion
- Nasolacrimal duct block.

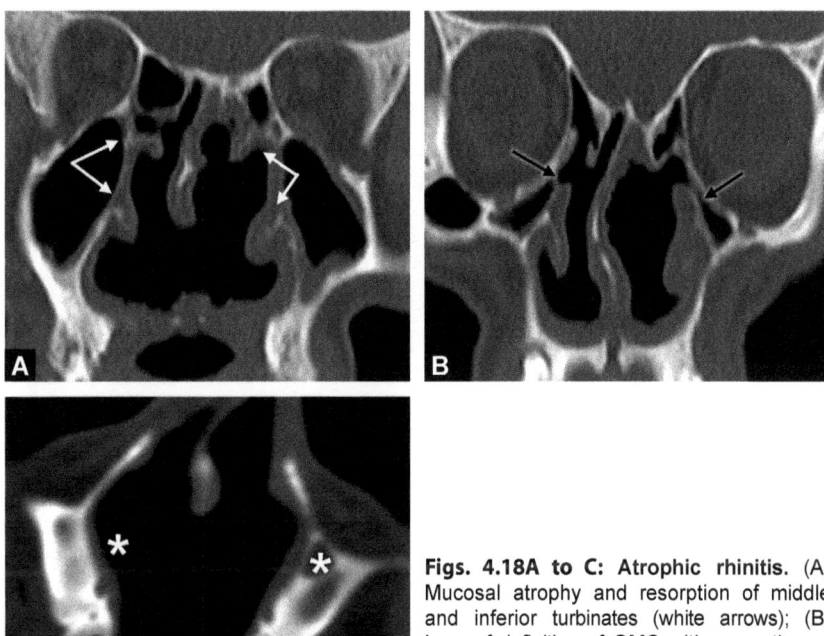

Figs. 4.18A to C: Atrophic rhinitis. (A) Mucosal atrophy and resorption of middle and inferior turbinates (white arrows); (B) Loss of definition of OMC with resorption of uncinate process (black arrows); (C) Roomy enlarged nasal cavities with outward bowing of lateral walls (asterisks).

Sinonasal Tuberculosis

- It is a rare entity and there is usually unilateral involvement
- Most common: Maxillary sinus involvement
- Pathological types:[9]
  - Mucosal disease with polyp formation
  - Bony involvement with fistula
  - Hyperplastic changes and tuberculoma formation
- Clinical and imaging features: Nonspecific
- Antral lavage examination: For AFB and culture for *Mycobacterium tuberculosis* is diagnostic.

Dental Infection and Sinusitis

- In those patients with sinusitis confined to a single maxillary sinus, especially with a recent/past history of tooth interventions, a dental cause for the infection should be suspected.
- Several of these patients have an oro-antral fistula (Figs. 4.19A and B) with discharge in the oral cavity (Further detailed in Chapter 24).

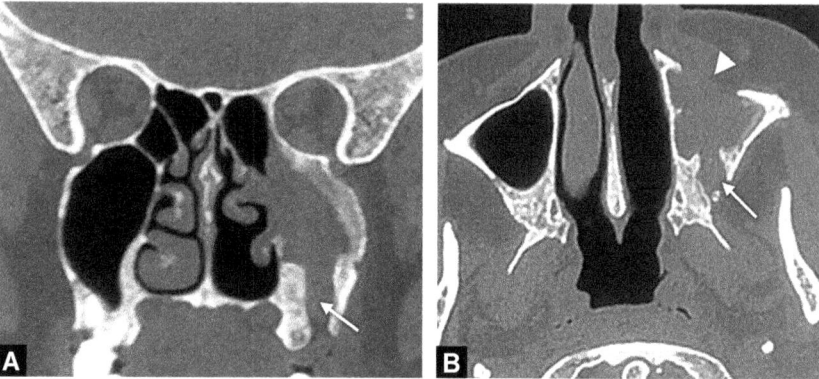

Figs. 4.19A and B: Oroantral fistula. Chronic left maxillary sinusitis and oroantral fistula (arrows) post-tooth extraction. Left antral anterior wall postoperative defect (post-Caldwell-Luc) (arrowhead).

DIFFERENTIAL DIAGNOSIS

Fungal Sinusitis

A. Acute Forms
- Difficult to differentiate complicated acute sinusitis of bacterial aetiology from acute invasive fungal sinusitis.
- However, if extra-sinus spread is seen into the orbit or perisinus soft tissues especially with intact sinus walls, suspect fungal aetiology.
- In immuno-compromised patients both pyogenic and fungal infections can be severe, but again possibility of fungal is always kept.

B. Chronic Forms
- Chronic inspissated secretions, mycetoma and chronic invasive sinusitis can all show hyperdensities in NCCT which appears hypointense on T2 weighted images. Hence, differentiating among these forms is difficult.
- Presence of bony erosions suggests chronic invasive fungal sinusitis among these.
- Invasive sinusitis also needs to be differentiated from malignancy.

Hypoplasia
- Is an important differential of silent sinus syndrome
- The key differentiating points are enlisted in Table 4.5 and detailed in Figures 4.20A to F.

CONCLUSION

Chronic rhinosinusitis is a common disease entity with varying patterns of involvement depending on the involvement of the sinus drainage pathways.

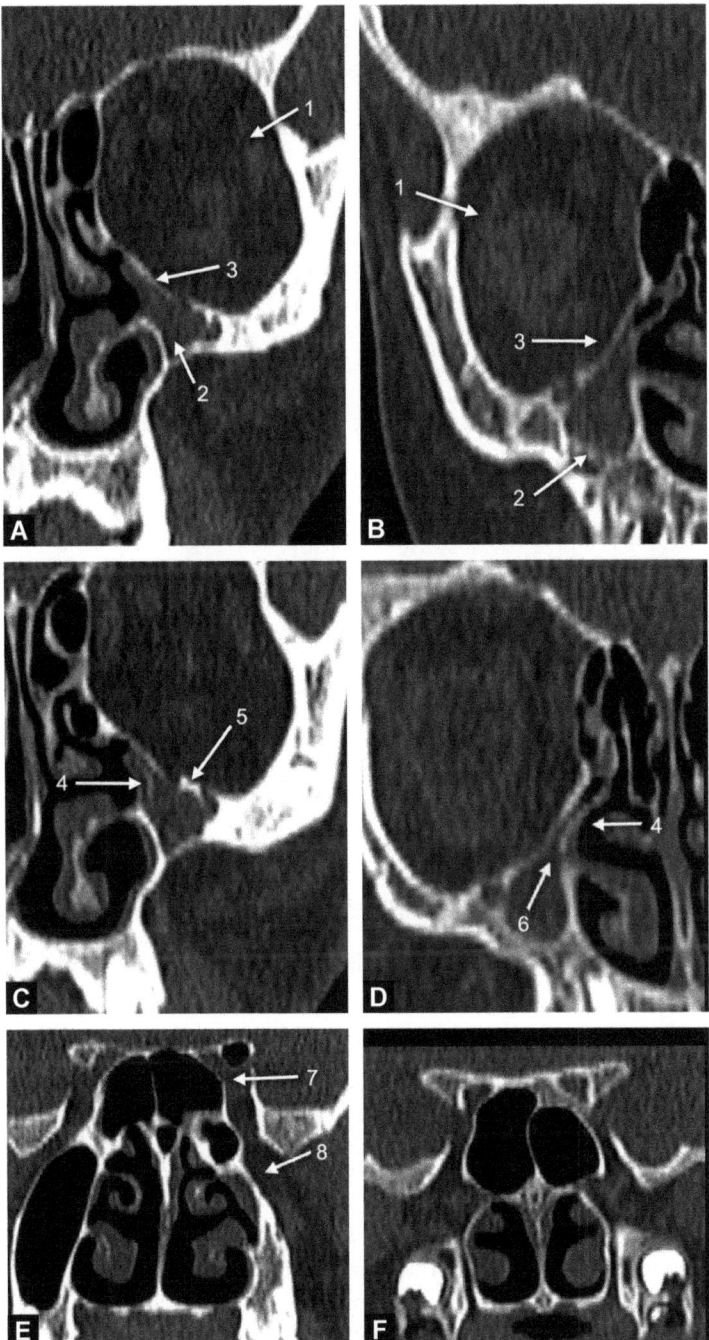

Figs. 4.20A to F: Hypoplasia (A, C, E) versus silent sinus syndrome (B, D, F). (1: enlargement of orbit; 2: small maxillary sinus; 3: infundibular occlusion and opaque sinus; 4: lateral retraction/displacement of uncinate process; 5: lateral displacement of infraorbital nerve canal; 6: inward retraction of sinus wall; 7: enlarged superior orbital fossa; 8: enlarged pterygopalatine fossa)

Table 4.5: Differentiating features of hypoplasia and silent sinus syndrome (Figs. 4.20A TO F).		
	Hypoplasia	Silent sinus syndrome
	Developmental: Due to poor pneumatization, extension into malar eminence laterally and alveolar ridge inferiorly does not happen	Acquired: Due to chronic ostial occlusion
Enlargement of Orbit	+	+
Lateral displacement of infraorbital nerve canal	+	-
Elevated canine fossa	+	-
Enlarged pterygopalatine fossa	+	-
Enlarged superior orbital fossa	+	-
Lateral retraction/displacement of uncinate process	+	+
Infundibular occlusion and opaque sinus	±	+
Inward retraction of sinus wall	-	+

REFERENCES

1. Mafee MF, Tran BH, Chapa AR. Imaging of rhinosinusitis and its complications: plain film, CT, and MRI. Clin Rev Allergy Immun. 2006:30;165-85.
2. Joshi VM, Sansi R. Imaging in sinonasal inflammatory disease. Neuroimag Clin N Am. 2015:25;549-68.
3. Broderick DF. The opacified paranasal sinus: approach and differential. Appl Radiol. 2015:44;9-17.
4. Whyte A, Chapeikin G. Opaque maxillary antrum: a pictorial review. Australas Radiol. 2005:49;203-13.
5. Babbel RW, Harnsberger HR, Sonkens J, et al. Recurring patterns of inflammatory sinonasal disease demonstrated on screening sinus CT. Am J Neuroradiol. 1992;13:903-12.
6. Sonkens JW, Harnsberger HR, Blanch GM, et al. The impact of screening sinus CT on the planning of functional endoscopic sinus surgery. Otolaryngol Head Neck Surg. 1991;105(6):802-13.
7. Bist SS, Bisht M, Purohit JP. Primary atrophic rhinitis: a clinical profile, microbiological and radiological study. ISRN Otolaryngol. 2012:404075.
8. Ssali CL. Atrophic rhinitis. A new curative surgical treatment (middle turbinectomy). J Laryngol Otol. 1973:87;397-403.
9. Kant S, Srivastava R, Verma AK, et al. Maxillary sinus tuberculosis: various presentations. Indian J Chest Dis Allied Sci. 2013;55:175-7.

5
CHAPTER

Imaging in Polyps and Mucoceles

Smita Manchanda, Ashu Seith Bhalla

- Introduction
- Nasal Polyps (Sinonasal Polyposis)
  - Etiology
  - Pathology
  - Imaging
- Choanal Polyps
  - Antrochoanal Polyp
  - Sphenochoanal Polyp
  - Ethmoidochoanal Polyps
- Retention Cysts
- Sinonasal Angiomatous Polyp (SAP) or Sinonasal Organized Hematoma
- Mucocele
- Large Air-filled Sinuses

INTRODUCTION

- Polyps are inflammatory, expansile masses of the sinonasal cavity.[1]
- They are the most common nasal cavity masses with frequent involvement of the ethmoid sinuses.
- Two forms of polyps are described:
  1. Nasal polyps [often associated with sinus involvement: sinonasal polyposis (SNP)]
  2. Choanal polyps.

NASAL POLYPS (SINONASAL POLYPOSIS)

Often bilateral disease with the involvement of nasal cavity and/or sinuses. These are more frequent in males.[1,2]

Etiology

- Multiple factors causing chronic mucosal inflammation may be responsible.
- Recurrent (acute/subacute) inflammation results in polypoidal changes.
- Associated with diverse etiologies including allergy, asthma, cystic fibrosis, aspirin intolerance, granulomatosis with polyangiitis, and allergic fungal rhinosinusitis.

- Chronic rhinosinusitis (CRS) is divided into two major phenotypes, i.e. (1) CRS with nasal polyps (CRSwNP) and (2) CRS without nasal polyps (CRSNP). Significant association between the form with polyps, and eosinophilia is seen.

Pathology (also see Chapter 10)
- Essentially polypoidal mucosal protrusions which are a consequence of accumulated fluid in the lamina propria.
- Mucosa shows either/combination of following changes: hypertrophic, polypoidal, fibrotic or atrophic.
- The surface of a polyp is mostly covered with ciliated pseudostratified columnar epithelium. However, the surface may have areas of transitional or squamous epithelium due to effects of air current. Mast cells are seen in most with neutrophils being present in the nonallergic forms, and eosinophils in the allergic form.

Imaging
- Polyps appear as as soft tissue masses in the nasal cavity/sinuses especially the ethmoids (Fig. 5.1A). Bilateral involvement is more frequent than unilateral involvement.
- Often expansile with thinning of overlying bony margin. Deossification of bone occurs mainly due to pressure erosions. Nasoethmoidal polyps lead to erosion of the septa, destruction of medial antral wall, and even skull base and lamina papyracea.
- Site of origin is thought to be the lateral nasal wall in the osteomeatal complex. Hence, the osteomeatal complex often shows changes with its widening (Fig. 5.1A), ballooning or erosion and destruction.
- CRSwNP may show areas of increased density due to "osteitis" (Fig. 5.1B).
- Sinonasal polyposis should hence be suspected (vs CRS alone) if there is expansion of the infundibulum or sinus expansion with bulging of lamina papyracea (Figs. 5.2A and B).

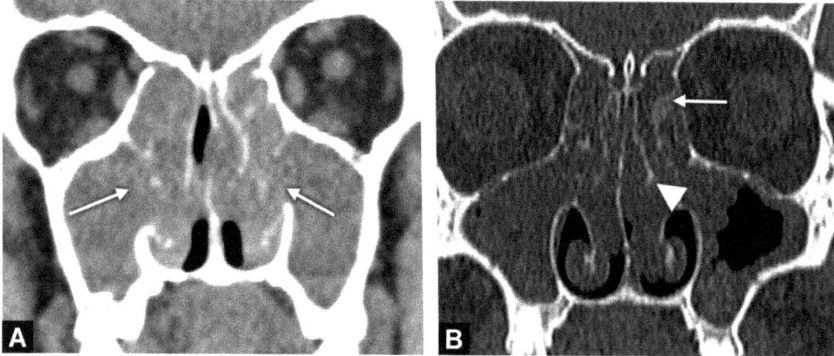

Figs. 5.1A and B: Sinonasal polyposis. (A) Expansile soft tissue masses in nasal cavity, bilateral maxillary, and ethmoid sinuses with widening of osteomeatal complex (arrows); and (B) Truncated middle turbinate (arrowhead). Increased bone density: "osteitis" (white arrow).

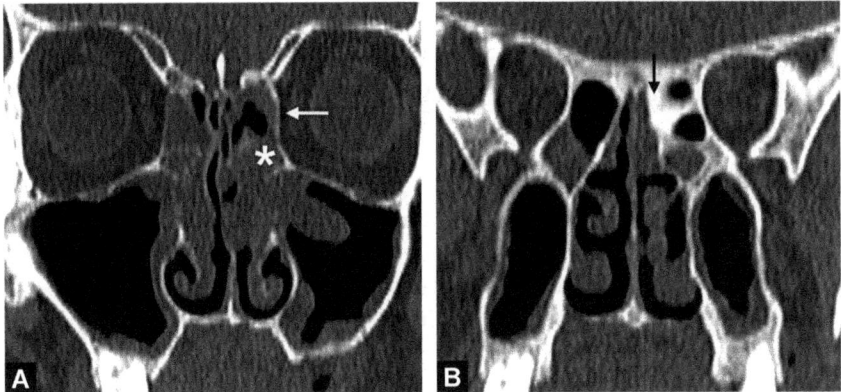

Figs. 5.2A and B: Nasoethmoidal polyposis. (A) Expansile polypoidal soft tissue bilateral ethmoids and nasal cavity. Bulging of lamina papyracea (arrow). Thinning of ethmoid trabeculae (asterisk); and (B) Osteitis left posterior ethmoid bony margins (black arrow).

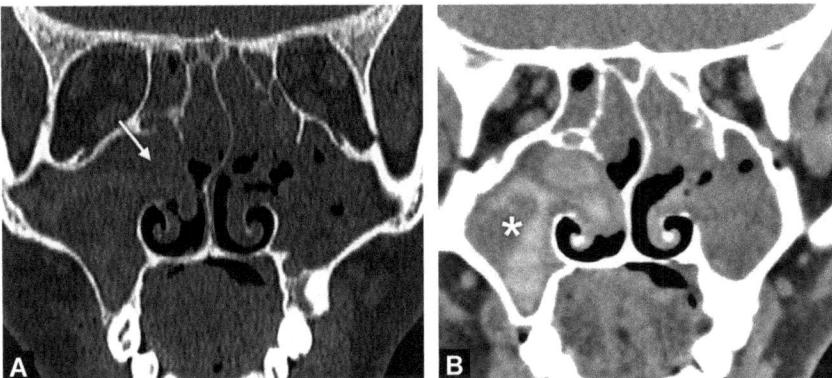

Figs. 5.3A and B: Polyposis with superadded fungal infection. (A) Expansile soft tissue masses in nasal cavity, bilateral maxillary and ethmoid sinuses. Widening of osteomeatal complex (arrow); and (B) Hyperdensity in right maxillary sinus: "double density sign" (asterisk).

- Sinonasal polyps may also be associated with a benign malformation called respiratory epithelial adenomatoid hamartoma. This causes expansion of the olfactory clefts adjoining the skull base with loss of volume of the olfactory bulbs. This subset of patients is associated with smell disturbances.
- Superadded fungal infection (noninvasive) may be present. This is suspected in the presence of the "double density sign" (Figs. 5.3A and B).
- The imaging appearance of the SNP may suggest the underlying etiology.[2] For example:
  - *Allergic fungal sinusitis*: Marked expansion often with central hyperdensities.
  - *Granulomatous disorders*: Septal destruction especially if associated with palate perforation.

> *Imaging Pearl*
> **When to suspect nasal polyposis in CRS?**
> When the middle turbinate is truncated with absence of its bulbous part.

CHOANAL POLYPS

- These are solitary, benign sinonasal masses which originate in a paranasal sinus and enter into the nasal cavity.
- These are typically unilateral and occur in young patients.
- *Imaging*: Variable density/signal intensity is characteristic.
- *Computed tomography (CT)*:
  - Polyps are of soft tissue density, however entrapped secretions may appear hypodense to hyperdense or even calcified (Figs. 5.4A and B). Foci of increased attenuation may also represent superadded fungal infection.
  - In case of multiple polyps there is entrapment of secretions between the polyps, and also in the crevices of the polyps.
  - Noncontrast computed tomography (NCCT) suffices in most, but in aggressive lesions mimicking malignancy, magnetic resonance imaging (MRI) is indicated.
- *Magnetic resonance imaging*:
  - Variable signal depending on the stage of the polyps.
  - Stages include initial edematous to glandular to cystic, and finally fibrous stage.[1] Similarly the entrapped secretions range from being mucoid to chronic desiccated.

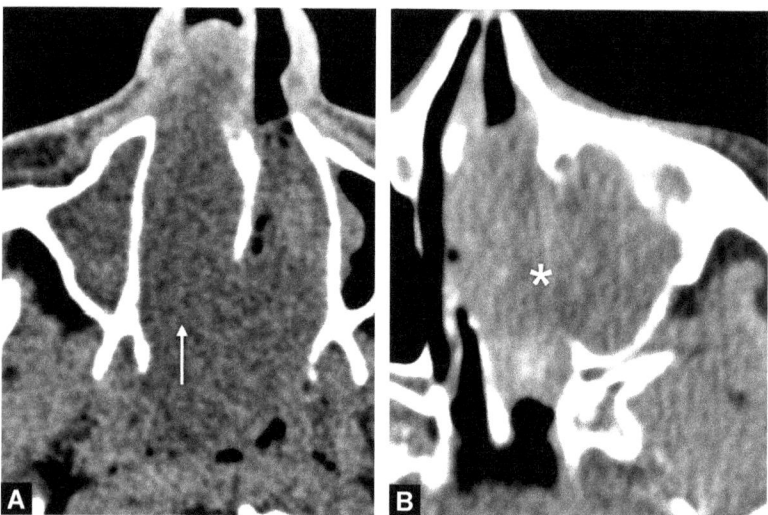

Figs. 5.4A and B: Polyps on noncontrast computed tomography (NCCT). Large expansile lesion in maxillary sinus and nasal cavity. Density varies according to the nature of entrapped secretions: hypodense (arrow) in (A) and soft tissue density (asterisk) in (B).

- This results in the polyp giving a variable appearance across different pulse sequences. This variation of signal intensities of various components of the polyps across different sequences aids in their distinction from tumors. Table 5.1 summarizes the basis of imaging appearance of polyp.
- Hence, variable signal intensity in different sequences is characteristic. Enhancement is intense with a layered appearance (Figs. 5.5A to C).
- Polyps may result in mucocele formation, and the distinction between the two can be difficult with the appearance resembling multiple polyps.
- *Differential diagnosis*:
  - Retention cyst shows rim enhancement, polyps demonstrate intense enhancement.

Table 5.1: Basis of imaging appearance of polyp.	
Stage of the hypertrophied mucosa: • Edematous • Glandular • Cystic • Fibrous	Content of the entrapped secretions (present between crevices and on surface): • CT: Hypodense initially → increasing concentration • MRI: Increasing T_1 signal, decreasing T_2 signal with increasing desiccation

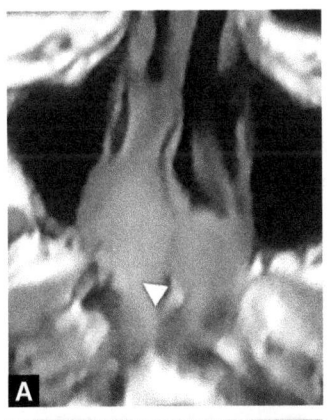
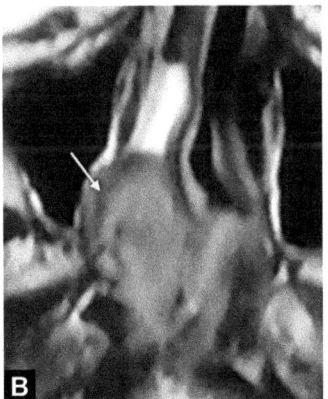
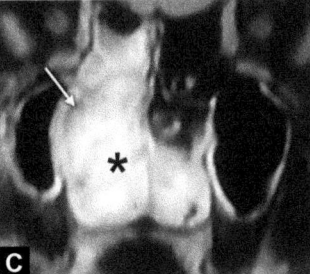

Figs. 5.5A to C: Polypoidal mass right ethmoidal cells, nasal cavity, choana. (A) Mass is hyperintense (arrowhead) on T1WI; (B) Intermediate signal on T2WI with hypointense rim (fibrotic part) (arrow); (C) Intense post contrast enhancement with a layered appearance (asterisk) and non-enhancing rim (arrow).

SI No	Types	Sinus of origin	Extension through	Extension to
			Table 5.2: Types of choanal polyps.	
1.	Antrochoanal	Maxillary sinus (antrum)	Maxillary infundibulum/ accessory ostium	Middle meatus and then to posterior choana
2.	Sphenochoanal	Sphenoid sinus	Sphenoid ostium	Sphenoethmoidal recess and then to choana
3.	Ethmoidochoanal	Ethmoid (posterior ethmoids) Bulla ethmoidalis	–	Choana

- *Types*:
  - The common types include antrochoanal, sphenochoanal and ethmoidochoanal (detailed in Table 5.2). The rare varieties are septochoanal (from the nasal septum) and those from the lateral wall of nose.[1,3]

Antrochoanal Polyp

- It is a subtype of polyp with a classical radiographic appearance and seen usually in young adults.
- Thought to develop from blocked mucous glands in the maxillary sinus forming retention cyst which enlarges and fills the maxillary sinus protruding through ostium into the nasal cavity. The mucous glands rupture resulting in inflammation. This chain of events occurs as a consequence of healing of acute sinusitis.
- *Imaging*: Unilateral, solitary lesions that extends from the maxillary sinus, through an expanded ostium (primary or accessory) into nasal cavity and nasopharynx (Figs. 5.6 and 5.7).
- *Differential diagnosis*:
  Inverted papillomas: Both entities look similar on NCCT. The key differentiating points are enlisted in Table 5.3.

SI No	Key feature	Antrochoanal polyp	Inverted papilloma
	Table 5.3: Key differentiating features between a antrochoanal and inverted papilloma.		
1.	Calcification	Rare	Characteristic but seen only in 10%
2.	Focal hyperostosis	Not seen	Characteristic
3.	Pattern of enhancement	Peripheral/layered	Cerebriform
4.	Site of origin	Maxillary sinus, hence fills sinus and extends through ostium	Lateral nasal wall near middle turbinate

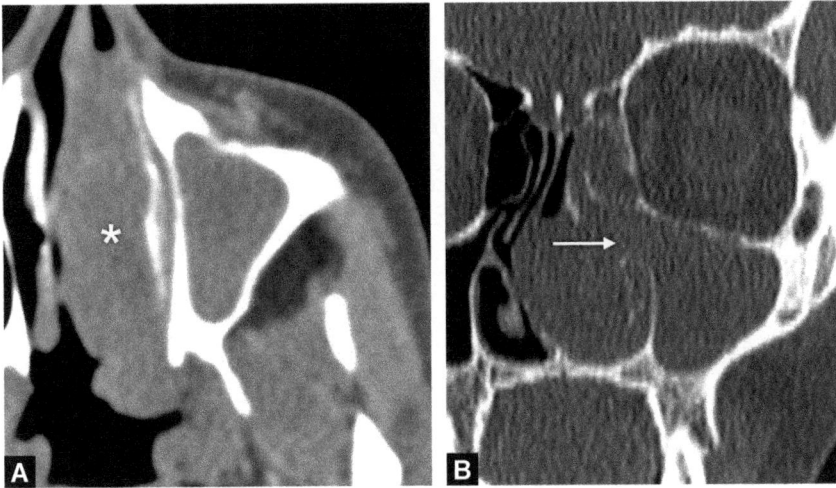

Figs. 5.6A and B: Antrochoanal polyp NCCT. (A) Soft tissue density mass left maxillary antrum and nasal cavity (asterisk); and (B) Widening of ostium (arrow).

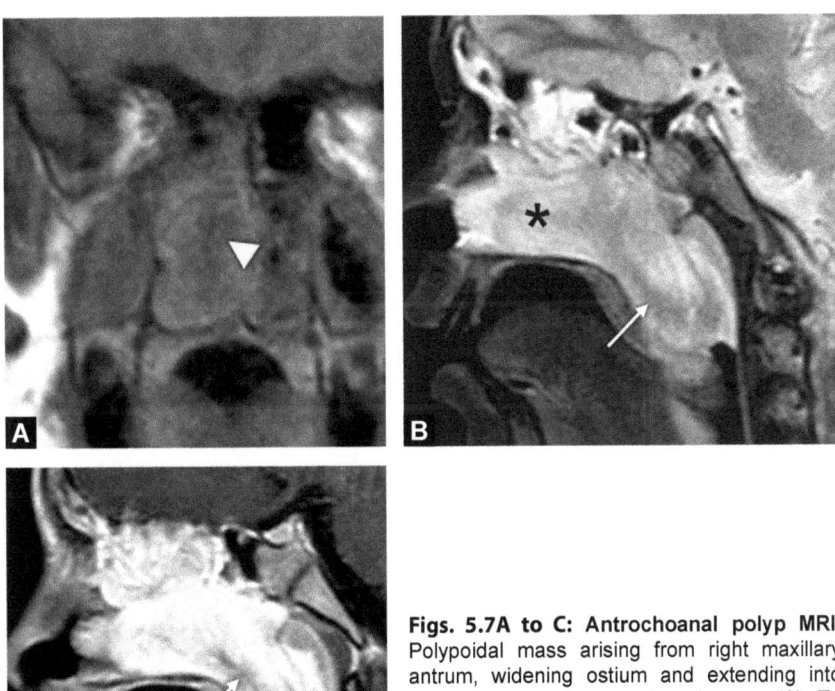

Figs. 5.7A to C: Antrochoanal polyp MRI. Polypoidal mass arising from right maxillary antrum, widening ostium and extending into nasal cavity and posterior choana. (A) T1 intermediate to hypointense (arrowhead), (B) T2 hyperintense (asterisk) with hypointense linear areas (arrow) (C) Intense enhancement with non enhancing linear areas (fibrotic part/ desiccated secretions) (arrow).

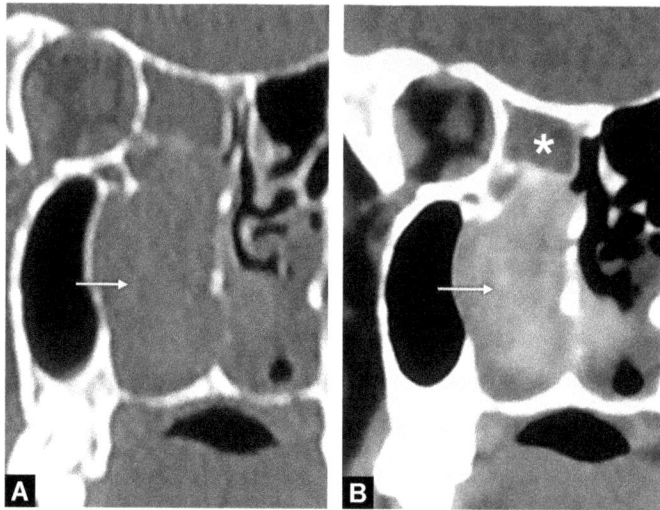

Figs. 5.8A and B: Ethmoidochoanal polyp. (A) Expansile (arrow) polypoidal mass right ethmoidal cells, nasal cavity, choana; (B) Mass is enhancing (arrow) with non-enhancing hypodense retained secretions in sphenoid sinus (asterisk).

Sphenochoanal Polyp

- Rare unilateral lesion which arises from the sphenoid sinus, extends through the sphenoid ostium into the sphenoethmoidal recess and then to choana.
- In the nasal cavity, it is seen to lie between the middle turbinate and nasal septum. This space, which is located medial to the middle turbinate, is not involved in antrochoanal polyp.[3]

Ethmoidochoanal Polyps

- Seen in young adults.
- Unilateral, expansile solitary lesions which extend from the ethmoid sinuses into nasal cavity and nasopharynx (Figs. 5.8A and B).

RETENTION CYSTS

- *Synonym*: Intramural sinus cyst.[3,4]
- Retention cyst (RC) may result from obstruction of serous or mucinous glands following inflammation. The contents may hence be predominantly serous or mucinous.
- Though these are nonsecreting cysts, they may enlarge enough to fill the sinus.
- Common finding seen in patients with CRS/as an incidental finding in asymptomatic individuals. Seen in almost 10% of healthy population.[1]
- Maxillary sinus is the most common site followed by the sphenoid sinus.
- There are two types of retention cysts: (1) mucous and (2) serous.

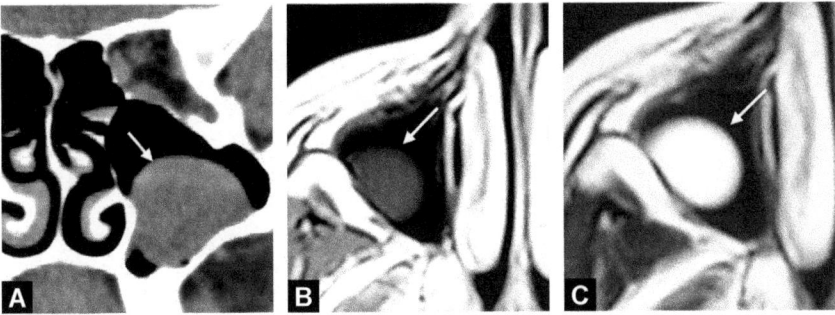

Figs. 5.9A to C: Retention cyst. (A) Well defined low density lesion along sinus wall (arrow); Outer margin is convex; (B) T1WI: Hypointense (arrow); and (C) T2WI: Hyperintense (arrow).

- *Mucous form*: Consequent to accumulation of mucous following obstruction of submucosal mucinous gland.
- *Serous form*: Due to collection of fluid in the submucosa.
- Both forms appear similar on imaging.
- *Imaging (Figs. 5.9A to C)*:
  - *CT*: Appears as well-defined, low-density lesion along the sinus wall with convex, outer margin.
  - *MRI*: Low signal intensity on T_1WI, and bright on T_2WI.

SINONASAL ANGIOMATOUS POLYP (SAP) OR SINONASAL ORGANIZED HEMATOMA

- Rare benign entity, referred to by various terms over the years.
- *Synonyms*: Sinonasal organized hematoma (SOH), pseudotumor, cavernous hemangioma, and cholesterol granuloma.
- Currently all these terms are thought to refer to the same/similar entities.
- *Most common site*: Maxillary sinus, medially near ostium.
- *Age group*: 20–40 years, can occur in children also.
- *Pathogenesis*: There are several hypotheses, two commonly proposed theories are:
  - When nasal polyps protrude through the maxillary ostium into the maxillary sinus, due to compression of the pedicle of the polyp there is vascular compromise. This leads to stasis, consequent edema and ischemia. Ischemia leads to venous infarction and subsequent neovascularization (SAP) and then fibrosis.
  - Formed due to development of a fibrous capsule around a hematoma (SOH). The fibrous capsule prevents resorption of the hematoma with SAP and recurrent hemorrhages within the lesion.
  - If cholesterol crystals deposit within the hematoma—resultant lesion is a "cholesterol granuloma".

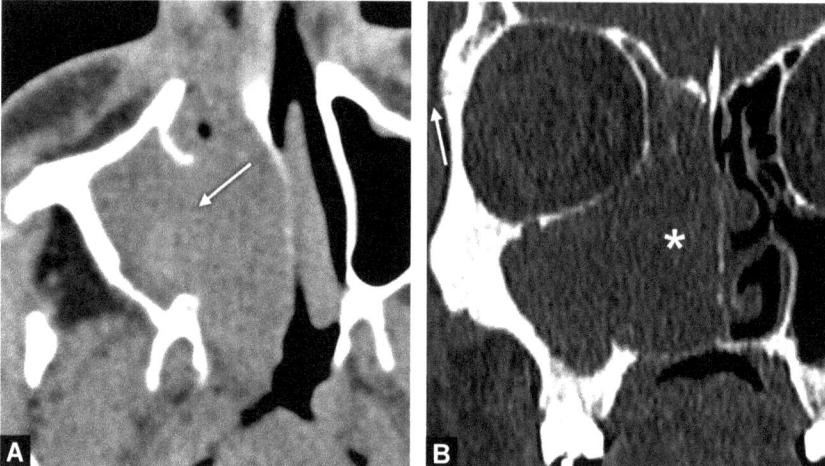

Figs. 5.10A and B: Sinonasal angiomatous polyp NCCT. (A) Mixed density, expansile lesion in right maxillary sinus and nasal cavity (arrow); and (B) Smooth demineralization of turbinates (asterisk) and lateral nasal wall.

- *Factors predisposing to hematoma:* Trauma, postsurgical, vascular lesions, coagulation disturbance or frequent nasal bleeds. Hence, common to both the entities is the neovascularization.
- *Most common presentation:* Recurrent epistaxis. Others: cheek swelling.
- *Imaging:* Reflects the numerous components of the lesion, i.e. soft tissue with hemorrhage in different stages, neovascularization with vascular proliferation and fibrosis.[5]
- *Computed tomography:*
  - NCCT (Figs. 5.10A and B): Mixed density/hyperdense on NCCT, expansile, smooth demineralization of bones especially uncinate process. Calcification: common.
  - Contrast-enhanced computed tomography (CECT): Characteristic papillary/frond like pattern of enhancement.
- *MRI (Figs. 5.11A to C):*
  - T1WI: Intermediate signal intensity (SI) with hyperintense foci.
  - T2WI: Heterogenous, surrounded by a hypointense rim (fibrous capsule). The magnetic resonance (MR) appearance is similar to polyps, however peripheral hypointense rim on T2WI is more consistently seen because of the fibrous capsule.
  - CEMRI: Hypointense linear septae which do not show enhancement.
- *Differential diagnosis:*
  - *Malignant mass:* The bony changes in malignancy are more erosive with less expansion of the sinus.
  - *Antrochoanal polyp:* SAP/SOH show more locally aggressive behavior (bone erosion). Also polyps appear more hypodense, while SAP/SOH is frequently hyperdense.

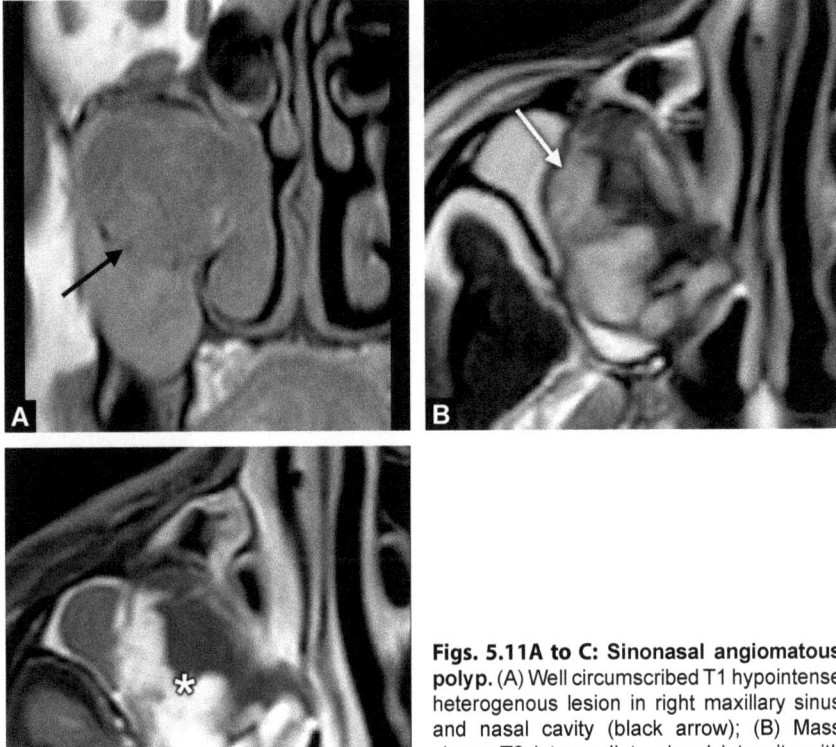

Figs. 5.11A to C: Sinonasal angiomatous polyp. (A) Well circumscribed T1 hypointense heterogenous lesion in right maxillary sinus and nasal cavity (black arrow); (B) Mass shows T2 intermediate signal intensity with T2 hypointense rim (arrow); and septa; (C) Lobular enhancement (asterisk) with no enhancement of the hypointense areas. Obstructive sinusitis in right maxillary sinus

MUCOCELE

- *Meaning*: "Collection of the mucous". It is the most common expansile sinus "mass".
- *Common location*: Frontal sinuses (approximately two-thirds); then ethmoids; with maxillary and sphenoid sinus involvement being infrequent.
- Obstruction of the drainage pathway of a sinus leads to accumulation of the secretions with marked expansion of the sinus. The lining is secretory respiratory columnar epithelium.
- Confined to a single sinus and in case a septum is present, then to a compartment of the sinus. May even occur within variants such as pneumatized anterior clinoid process, an Onodi cell or even in concha bullosa.[2]
- *Causes*: Inflammatory, traumatic, repeated surgeries, and tumors (such as ossifying fibroma or fibrous dysplasia).
- Clinical presentation is due to compression of the adjoining structures, optic nerve compression can result in diminution of vision.

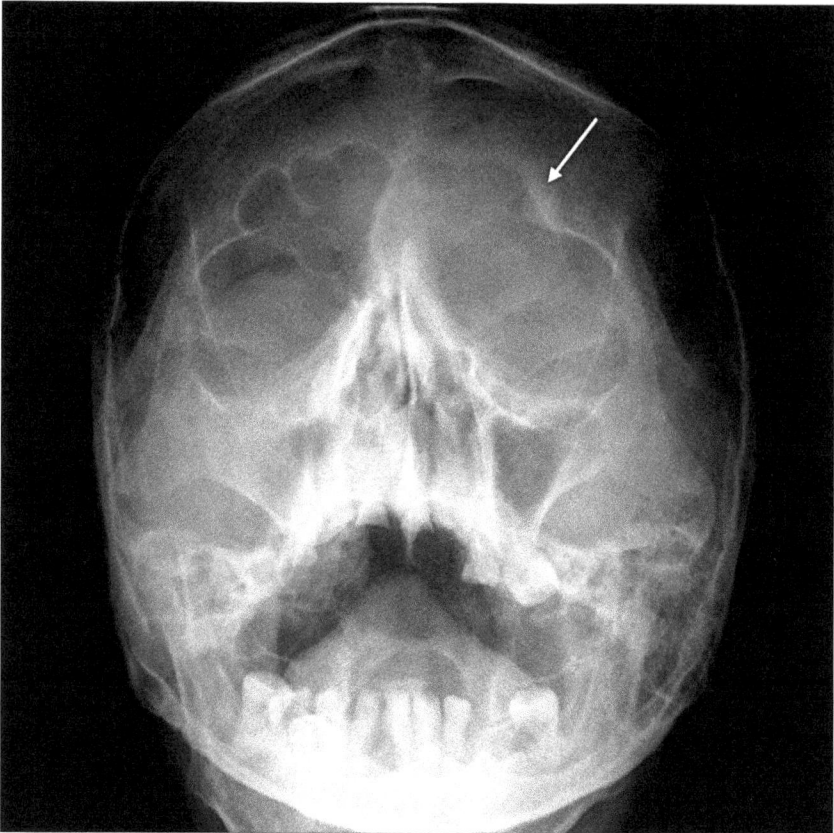

Fig. 5.12: Frontal mucocele (Water's view). Opacification with expansion of left frontal sinus (arrow).

- *Imaging:*[2,3]
  - *Plain radiographs* reveal opacification of the sinus with expansion, often marked (Fig. 5.12).
  - *CT:* The expanded sinus contains secretions and is hence hypodense/isodense to brain parenchyma and homogenous. Appears hyperdense if inspissated secretions. Peripheral calcification may be seen.
  - Cause slow expansion with remodeling of the sinus walls and there may be scalloping of the adjoining borders (Figs. 5.13A and B).
  - Usually there is thinning and deossification of sinus walls, but uncommonly they may show a more aggressive behavior with bone destruction and intracranial/orbital extension. Focal areas of lysis or large defects may be seen.
  - In frontal mucocele, the intactness of the posterior wall is critical to evaluate (Fig. 5.14).
  - Wall erosion may be seen in sphenoid mucocele particularly when associated with a mycetoma. A concurrent mycetoma should be

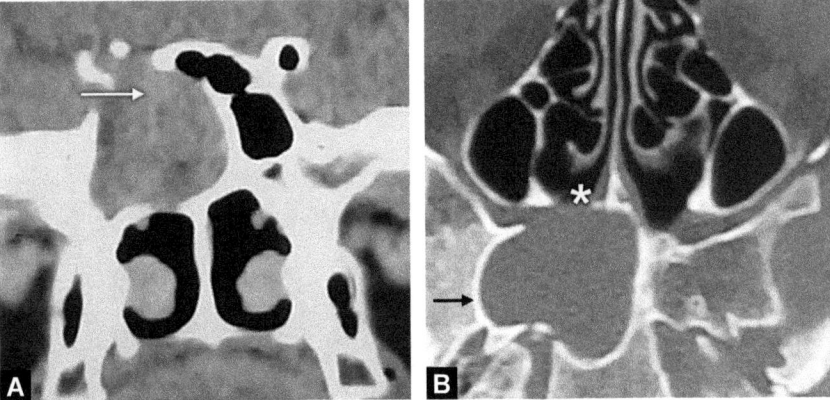

Figs. 5.13A and B: Sphenoid mucocele. (A) Expansion of right sphenoid sinus with hyperdense contents (arrow); (B) with thinning and scalloping of bony margins (black arrow). Right sphenoethmoidal recess blocked by inflammatory mucosal thickening (asterisk) resulting in sphenoid mucocele.

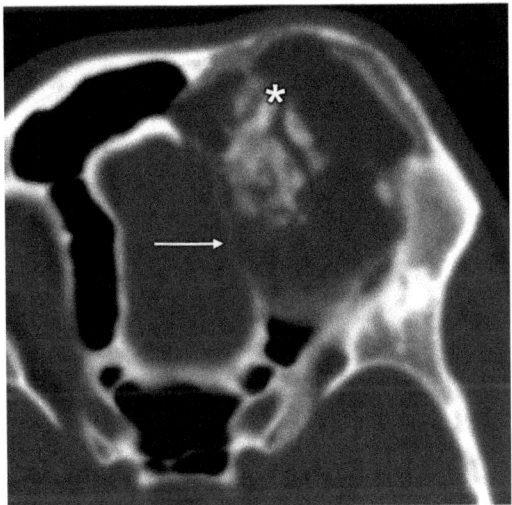

Fig. 5.14: Frontal Mucocele: posterior wall assessment. Expansion of left frontal sinus with some internal ossified contents (ossifying fibroma) (asterisk). Deossification of the posterior wall (arrow) and thickening of the anterior wall.

suspected in a mucocele in presence of central hyperdensity with scattered (linear or round) calcifications. MRI shows hypointense signal on T2WI.
- *MRI*: Appearance of secretions on imaging (Figs. 5.15 and 5.16) depends on the protein content of the secretions as detailed in Chapter 4. Hence, they may give similar appearance to CRS or fungal sinusitis.
- On contrast administration only the mucosal lining enhances giving appearances of rim enhancement (vs tumors).

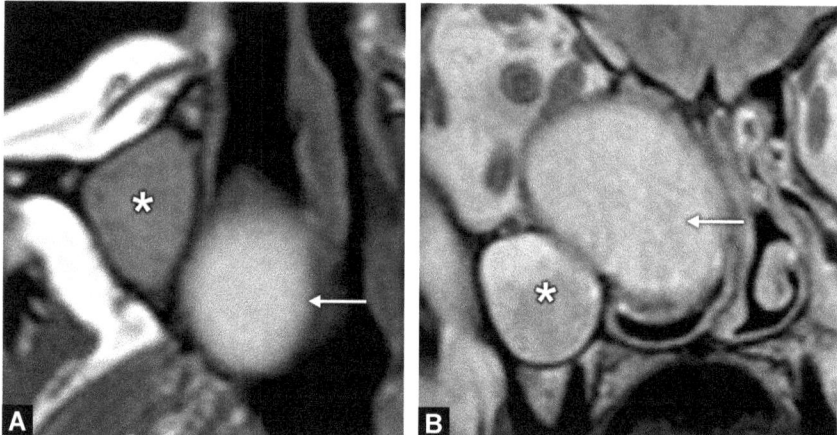

Figs. 5.15A and B: Ethmoidal mucocele. Mucocele shows T1 (A) and T2 (B) hyperintense signal intensity (arrow), obstructive right maxillary sinusitis (asterisk) shows intermediate SI on T1WI and heterogenous, predominant hypointensity on T2WI (retained secretions).

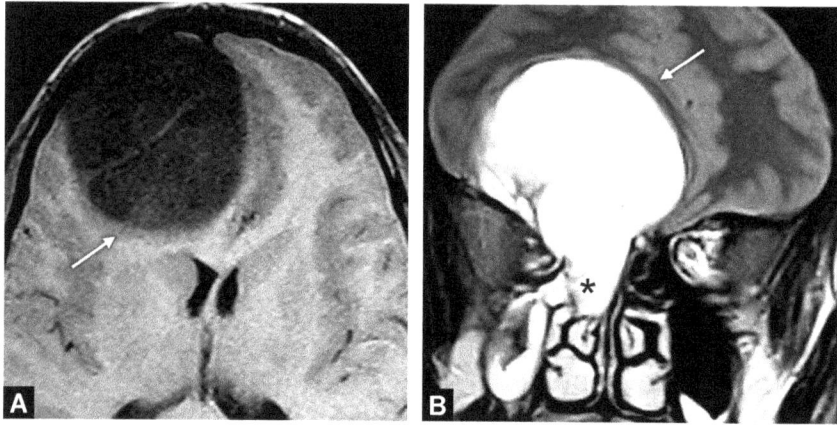

Figs. 5.16A and B: Large right frontal mucocele: extradural extension. Expansile lesion right frontal sinus with blockage of frontonasal drainage pathway (asterisk), T1 hypointense (A) and T2 hyperintense (B) contents; with buckling of gray white matter interface in right frontal lobe (arrow).

- The intracranial (Figs. 5.16A and B)/orbital extension is also well documented.
- On CT and MRI, it is important to look for the *cause of the mucocele*. The drainage pathway of the obstructed sinus should be meticulously reported. The cause may be *inflammatory mucosal thickening (see Figs. 5.13A and B), post-traumatic and postoperative*. Though less frequent, it is important to exclude a *tumor* (Figs. 5.17A to C) as a cause for the obstruction. This may be challenging and requires contrast

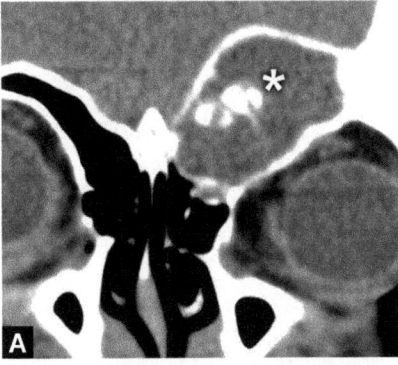
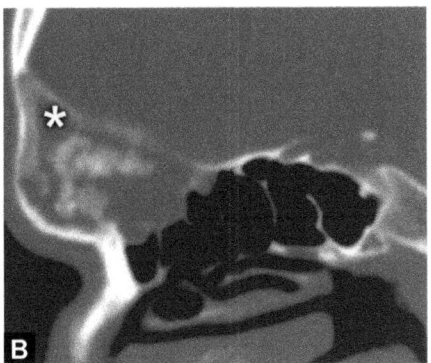
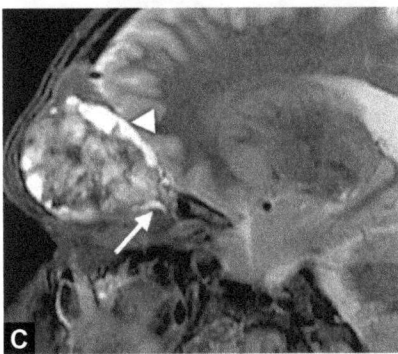

Figs. 5.17 A to C: Secondary Mucocele in a case of Ossifying Fibroma (OF): Role of MRI (A and B) CT: Expansion of left frontal sinus with soft tissue density contents with small internal ossific component (asterisk). Distinction between tumor and mucocele cannot be made. (C) MRI: Nonossified component of the tumor is also well seen on the T2WI: heterogeneous signal mass (arrow) blocking the left frontal ostium. Peripheral T2 hyperintensity on MRI represents the secretions in the mucocele (arrowhead).

administration. In addition, both CT and MR should be reviewed together.[2,3]

- *Differential diagnosis*:
  - *Obstructed sinus*: Obstruction with retained secretions in absence of expansion
  - *Retention cysts*: Borders are non-scalloped
  - *Tumors*: Solid pattern of enhancement in tumors
  - *Cephaloceles*: Skull-base defects with herniation of meninges/CSF (cerebrospinal fluid).

LARGE AIR-FILLED SINUSES

- Pneumatization of the sinuses is variable and occasionally large air-filled sinuses may be seen. This condition has been most frequently described for frontal sinus. While it may be a normal variant, it may also result from ball valve mechanism (partial obstruction of frontal sinus drainage pathway due to mucosal edema), or even following the spontaneous drainage of a mucocele. The various terms used are:[6]
  - *Pneumosinus/hypersinus*: Large frontal sinus (normal variant).
  - *Pneumosinus dilatans*: Abnormal expansion of the sinus which encroaches on the surrounding structures. The sinus walls are however

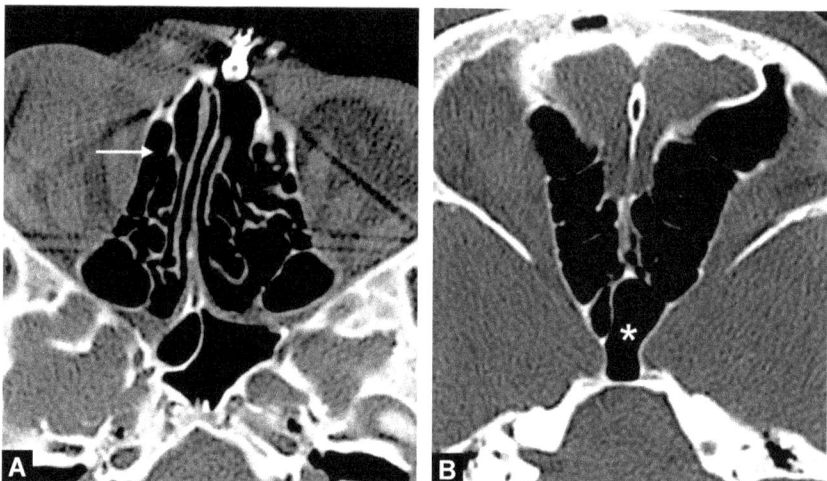

Figs. 5.18A and B: Pneumosinus dilatans in a case of Crouzon Syndrome. (A) Large air filled ethmoid sinuses (arrow) with mid-face hypoplasia; (B) Small sphenoid bone (asterisk).

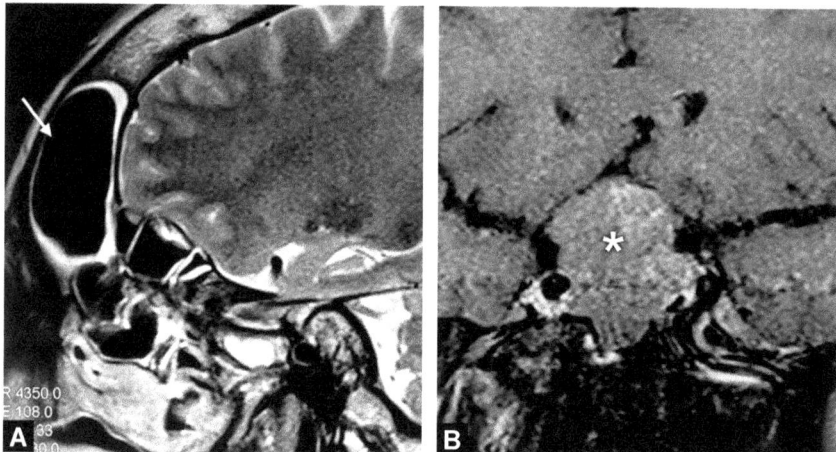

Figs. 5.19A and B: Pneumosinus dilatans in acromegaly. (A) Abnormally expanded air-filled frontal and ethmoid sinuses (arrow); and (B) Heterogenously enhancing large sellar mass s/o pituitary macroadenoma (asterisk).

of normal thickness. Initially used for frontal sinus but any sinus may be affected (Figs. 5.18 and 5.19).
- *Pneumocele*: Abnormal expansion with thinning/demineralization of the walls of the sinus.
- *Complications*:
  - Rupture of such sinus can result in pneumocephalus.
  - Compression of the optic nerve in the optic canal can result in diminution of vision.

- *Causes*:
    - Acromegaly
    - Anterior skull base meningioma
    - Anterior skull base arachnoid cyst
    - Fibrous dysplasia.
- *Management*: If symptomatic, endoscopic decompression is required.

CONCLUSION

Polyps and mucoceles are common expansile masses of the sinonasal cavity. In case of mucoceles, imaging evaluation should be done to look for an underlying cause.

REFERENCES

1. Mafee MF, Tran BH, Chapa AR. Imaging of rhinosinusitis and its complications: plain film, CT, and MRI. Clin Rev Allergy Immun. 2006;30:165-86.
2. Joshi VM, Sansi R. Imaging in sinonasal inflammatory disease. Neuroimag Clin N Am. 2015;25:549-68.
3. Broderick DF. The opacified paranasal sinus: approach and differential. Appl Radiol. 2015;44:9-17.
4. Whyte A, Chapeikin G. Opaque maxillary antrum: a pictorial review. Australas Radiol. 2005;49:203-13.
5. Zou J, Man F, Deng K, et al. CT and MR imaging findings of sinonasal angiomatous polyps. Eur J Radiol. 2014;83:545-51.
6. Urken ML, Som PM, Lawson W, et al. Abnormally large frontal sinus. II. Nomenclature, pathology, and symptoms. Laryngoscope. 1987;97:606-11.

6
CHAPTER

Chronic Rhinosinusitis: Clinical Aspects

Arvind Kumar Kairo, Hitesh Verma

- Introduction
- Allergic Rhinosinusitis
  - Diagnosis
  - Treatment
- Infectious Rhinosinusitis
- Chronic Infectious Rhinosinusitis
  - Treatment
- Polyposis
  - Diagnosis
  - Treatment

INTRODUCTION

- Rhinosinusitis (RS) is defined as inflammation of the mucosa of nose and paranasal sinuses.
- Rhinosinusitis is broadly classified into allergic, infectious, and other groups (such as hormonal, occupational, drug, food related and emotional).

ALLERGIC RHINOSINUSITIS

- The prevalence of allergic rhinosinusitis is between 10% and 20% of population with a male predominance and it is more common in young adults. It is frequently associated with other allergic conditions such as asthma, conjunctivitis as a part of the "allergic march".
- If the symptoms last for less than 4 days a week, for less than 4 weeks, RS is called "intermittent".
- If the symptoms last for more than 4 days a week and for more than 4 weeks, RS is called "persistent".

Diagnosis

- *Diagnostic provocative tests*:
  - *Allergy testing:* Skin prick test (SPT), serum specific immunoglobulin E (IgE) [as radioallergosorbent test (RAST)]
  - Allergen, lysine aspirin and methacholine nasal challenge test
- Radiology
- Nasal airway can be assessed by rhinomanometry or acoustic rhinometry.

Treatment

- Primary prevention is by restriction of allergen exposure.
- *Pharmacotherapy*:
  - *Antihistaminics*: These helps in relieving symptoms in the initial hours of exposure such as running of nose, itching, and sneezing.
  - *Topical glucocorticosteroids*: The onset of action is slow and starts after 6-12 hours, reaches its maximum level after a few days. It is the most effective treatment for allergic rhinosinusitis. It acts on all the forms of symptoms.
  - *Topical nasal decongestants*: These act by reducing nasal obstruction. Persistent use for more than 3 to 7 days (J Investig Allergol Clin Immunol 2006; Vol. 16(3): 148-155) can cause rhinitis medicamentosa.
  - Spray form of sodium cromoglycate and ipratropium bromide are also useful but have limited compliance.
  - *Systemic corticosteroids*: Tapering dose of oral steroids is indicated in patients with severe symptoms not responding to above medications.
  - *Immunotherapy*: Immune tolerance is created by repeated exposure to the allergen extract. Immunotherapy may be considered in patients with limited spectrum of allergies, with severe disease and failure to response to usual treatment as it can cause serious systemic reaction, and the treatment is cumbersome.
  - *Surgical indication* in allergic rhinosinusitis is the presence of gross septal deviation and thick turbinates which can affect use of topical medication.

INFECTIOUS RHINOSINUSITIS

- A variety of viruses can cause acute rhinitis. The sinus may be involved by secondary bacterial infection. *Streptococcus pneumoniae* and *Haemophilus influenzae* are the most common bacteria causing rhinosinusitis. The fungi and bacteria causing RS are discussed in Chapter 4. Infectious rhinosinusitis is further classified into four subtypes based on clinical presentation.[1]
  - *Acute infectious RS*: The duration of symptoms is less than 12 weeks with complete resolution of symptoms.
  - *Recurrent acute infectious RS*: The number of acute episodes is less than 4 per year, with 8 weeks symptom-free period without treatment.
  - *Chronic infectious RS*: The duration of symptoms is more than 12 weeks, or incomplete resolution on radiology for more than 4 weeks after starting medical therapy.
  - *Acute exacerbations of chronic RS*: The patient is presents with newer symptoms or worsening of existing symptom.

Chronic Infectious Rhinosinusitis

Diagnosis of infectious rhinosinusitis is based on following criteria which were given by the Rhinosinusitis Task Force of the American Academy of

| Table 6.1: Diagnostic criteria of infectious rhinosinusitis. ||
Major criteria	Minor criteria
Facial pain/pressure/fullness Nasal obstruction/blockage Nasal or postnasal discharge/purulence (by history or physical examination) Hyposmia/anosmia Fever (in acute rhinosinusitis only)	Headaches Fever (other than acute rhinosinusitis) Halitosis Fatigue Dental pain Cough Ear pain/pressure/fullness

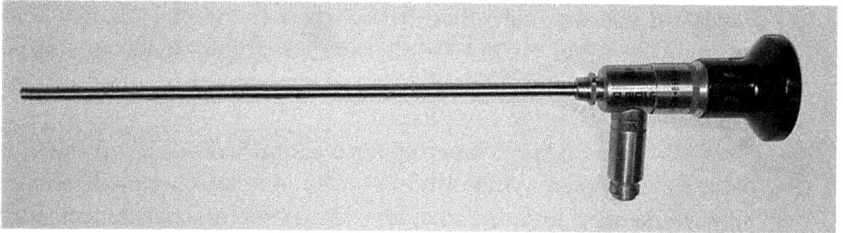

Fig. 6.1: 0° sinoscope.

Otolaryngology—Head and Neck Surgery in 1997. The symptoms are divided into major and minor type to evaluate severity of disease.[1] To diagnose RS, patient must have two major, or one major with two minor criteria (Table 6.1).

- *Nasal endoscopy*: It is indicated in patients with unreliable history or sinusitis is not responding to medical management, postoperative cavity care and in patients with unreliable history. The 0°, 30°, 45° and 70° endoscopes with diameter of 4 mm (adult) (Fig. 6.1) and 2.7 mm (pediatric) are used to examine nasal cavity and sinus drainage pathways. To facilitate examination, high intensity light source and light cable is required. The prerequisites for nasal endoscopic examination are consent, position, and application of local anesthetic with decongestants.
- The procedure is documented in the form of three passes:
  1. First pass includes examination of floor of nasal cavity along with inferior meatus and nasopharynx.
  2. Second pass entails finding the space in between inferior and middle meatus, and sphenoethmoidal recess is documented here.
  3. *Third pass*: The examination of deeper part of middle meatus such as uncinate process, ethmoidal infundibulum, hiatus semilunaris, and bulla ethmoidalis are documented here.

Treatment

- Hydration maintenance to maintain sol-gel ratio in mucous for proper mucociliary clearance.
- *Antibiotics*: The duration of treatment is from 7 to 14 days and first-line management for acute rhinosinusitis is beta lactam or fluoroquinolone

groups. In non-responding cases with usual treatment, culture based antibiotics are indicated.
- A long course of macrolide group antibiotic is added along with topical steroid to avoid relapse as both have anti-inflammatory response.
- In cases where medical management is not working, ostia of involved sinus can be targeted with preservation of mucosa. Such endoscopic sinus surgery is called Functional Endoscopic Sinus Surgery (FESS). The goal of this procedure is to reestablish sinus ventilation and normal function.
- Nasal endoscopy is used to give post operative care.
- Alkaline nasal douches—nasal douches are indicated in rhinitis patients and as a part of postsurgery cavity management. It improves quality of life to great extent.

Polyposis
- Patients with nasal polyposis presents with gradually progressive nasal obstruction along with all other symptoms of chronic rhinosinusitis.
- It becomes persistent over a period of time with more viscous nasal secretion.
- Patients may have abnormality of sense of smell and taste when polyposis covers the area of olfaction.

Diagnosis
- Endoscopic staging system used for nasal polyposis is (*The Lund and Mackay staging system*)[2]
  - Stage 1: No polyp
  - Stage 2: Polyp confined to middle meatus
  - Stage 3: Polyp extending below middle meatus
  - Stage 4: Massive polyposis
- There are numerous secondary causes of polyposis which should be suspected in presence of multiple and persistent polyps and excluded (*see* Chapter 5).

Treatment
- Intranasal and systemic corticosteroids are the first-line management for nasal polyposis. Other drugs have limited effect and can be prescribed in addition.
- Systemic steroids for 10–14 days can correct early stage polyposis. In massive polyposis appropriate treatment is surgery and steroids can be a part of treatment.
- In cases of nasal polyposis with irreversible mucosal disease, the treatment plan is FESS. It is a minimally invasive technique in which paranasal sinus ostia are opened under direct visualization. Open surgery is occasionally indicated for disease inaccessible through endoscopy.
- Different surgeries used for chronic rhinosinusitis are mentioned in Table 6.2.

Table 6.2: Surgeries for chronic rhinosinusitis.		
Endoscopic surgeries	Surgeries with invisible incision	Open surgeries
Draf I to III	Antral washout	Frontoethmosphenoidectomy
Middle meatal Antrostomy	Caldwell–Luc	Lothrop
Endonasal drainage	Intranasal antrostomy	Osteoplastic flap
Uncinectomy	Trephination (of the frontal sinus)	Cranialization (of the frontal sinus)
Ethmoidectomy	Transantral ethmoidectomy	

REFERENCES

1. Hadley JA, Schaefer SD. Clinical evaluation of rhinosinusitis: history and physical examination. Otolaryngol Head Neck Surg. 1997;117:S8-11.
2. Lund VJ, Mackay IS. Staging in rhinosinusitis. Rhinology. 1993;31:183-4.

Imaging in Fungal Sinusitis

Ashu Seith Bhalla, Smita Manchanda

- Introduction
- Classification
  - Noninvasive
  - Invasive
- Imaging Modalities
  - Computed Tomography
  - Magnetic Resonance Imaging
- Types
  - Noninvasive Forms
    - Allergic Fungal Sinusitis
    - Fungal Ball/Mycetoma
  - Invasive Fungal Sinusitis
    - Acute Invasive
    - Chronic Invasive Fungal Sinusitis

INTRODUCTION

Fungal sinusitis is frequently encountered in Asia and has protean clinical and radiological manifestations. The most frequent pathogen is the *Aspergillus* species.

CLASSIFICATION

The classification of fungal sinusitis is based on histopathology. The International Society for Human and Animal Mycology group classification[1] divides fungal sinusitis into the following groups/forms.

Noninvasive
- Allergic fungal sinusitis
- Mycetoma

Invasive
- Acute
- Chronic (nongranulomatous and granulomatous)

IMAGING MODALITIES

Noncontrast computed tomography (NCCT) is the initial imaging modality of choice. Contrast-enhanced magnetic resonance imaging (CEMRI) is required for extent of invasive disease.[2]

Computed Tomography

- Initially when the secretions are watery, these appear low attenuation on NCCT (similar to all forms of rhinosinusitis).
- Over a period of time, the fluid content of the secretions decreases and calcium and magnesium salts get deposited. Iron, magnesium and manganese accumulate in fungal sinusitis as these are thought to be essential for amino acid metabolism of the fungus. This results in the appearance of high attenuation on NCCT (Fig. 7.1).

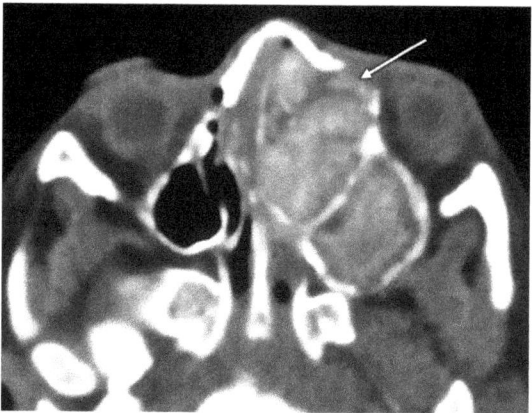

Fig. 7.1: Noncontrast computed tomography (NCCT) allergic fungal sinusitis. Central hyperdense contents (arrow) in expanded left maxillary and ethmoid sinuses; and nasal cavity.

Magnetic Resonance Imaging

- Signal intensity on MRI is governed by the viscosity of secretions, their protein content (as in other forms of rhinosinusitis) and the deposition of salts. Characteristic T2 hypointensity (Fig. 7.2) is seen due to the presence of iron and magnesium salts.

TYPES

Noninvasive Forms

Allergic Fungal Sinusitis

- Allergic fungal sinusitis (AFS) is the most common form and is an allergic response to colonized fungi.
- AFS is the commonest form and is an allergic response to colonized fungi.
- It is seen in young, immunocompetent patients with history of atopy.

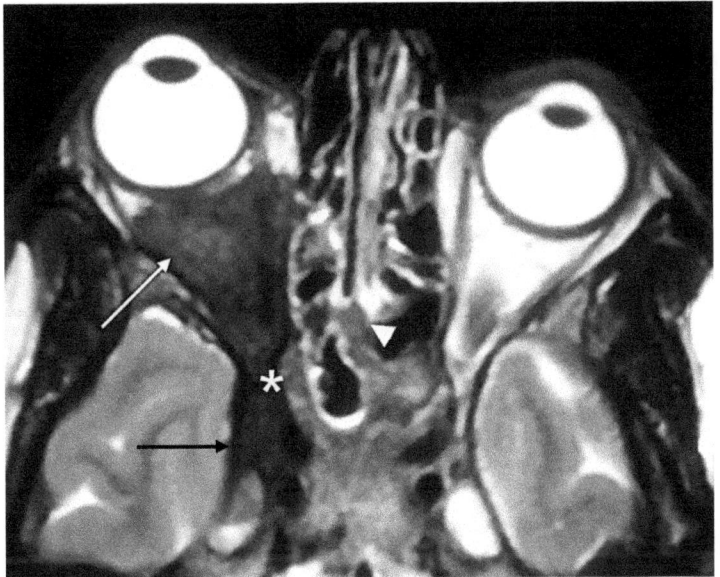

Fig. 7.2: Magnetic resonance imaging (MRI) rhino-orbito-cerebral mucormycosis. Axial T2WI: markedly T2 hypointense soft tissue in right orbit (white arrow), orbital apex (asterisk) and cavernous sinus (black arrow). Intermediate signal contents in bilateral ethmoid sinuses (arrowhead).

Pathology:
- Pathology is similar to allergic bronchopulmonary aspergillosis (ABPA).
- Histopathology reveals mucus impaction, cellular debris, fungal elements, inflammatory response.

Imaging:
- Involvement is unilateral; or if bilateral, it is then asymmetric.
- Multiple sinuses are affected with maxillary and ethmoid sinuses being the most frequent.
- In about 30% patients AFS may erode the skull base.[3]
- *NCCT (Figs. 7.3A and B):*
  - Central hyperdensity and peripheral hypodensity outlining in the sinus wall (due to inflamed mucosa)
  - Expansion of sinuses, remodeling and thinning/erosion of bony sinus walls.
- *MRI (Figs. 7.4A to C):*
  - Variable depending on the content of the secretions as has been described in chronic rhinosinusitis (*see* Chapter 4)
  - *T1, T2 signal:* Iso/hypointense or profoundly hypointense (signal void)
  - *Contrast-enhanced magnetic resonance (CEMR):* Mucosal thickening and enhancement. Minimal spread to extra sinus soft tissues.
  - *Pitfall:* There is underestimation of the extent of involvement on MRI, and hence it should always be correlated with CT.

Section 2 Inflammatory Nasal Conditions

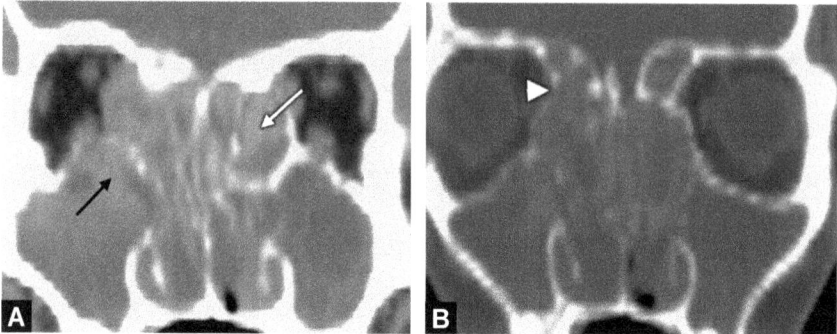

Figs. 7.3A and B: Allergic fungal sinusitis. (A) Sinus window: expansion of bilateral maxillary, ethmoid sinuses; central hyperdensity, peripheral hypodensity (white arrow), remodeling and thinning of walls (black arrow); and (B) Bone window. Erosion of lamina papyracea, intraorbital extension (arrowhead).

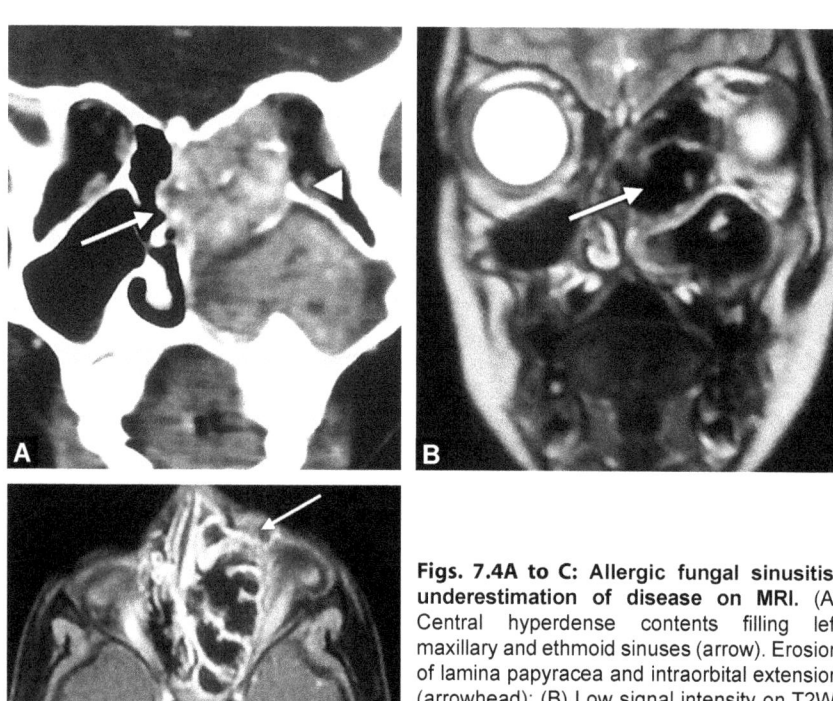

Figs. 7.4A to C: Allergic fungal sinusitis: underestimation of disease on MRI. (A) Central hyperdense contents filling left maxillary and ethmoid sinuses (arrow). Erosion of lamina papyracea and intraorbital extension (arrowhead); (B) Low signal intensity on T2WI in maxillary and ethmoid sinuses (arrow) mimics normal aerated sinuses; and (C) Enhancing mucosal lining and extrasinus soft tissue (arrow).

Fungal Ball/Mycetoma

- *Synonym:* Aspergilloma
- A mass like noninvasive lesion composed of fungal hyphae forms within the sinus.

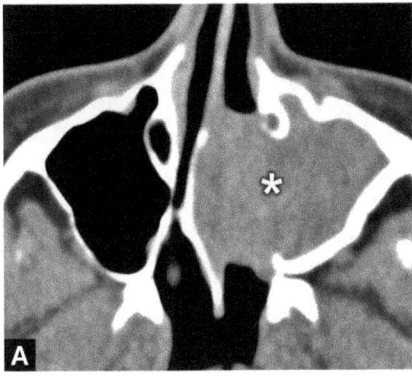 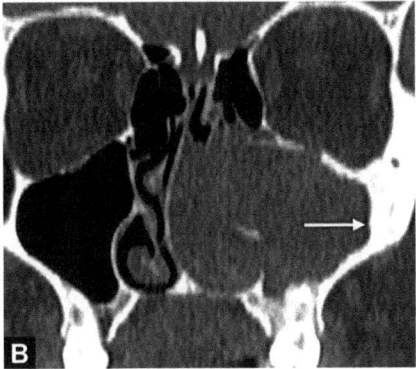

Figs. 7.5A and B: Mycetoma: NCCT. (A) Soft tissue opacification of left maxillary sinus and nasal cavity (asterisk); and (B) Mild thickening and sclerosis of bony walls (arrow).

- It is seen in immunocompetent patients, not atopic, more common in women, and older age.
- Mostly single sinus is involved and maxillary sinus is most commonly affected. Less frequently sphenoid, frontal and ethmoid sinuses are involved in that order.[4]
- *Organism*: *Aspergillus fumigatus* is most frequently responsible.
- *Histopathology*: Fungal hyphae are seen with no background of allergic mucin (versus AFS), deposits of calcium oxalate may be present.
- *NCCT (Figs. 7.5A and B)*:
  - Soft tissue opacification of involved sinuses
  - Central hyperdensities with or without calcifications
  - Pattern of calcification is fine, round or linear
  - Peripheral, hypodense inflamed mucosa may be seen
  - Sinus cavity volume is normal or decreased; expansion with thin walls is far less frequent
  - Bony walls show thickening and sclerosis.
- *MRI (Figs. 7.6A and B)*:

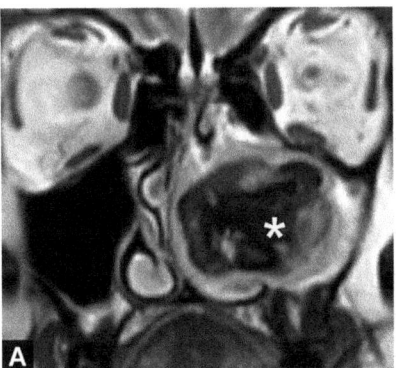 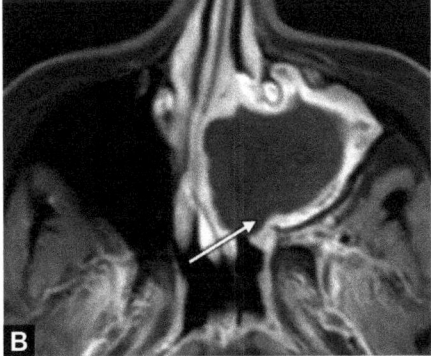

Figs. 7.6A and B: Mycetoma: MRI (same patient as in Figs. 7.5A and B). (A) Mass like heterogenous lesion with central T2 hypointensity (asterisk); and (B) Non-enhancing mass with only mucosal enhancement (arrow).

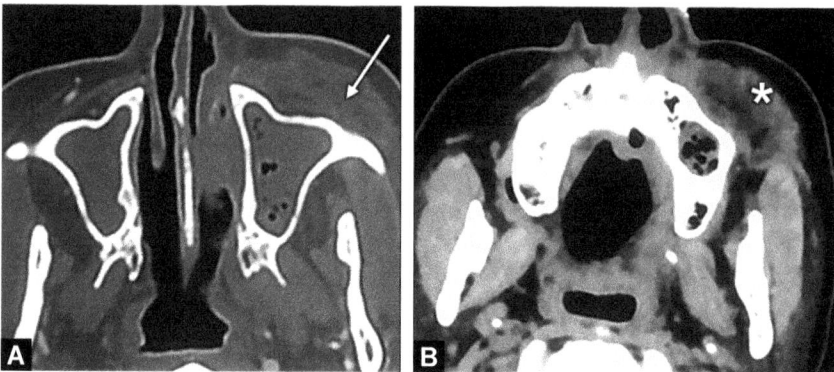

Figs. 7.7A and B: Acute invasive fungal sinusitis (mucormycosis). (A) Bilateral maxillary sinusitis. Left premaxillary soft tissue with intact bony margins (arrow); (B) Necrosis in the extrasinus soft tissues (asterisk).

- *T1*: Heterogenous, predominantly low signal intensity
- *T2*: Also low signal intensity (due to calcium, magnesium and manganese salts)
- *CEMRI*: Mild/no enhancement of the sinus contents.
- *Differential diagnosis*:
  - Chronic obstructed sinus (non-fungal) with inspissated secretions: cannot be differentiated on imaging.

Invasive Fungal Sinusitis

Acute Invasive

- *Synonym*: Rhino-sino-orbito-cerebral mycosis
- Acute onset, rapidly progressive fungal infection with invasion of the vessels and surrounding soft tissues.[5]
- Mostly immunocompromised patients, occasionally in immunocompetent.
- Acute clinical illness, rapidly progressive with high mortality.
- *Fungi responsible*:
  - *Aspergillus sp.* (more frequent in neutropenic patients)
  - Mucoraceae family (*Mucor, Rhizopus,* and *Absidia*) more common in diabetics especially poorly controlled ones.
- *Symptoms:* Nonspecific, fever, rhinorrhea, facial pain, headache, and diplopia.
- *Frequent sites*: Maxillary and ethmoid sinuses.[2]
- *CT*
  - Mucosal thickening/opacification of affected sinuses
  - Hyperdense areas within
  - Adjoining soft tissue thickening may be seen despite intact bony sinus walls (Figs. 7.7A and B).

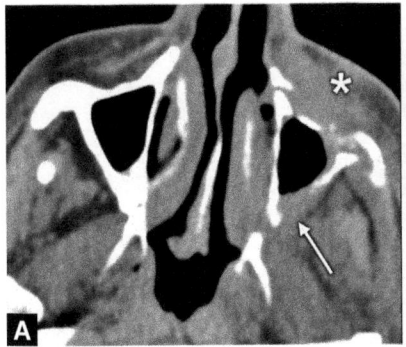
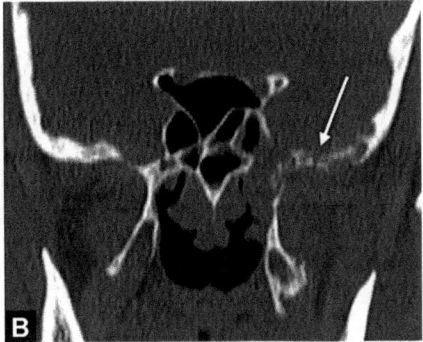

Figs. 7.8A and B: Acute invasive fungal sinusitis with bone erosions. (A) Mucosal thickening left maxillary sinus. Erosion of sinus walls with premaxillary (asterisk) and retroantral (arrow) soft tissue; and (B) Permeative lysis of sphenoid bone (arrow) with extrasinus soft tissue in infratemporal fossa.

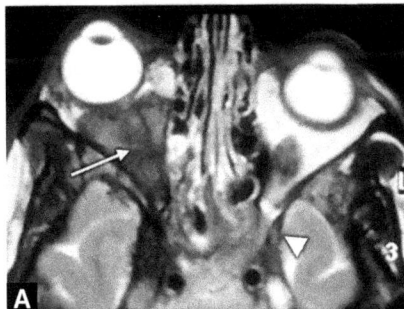
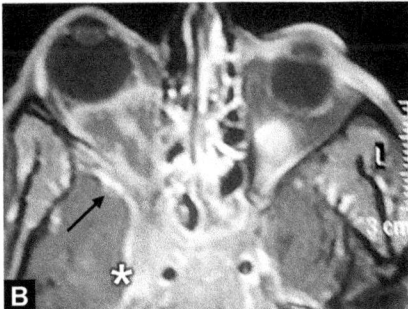

Figs. 7.9A and B: Acute invasive fungal sinusitis magnetic resonance imaging (MRI). (A) Intermediate to hypointense signal intensity soft tissue in right orbit (arrow), orbital apex and cavernous sinus (arrowhead); and (B) Abnormal mucosal enhancement in ethmoid sinuses, right orbit, dura along temporal fossa (black arrow) and cavernous sinus (asterisk).

- This extrasinus spread is thought to occur through microvascular channels in the bone. The presence of soft tissue edema/infiltration is a poor prognostic indicator.
- Sites of extrasinus spread include: premaxillary tissues, retroantral fat as well as pterygopalatine fossa.
- Bony erosions are seen in the more severe forms (Figs. 7.8A and B).
- MRI
  - Opacified sinuses may appear hypointense on both T1 and T2 weighted images (T2WIs).
  - As stated earlier, MRI can underestimate the extent of involvement and should always be correlated with the CT.
  - CEMRI is superior to CT for demonstrating the soft tissue, intracranial and intraorbital extension (Figs. 7.9A and B).
  - *Soft tissue edema*: T1WI shows replacement of fat in affected areas with soft tissue, hyperintense on T2WI with contrast enhancement.

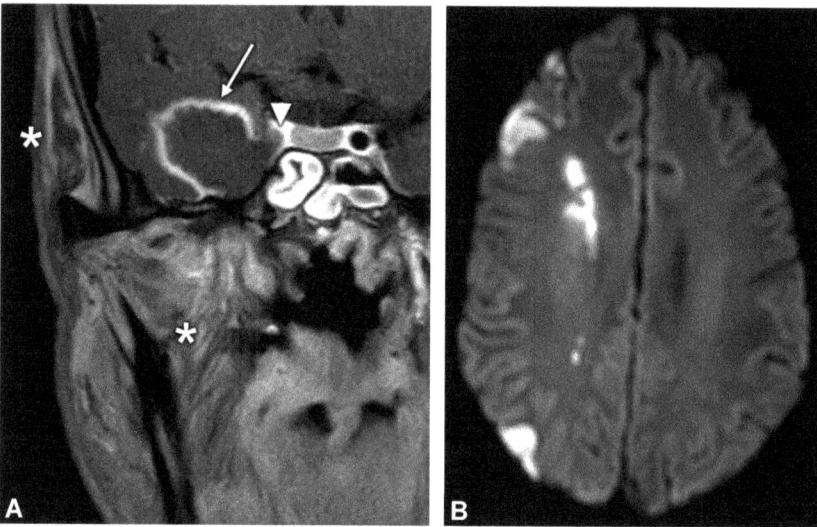

Figs. 7.10A and B: Complicated fungal sinusitis. (A) Rim enhancing abscess right temporal lobe (arrow) and abnormal enhancing soft tissue in the temporalis muscle and infratemporal fossa (asterisk). Thrombosis of right cavernous internal carotid artery (ICA) (arrowhead); and (B) Diffusion-weighted imaging (DWI) image showing multiple infarcts right middle cerebral artery (MCA) and watershed territory.

- *Characteristic sign*: "Black turbinate sign"—refers to absence of enhancement in areas, which normally enhance such as nasal mucosa and the turbinates. Lack of enhancement implies tissue necrosis and is highly suggestive of angioinvasive fungal sinusitis.[2]
- Critical areas of extension to be mapped: orbit, intracranial extension including cavernous sinus.
- Involvement of the internal carotid artery in its cavernous part in the form of thrombosis, mycotic pseudoaneurysm formation or even dissection should be looked for (Figs. 7.10A and B).
- *Aspergillosis versus Mucormycosis:* It is difficult to differentiate aspergillosis from mucormycosis and biopsy is essential. Some characteristic features described for mucormycosis include:
  - The earliest signs described by Green et al.[6] were nodular mucosal thickening, with no air-fluid levels and patchy erosion of the bony sinus walls. These signs however are not pathognomonic for mucormycosis.
  - Characteristic distribution of mucormycosis is the involvement of nasal cavity, sinuses, and orbit.
  - Periosteitis and osteitis are typically present along with lowdensity areas within soft tissues suggesting necrosis in mucormycosis (*see* Figs. 7.7A and B).
  - Mucor may also cause adjacent skull base osteomyelitis with lysis and sequestrum formation (Fig. 7.11).

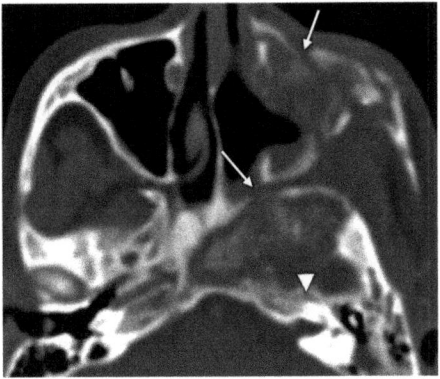

Fig. 7.11: Invasive fungal sinusitis (mucormycosis). Post-functional endoscopic sinus surgery (FESS), residual mucosal thickening left maxillary and sphenoid sinus. Osteitis of maxilla and sphenoid (arrows) with sequestrum formation (arrowhead).

- *Differential diagnosis*:
    - It is difficult to differentiate fungal sinusitis from invasive bacterial forms.
    - As fungal infection has a propensity to infiltrate the vessels, on intracranial spread these are more likely to cause thrombosis and resultant infarctions, hemorrhages and even pseudoaneurysms.
    - Hypointense signal on T2WIs suggests a fungal etiology.

Chronic Invasive Fungal Sinusitis

- The term chronic is used for the more indolent form of the disease (duration more than 4 weeks)
- It is of two forms *(Table 7.1)*: With or without granulomas, with the former being called chronic granulomatous invasive fungal sinusitis.[2]
- The comparison between AFS and chronic invasive fungal sinusitis has been detailed in Table 7.2[7] and illustrated in Figures 7.12A to F.

Chronic granulomatous invasive fungal sinusitis:
- Slow, protracted course similar to the nongranulomatous form.
- Occurs in immunocompetent patients and the symptoms are similar to chronic sinusitis.

Table 7.1: Chronic invasive fungal sinusitis: granulomatous versus nongranulomatous disease.		
	Granulomatous	*Nongranulomatous*
Patient profile	Immunocompetent	Immunocompromised
Endemic areas	Southeast Asia and Africa	–
Organism	*Aspergillus flavus*	*Aspergillus fumigatus*
Imaging	• Usually localized to one or two sinuses • Extrasinus soft tissue often more than intrasinus soft tissue	• Similar to acute invasive fungal sinusitis • Calcification more frequent and more dense

Table 7.2: Comparison between allergic fungal sinusitis and chronic invasive fungal sinusitis.[7]

Key features	Allergic fungal sinusitis	Chronic invasive fungal sinusitis
Clinical presentation	Nasal/Sinus symptoms predominate	Maybe present/absent
	Diplopia/decreased vision maybe seen	Proptosis/decreased vision/diplopia
	Facial swelling not seen	Facial swelling; decreased sensation
	Cranial spread infrequent	Seizures/altered sensorium more frequent
Examination	Nasal polyps	Maybe present/absent
Organism	*Aspergillus flavus*	*A. flavus*
HPE	Allergic mucin, Charcot Leyden crystals, eosinophilic debris, fungal hyphae, no invasion	Inflammatory infiltrate, neutrophilic, fungal hyphae with invasion
Distribution	Bilateral with involvement of multiple sinuses more frequent	More often unilateral with involvement of few sinuses
Expansion of involved sinus	Seen	Normal size sinus
Bone erosion	Expansion with thinning of overlying cortex, Demineralization of thinned cortex appears as erosion	Bone erosions seen at limited sites corresponding to the site of extrasinus extension
Extrasinus spread	Limited, focal	Extensive. Extrasinus soft tissue often exceeds that within the sinus
CT morphology	Heterogenous Central hyperdense areas with peripheral low density	Homogenous Hyperdensities seldom seen
MRI		
T1WI	Intermediate	Low
T2WI	Low	Low
Post-contrast T1WI	Mucosal enhancement seen	Entire soft tissue enhances

(CT: Computed tomography; MRI: Magnetic resonance imaging; T1WI: T1 weighted image).

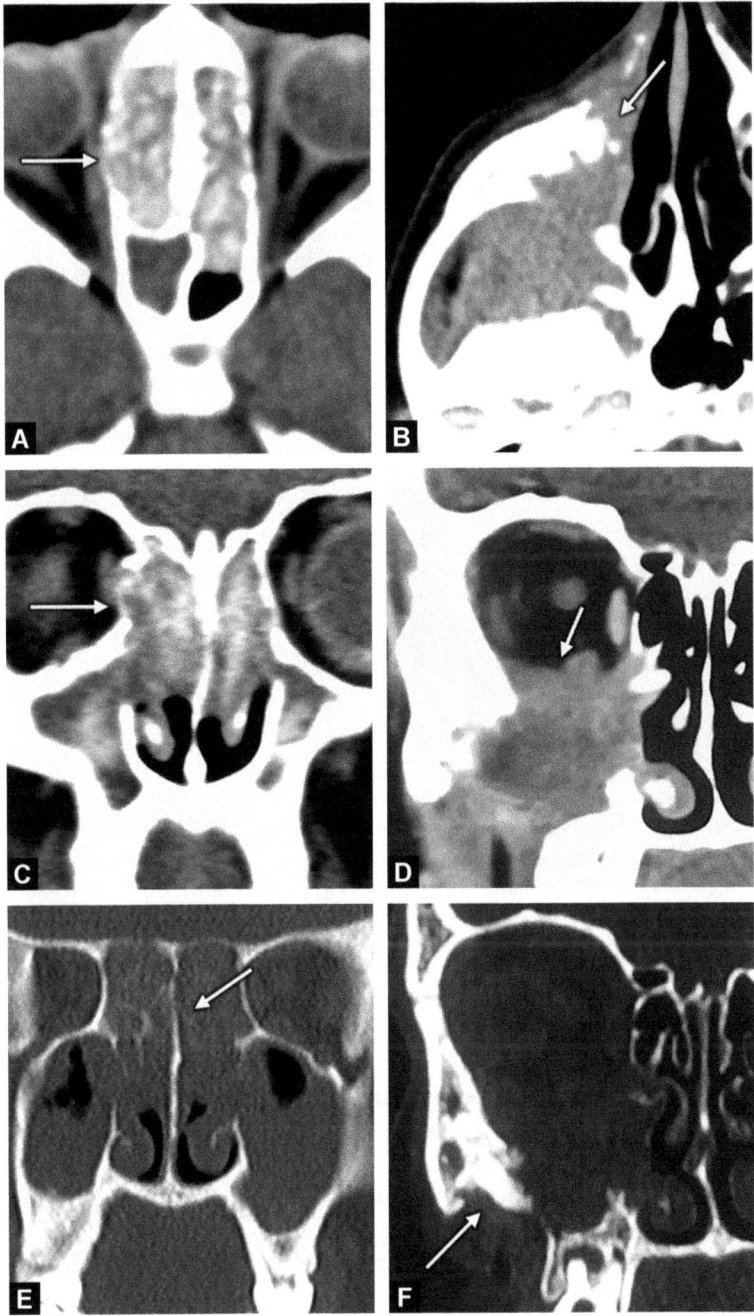

Figs. 7.12A to F: Allergic fungal sinusitis (AFS) (A, C, and E) versus chronic invasive fungal sinusitis (CIFS) (B, D, and F). Bilateral and hyperdense contents (arrow in A) in AFS; Unilateral and soft tissue density (arrow in B) in CIFS. Limited extrasinus spread (arrow in C) in AFS; Extensive soft tissue spread to orbit and infratemporal fossa (arrow in D) in CIFS. Mild expansion with demineralization of ethmoid trabeculae (arrow in E) in AFS; Erosion of maxillary bone with reactive sclerosis of zygomatic bone (arrow in F) in CIFS.

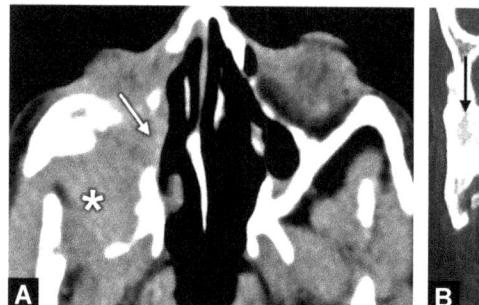
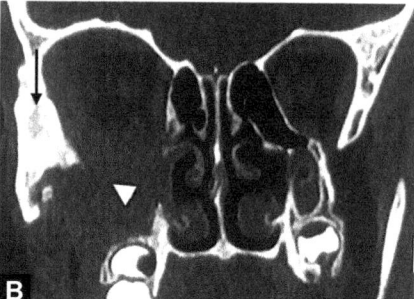

Figs. 7.13A and B: Chronic granulomatous invasive fungal sinusitis (*Mucorale sp.*). (A) Soft tissue in right maxillary sinus (arrow). Extrasinus spread to orbit, retroantral fat and masticator space (asterisk); and (B) Erosion of bony margins (arrowhead) and sclerosis of zygomatic bone (black arrow).

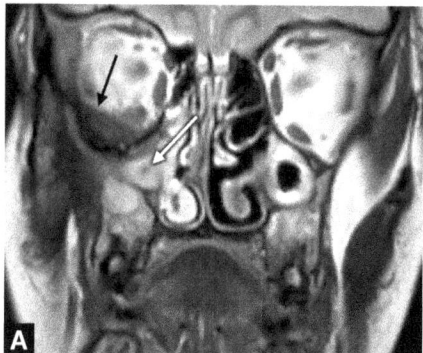
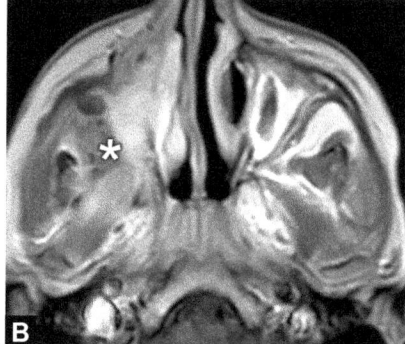

Figs. 7.14A and B: Chronic Granulomatous invasive fungal sinusitis: magnetic resonance imaging (MRI) (same patient as in Figs. 7.12A to E). (A) Sinus soft tissue is intermediate signal intensity (white arrow). Extrasinus soft tissue (orbit and infratemporal fossa): T2 hypointense (black arrow) (B) with contrast enhancement (asterisk).

- Highest reported prevalence is in Southeast Asia and Africa
- *Causative agents*: *Aspergillus sp.*; most frequent being *Aspergillus flavus*
- Histopathology shows noncaseating granulomas with findings of fungal invasion.
- *Imaging findings*:
  - Similar to other forms of chronic invasive fungal sinusitis.
  - Nonspecific appearance.
  - *Distribution*: Usually a single or two sinuses involved.
  - No sinus expansion seen.
  - Bone erosion more localized but often extrasinus involvement of the disease is more extensive than the intrasinus extent (Figs. 7.13A and B).
  - *MRI*: Better delineates the soft tissue extension (Figs. 7.14A and B). Low signal intensity on T2WIs is characteristic.

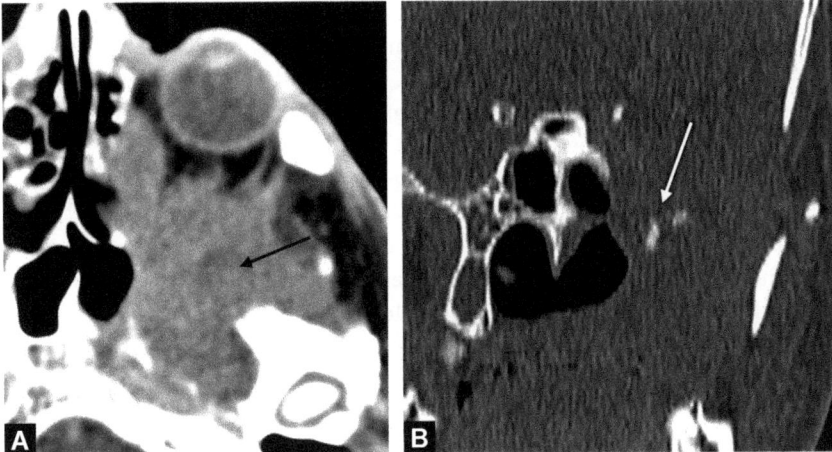

Figs. 7.15A and B: Chronic nongranulomatous invasive fungal sinusitis (aspergillosis). (A) Postoperative case of invasive aspergillosis. Extrasinus homogenous soft tissue in left orbit, infratemporal fossa (black arrow); and (B) Lytic destruction of left sphenoid bone (white arrow).

Chronic nongranulomatous invasive fungal sinusitis:
- This form also primarily occurs in immunocompromised patients.
- Symptoms are similar to non-fungal chronic rhinosinusitis but showing a poor response to treatment.
- May present with orbital apex syndrome.
- *Common agents*: *Aspergillus sp.* (especially *A. fumigatus*).
- *Imaging*:
  - Findings are similar to the acute invasive forms. Extrasinus extension may also be seen (Figs. 7.15A and B).
  - However, calcification if seen is different in the two forms; with punctate calcifications being seen in the acute forms, while more dense and coarse calcification is seen in the chronic form. Also, it is seen more frequently in the chronic disease.

CONCLUSION

Fungal sinusitis has protean manifestations but with several highly suggestive radiological signs.

REFERENCES

1. Chakrabarti A, Denning DW, Ferguson BJ, et al. Fungal rhinosinusitis: a categorization and definitional schema addressing current controversies. Laryngoscope. 2009;119:1809-18.
2. Raz E, Win W, Hagiwara M, et al. Fungal Sinusitis. Neuroimaging Clin N Am. 2015;25:569-76.

3. Connor SE. The skull base in the evaluation of sinonasal disease: role of computed tomography and MR imaging. Neuroimaging Clin N Am. 2015;25: 619-51.
4. Aibandi M, McCoy VA, Bazan C III. Imaging features of invasive and noninvasive fungal sinusitis: a review. Radiographics. 2007;27:1283-96.
5. Mafee MF, Tran BH, Chapa AR. Imaging of rhinosinusitis and its complications: plain film, CT, and MRI. Clin Rev Allergy Immunol. 2006;30:165-86.
6. Green WH, Goldberg HI, Wohl GT. Mucormycosis infection of the cranio-facial structures. Am I Roentgenol Radium Ther Nucl Med. 1967;101:802-6.
7. Reddy CEE, Gupta AK, Singh P, et al. Imaging of granulomatous and chronic invasive fungal sinusitis: comparison with allergic fungal sinusitis. Otolaryngol Head Neck Surg. 2010;143:294-300.

CHAPTER 8

Fungal Diseases of Nose and Paranasal Sinuses: Surgical Aspects

Suresh C Sharma, Kapil Sikka

- Introduction
- Classification
  - Mycetoma (Fungal Ball)
  - Allergic Fungal Rhinosinusitis
  - Invasive Fungal Rhinosinusitis
- Clinical Characteristics
  - Allergic Fungal Rhinosinusitis
  - Invasive Fungal Sinusitis
  - Chronic Invasive Rhinosinusitis
- Diagnosis
- Treatment
  - Mycetoma
  - Allergic Fungal Rhinosinusitis
  - Invasive Fungal Sinusitis

INTRODUCTION

- Fungal sinusitis is a common disease in the Indian subcontinent, and elsewhere especially in the developing world.
- These are common in North and Northwest India.
- The disease encompasses a heterogeneous spectrum.
- Careful interpretation of clinical and radiological findings is paramount as management of various spectra is different and some drugs, such as steroids may be treatment of choice in one form and highly counterproductive in other.

CLASSIFICATION

- The disease has been classified largely on the basis of immune status of the host and the immune response to the fungus. Some overlap exists between various subtypes.
- The more deficient the immune system, the more aggressive is the disease.

Broadly, fungal sinusitis is classified as:
- *Noninvasive*:
  - Fungus balls (also called as mycetoma)
  - Allergic fungal rhinosinusitis (AFRS)

- *Invasive*:
  - Acute invasive
  - Chronic invasive (further classified into granulomatous and non-granulomatous).[1]

Mycetoma (Fungal Ball)

- This is the benign presence of "tangled mats" of hyphae in typically one sinus.
- Frequently detected incidentally or by vague nasal symptoms.

Allergic Fungal Rhinosinusitis

- The disease, though common, is poorly understood.
- The mechanisms of occurrence are presumably similar to allergic bronchopulmonary aspergillosis mediated by both type 1 [immunoglobulin E (IgE)] and type III (IgG-antigen immune complexes).
- The disease is hence an immune response to fungi rather than direct infection.
- Polypi are the hallmark of AFRS disease. There is gradual accumulation of allergic mucin.
- Bent and Kuhn have outlined the major and minor clinicopathologic features for diagnosis of AFRS (Table 8.1).[2]

The criteria, though not pathognomonic, are a guide to the diagnosis of AFRS. Some, such as bone erosion have hence been modified as the same is not a hallmark of AFRS but of invasive fungus.

Invasive Fungal Rhinosinusitis

- The hallmark of this type of fungal infection is tissue invasion which clinicoradiologically differentiates it from AFRS.
- Acute invasive rhinosinusitis is a term used for a fulminant infection where the patient is usually immunocompromised and the time course is less than 4 weeks. Vascular invasion is prominent histologically. Most patients are immunocompromised.
- Chronic invasive rhinosinusitis patients have a more protracted disease course (more than 4 weeks) and have minimal or no vascular invasion, and immune compromised states.

Table 8.1: Diagnostic criteria of allergic fungal rhinosinusitis (AFRS).	
Major criteria	Minor criteria
Evidence of type 1 (IgE-mediated) hypersensitivity	Asthma
Nasal polyposis	Unilateral predominance
Characteristic CT findings	Radiographic bone erosion
Eosinophilic mucus	Fungal culture
Positive fungal smear	Charcot Leyden crystals
	Serum eosinophilia

(IgE: Immunoglobulin E; CT: Computed tomography).

CLINICAL CHARACTERISTICS

Allergic Fungal Rhinosinusitis

- As already mentioned, AFRS is the immune-mediated hypersensitivity to fungus.
- The clinical features are result of accumulation of allergic fungal mucin, consisting of eosinophils, Charcot-Leyden crystals and fungal hyphae. The resulting expansion of sinuses leads to bone remodeling and decalcification. Polypi, as already mentioned are universally present.
- Sinus remodeling, can lead to orbital symptoms like proptosis and visual loss (Fig. 8.1).

Invasive Fungal Sinusitis

- The symptoms of acute and chronic sinusitis are largely as a result of tissue invasion by fungus, the former being more fulminant and florid. Since vascular invasion is key feature of acute invasive fungal sinusitis, tissue necrosis is an early feature.
- Fever may be seen in 50% cases and most patients present with discoloration of cutaneous and mucosal areas of nose and palate. Since most patients of acute invasive sinusitis are immune compromised (diabetics being most common), features of primary disease are mostly present (Fig. 8.2).
- Extensive rapid spread of disease is common and patients frequently present with symptoms of intracranial spread, cavernous sinus thrombosis and fungal meningitis.

Chronic Invasive Rhinosinusitis

- Generally occurs in immune competent individuals and mimics other sinonasal disorders like sinusitis, neoplasms and granulomatosis with polyangiitis.
- Nasal obstruction, headache, proptosis, and visual loss are common presenting symptoms.
- Pain, with neuralgic characteristics is frequent and very difficult to treat. It indicates neural invasion and a guarded prognosis.

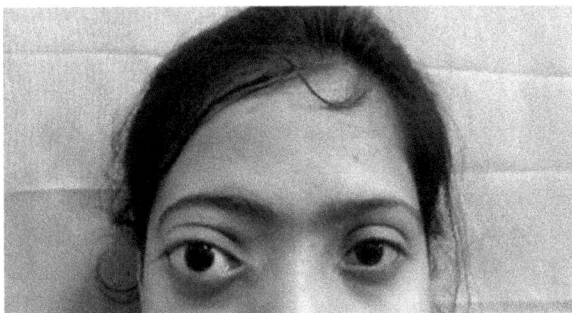

Fig. 8.1: Allergic fungal rhinosinusitis, right eye proptosis.

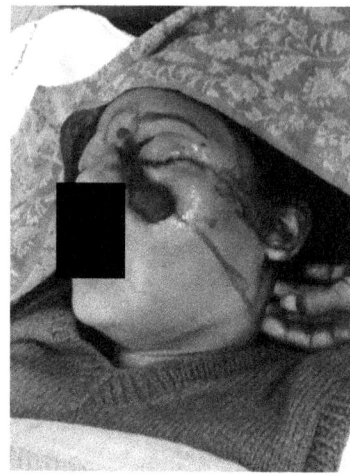

Fig. 8.2: Patient presenting with acute invasive fungal sinusitis, with blackening of skin and surrounding edema.

DIAGNOSIS

- Mode of diagnosis of various fungal disease subtypes is different. Mycetoma and AFRS can be readily diagnosed clinicoradiologically and tissue diagnosis is generally confirmed only after therapeutic excisions.
- Most frequent pathogens in AFRS are the *Aspergillus* and dematiaceous molds (*Alternaria* and *Bipolaris*).
- Acute invasive rhinosinusitis, however, is generally caused by zygomycete fungi frequently being *Mucor* and *Rhizopus*. Though clinically evident in most cases, rapid testing with 10–20% potassium hydroxide and microscopic examination can provide valuable clue to diagnosis. Since early initiation of treatment is vital, this information can provide ground for management.

TREATMENT

Mycetoma

Simple surgical excision is curative. Antifungal drugs are not indicated.

Allergic Fungal Rhinosinusitis

- Surgery is routinely required in these cases to alleviate symptoms and also reduce fungal and mucin load. Most cases can now be managed by endoscopic surgery.
- Follow-up protocols vary among institutes. Steroids are mainstay of postoperative management. Topical and oral steroids may be used till normal mucosa is obtained and followed up for many years.
- Antifungals have debatable efficacy.

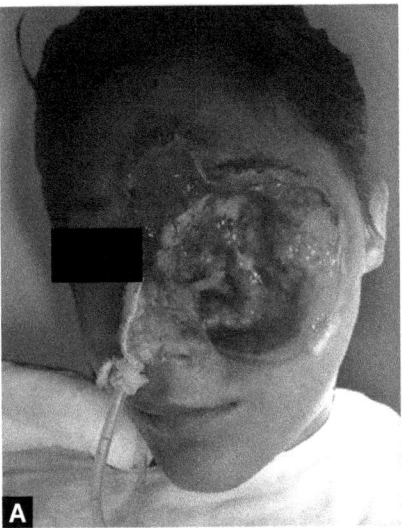
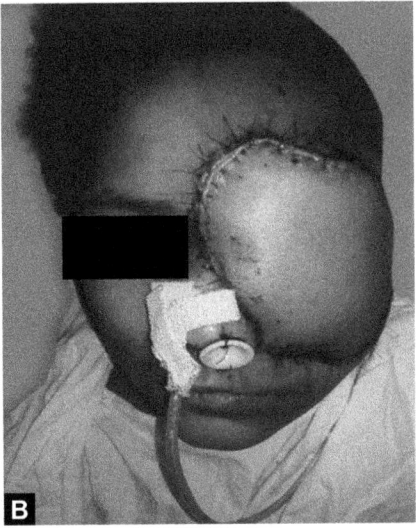

Figs. 8.3A and B: Patient in Figure 8.2 after debridement and the defect (A) and after reconstruction with anterolateral thigh free flap (B).

Invasive Fungal Sinusitis

- Treatment depends on various factors. Chronic invasive sinusitis patients, who are immune competent may be managed by debridement and oral azole antifungals (Itraconazole and Voriconazole).
- Acute invasive fungal sinusitis, however requires very aggressive and early management. The immune compromised situation needs early reversal and acidosis requires rapid control.
- Mainstay of treatment is systemic amphotericin and surgical debridement. Amphotericin is toxic in causing renal and hematological adverse effects and require close monitoring. Liposomal formulations of amphotericin have enabled rapid build-up of antifungal concentrations and are less toxic.
- Debridement at times needs to be extensive and mandates removal of necrotic bones and soft tissues of face, orbit, and nose. Defects can at times be very debilitating and require reconstruction with flaps when patient is cured (Figs. 8.3A and B).

REFERENCES

1. Ferguson BJ. Fungal rhinosinusitis: a spectrum of disease. In: Ramanathan Jr, Mims JW. The Otolaryngologic Clinics of North America. Masson SAS; Elsevier; 2017. pp. 227-454.
2. Flint PW, Haughey BH, Lund VJ, et al. Cummings Otolaryngology: Head and Neck Surgery, 6th edition. Canada: Saunders-Elsevier; 2015.

CHAPTER 9

Pre- and Post-Functional Endoscopic Sinus Surgery Imaging

Ankur Goyal, Ashu Seith Bhalla, Arvind Kumar Kairo

- Terminology
- Functional Endoscopic Sinus Surgery (FESS)
  - Indications
  - Basic Principles
  - Steps of Surgery
- Pre-Functional Endoscopic Sinus Surgery (Pre-FESS) Imaging
  - Structured Reporting
    - Mapping Sinus Involvement
    - Detailing Drainage Pathways
    - Anatomic Variants
- Post-Functional Endoscopic Sinus Surgery (Post-FESS) Appearance
- Complications of FESS
  - Immediate/Early Complications
    - Cerebrospinal Fluid Rhinorrhea
    - Orbital Complications
    - Vascular Complications
  - Late Complications
    - Recurrence
    - Empty Nose Syndrome
    - Rare Complications
    - Lipogranuloma

TERMINOLOGY

- *Endoscopic sinus surgery (ESS)*: Generic term for all sinus surgeries performed through the endoscopic route.
- Besides diseases of the paranasal sinuses, endoscopic trans-sinus route provides a way to surgically approach lesions of the orbit and anterior skull base (ASB) [e.g. repair for cerebrospinal fluid (CSF) leak].
- *Functional endoscopic sinus surgery (FESS)*—is a type of endoscopic sinus surgery which refers to minimally invasive treatment to restore sinus ventilation and normal function. It is done only for non-neoplastic mucosal diseases.

FUNCTIONAL ENDOSCOPIC SINUS SURGERY (FESS)

Goal of functional endoscopic sinus surgery is to reestablish the normal mucociliary clearance and normal ventilation in cases of refractory rhinosinusitis. Every sinus has its own natural pattern of drainage and innate mucociliary clearance pattern. Obstruction in the paths of these pathways inhibits proper clearance.

Indications

- Refractory sinus obstruction, not responding to medical therapy
- Polyps
- Mucoceles.

Basic Principles

- The procedure involves removing the diseased mucosa, preserving the maximum normal mucosa and optimally widening the natural ostia of the sinuses.
- Osteomeatal complex (OMC) is the main area to be operated in FESS since even minimal inflammation can lead to obstruction of drainage and ventilation of maxillary, anterior ethmoid and frontal sinuses.
- If FESS is done from anterior to posterior direction, then it is called *Messerklinger technique* and the reverse is known as *Wigand technique*.
- 0 and 30 degree endoscopes (sinuscope) are must for FESS.
- 45, 70, and 90 degree sinuscopes are also available to visualize hidden areas.

Steps of Surgery

It is not necessary to open every sinus ostia; thus, surgery is tailor-made for each case according to requirement/scenario. The common sequence of steps is as follows:

1. Medialization of middle turbinate to open up middle meatal area.
2. *Uncinectomy*—removal of uncinate process. Incomplete removal of uncinate is a common cause of failure of FESS as it plays key role in OMC formation.
3. *Middle meatal antrostomy*: Identification and enlargement of the natural opening of the maxillary sinus into the middle meatus.
4. *Frontal sinusotomy* and clearance of the frontal recess.
5. *Anterior ethmoidectomy*: Opening the ethmoid bulla.
6. *Posterior ethmoidectomy and sphenoidotomy*: Breaching the basal lamina.

PRE-FUNCTIONAL ENDOSCOPIC SINUS SURGERY (PRE-FESS) IMAGING

- Multidetector computed tomography (MDCT) images should be viewed on a workstation in all the three planes [(1) axial, (2) coronal, and (3) sagittal] (Table 9.1).
- Additional oblique planes may also be used as and when required.

Plane	Structures best delineated
\multicolumn{2}{c}{**Table 9.1: Utility of the different planes in multidetector computed tomography (MDCT).**}
Coronal	• Osteomeatal complex (OMC) • Frontal sinus drainage pathway • Cribriform plate • Lamina papyracea • Nasal septum deviation and spurs • Vertical attachment of the middle turbinate
Axial	• Basal lamella (dividing anterior from posterior ethmoidal cells) • Sphenoethmoidal recess • Sphenoid ostium
Sagittal	• OMC • Frontal sinus drainage pathway (parasagittal images) • Frontal recess • Bulla ethmoidalis • Uncinate process • Ethmoidal air cells drainage: Anterior → middle meatus Posterior → sphenoethmoidal recess • Agger nasi cells • Sphenoid ostia

Structured Reporting

- It is important to use a structured reporting format for reporting CT scans of paranasal sinus diseases (Table 9.2 and Figs. 9.1A to F).
- The preprocedural radiology report should encompass following components:
  - Mapping sinus involvement
  - Detailing drainage pathways
  - Anatomic variants especially critical variants (for instance uncinated process, olfactory fossa, Heller cell, and Onodi cell)
  - Relevant details of surrounding structures (orbit, cranium, and oral cavity)
  - Incidental findings, if any.

Mapping Sinus Involvement

- This involves detailing the extent of disease and complications.
- Listing of sinuses involved and assigning pattern.
- Comment on attenuation of secretions—hyperdense secretions should be specifically mentioned.
- Status of sinus walls—mucoperiosteal thickening/erosion
  - *Hyperostosis*: Extensive drilling required and there is a need to rule out alternative etiology
  - *Dehiscence*: Risk of penetration.
- Caution—exclude tumor as a cause for obstruction.

Detailing Drainage Pathways

- Since the aim of FESS is to restore drainage pathways, detailing the involvement of these is critical.

Anatomic Variants

- These may contribute to obstruction of drainage pathways and/or pose a surgical risk. Hence the need of detailing them in radiology reports.
- The structure wise anatomic variants are detailed in Chapter 2.
- The anatomic variants can be classified into three categories:
    1. Those obstructing the drainage pathways: refer Chapter 2.
    2. Those posing a surgical risk and may require alterations in surgical technique (Table 9.3 and Figs. 9.2A to F).
    3. Those responsible for recurrent disease are enlisted in Table 9.4.

Table 9.2: Structured reporting format.

Admitting diagnosis: Nasal obstruction

Report	RT	LT
1. Opacification of sinuses (present/absent)		
Frontal sinus	A	A
Ethmoid sinus	A	A
Maxillary sinus	A	P
Sphenoid sinus	A	A
2. Mucoperiosteal thickening of sinuses (present/absent)		
Frontal sinus	P	P
Ethmoid sinus	P	P
Maxillary sinus	P	P
Sphenoid sinus	P	A
3. Any hyperdense contents (mention site)	No	No
4. Pneumatization of sinuses (normal/hypoplastic)		
Frontal sinus	N	N
Ethmoid sinus	N	N
Maxillary sinus	N	N
Sphenoid sinus—sellar	N	N
Sphenoid sinus—presellar	H	H

Contd...

Contd...

	RT	LT
5. Bone expansion (mention site)	A	A
6. Bone erosion (mention site)	A	A
7. Bone sclerosis (mention site)	A	A
8. Nasal septum—deviated/midline	Deviated to left	
9. Middle turbinate anatomy (normal/abnormal)	N	N
10. Uncinate process insertion	Lamina papyracea	Lamina papyracea
11. Osteomeatal complex	Obstructed	Obstructed
12. Frontal nasal duct pathway	Obstructed	Obstructed
13. Sphenoethmoidal recess	Obstructed	Patent
14. Inferior turbinate	Hypertrophied	Hypertrophied
15. Infraorbital ethmoidal (Haller) cell	Absent	Absent
16. Sphenoethmoidal (Onodi cell)	Absent	Absent
17. Anterior clinoid process pneumatization	Absent	Absent
18. Lamina papyracea integrity	Intact	Intact
19. Cribriform plate anatomy (Keros classification I/II/III)	II	II
20. Ethmoid skull base integrity	Intact	Intact
21. Optic nerve anatomy (covered by bone or not)	Yes	Yes
22. Internal carotid artery (ICA) anatomy (covered by bone or not)	Yes	Yes
23. Orbit	N	N
24. Nasopharynx	N	N
25. Visualized brain parenchyma	N	N
26. Additional findings	Nil	Nil

Impression:
- Mucoperiosteal thickening in bilateral, frontal, ethmoid and right sphenoid sinus, partial.
- Opacification of left maxillary sinus, bilateral obstructed osteomeatal complex (OMC) and deviated nasal septum (DNS) to left with B/L inferior turbinate hypertrophy suggestive of pansinusitis.
- No anatomical variant suggestive of posing surgical risk identified.

Chapter 9 Pre- and Post-Functional Endoscopic Sinus Surgery Imaging 123

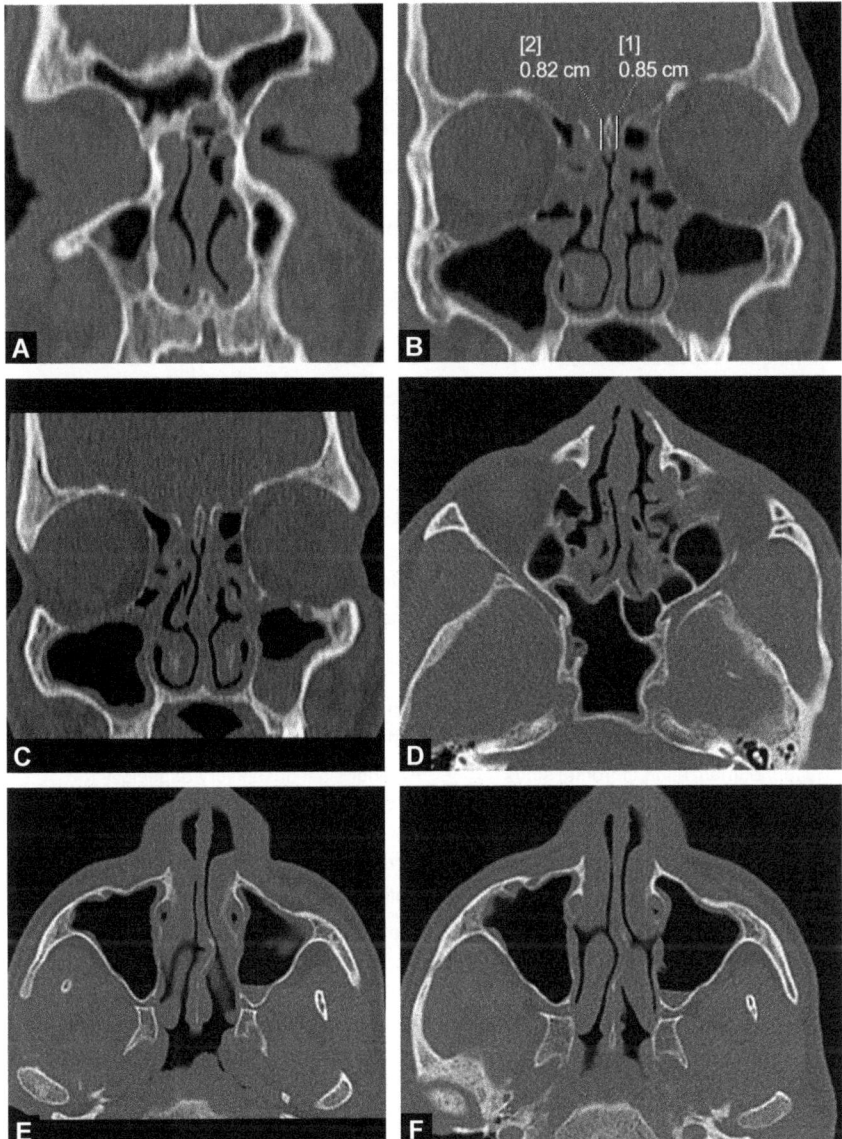

Figs. 9.1A to F: Example of structured reporting format.

Table 9.3: Anatomical variants having surgical relevance.

Anatomic variants posing surgical risk	Modification of technique required
Deviated nasal septum	Septoplasty may be required to improve access
Uncinate process—acute angle of lamina papyracea attachment	Orbital injury more likely
Maxillary sinus hypoplasia	Orbital injury due to close approximation of medial walls of the sinus and orbit
Small bulla ethmoidalis → medial projection of LP (torus lateralis)	Orbital injury
LP defects (especially in posterior part due to less orbital fat)	Orbital injury
Medially placed LP [compared with osteomeatal complex (OMC)—usually in same plane]	Orbital injury
Dehiscent infraorbital nerve (along maxillary roof)	Risk of nerve injury
Frontal cell	Anterior skull base penetration
Decreased vertical distance between maxillary sinus roof and anterior skull base	Anterior skull base injury
Areas of dehiscence in posterior wall of frontal sinuses	Risk of meningitis (as sinus washes done during procedure)
Hypopneumatization of frontal sinus	Anterior skull base injury especially if external approach planned [done for disease in lateral part of frontal sinuses (FS)] as trephination is done
Onodi cells	Optic nerve injury
Hyperpneumatization of sphenoid sinus Focal dehiscence may be seen lateral wall	Internal carotid artery (ICA), optic nerve, V2 in foramen rotundum, vidian artery in vidian canal
Supaorbital ethmoidal cells	Mistaken for frontal sinus Anterior ethmoidal artery also displaced posteriorly
Pneumatized basal lamella	Mistaken for posterior ethmoidal cells
Type III Keros anterior skull base configuration	Intracranial penetration
Deficient bony canal of anterior ethmoidal artery	

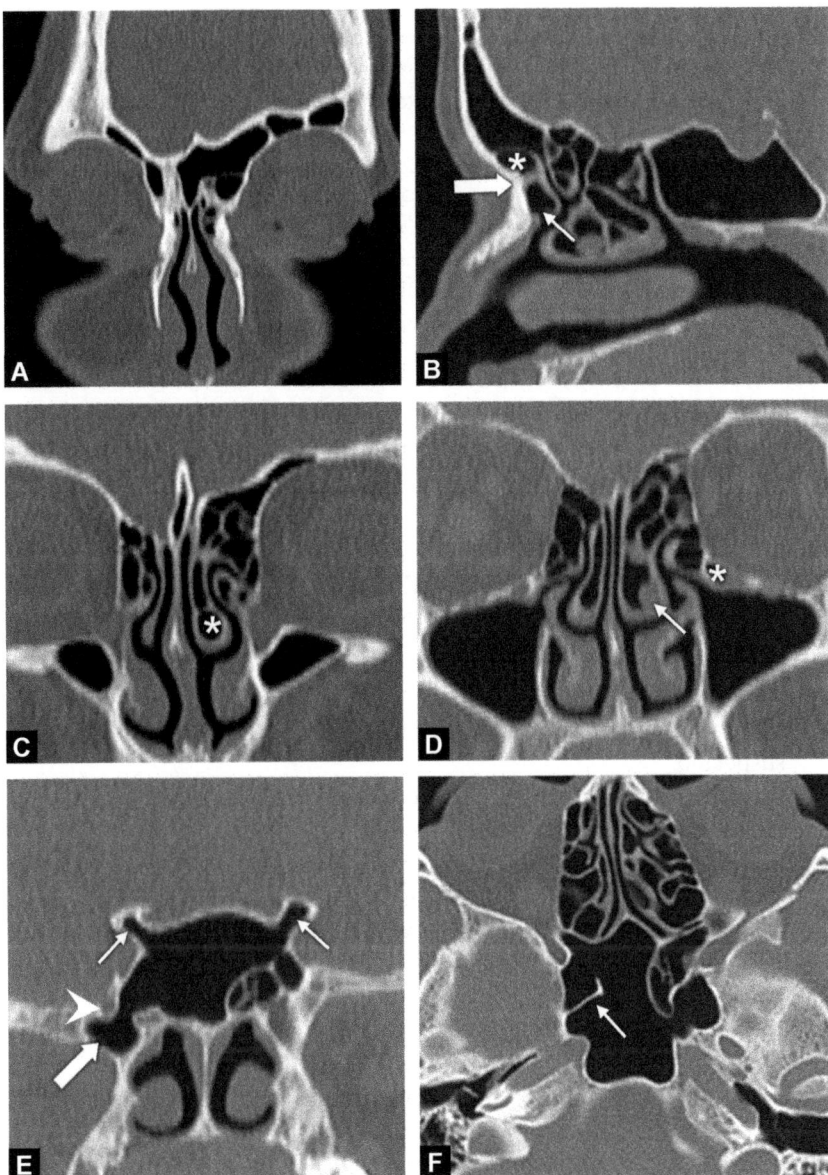

Figs. 9.2A to F: Anatomic variants posing surgical risk. (A) Hypopneumatization of RT frontal sinus; (B) Type 3 frontal cell (asterisk) projecting above the frontal beak (solid arrow). Agger nasi is shown by thin arrow; (C) Asymmetric depth of olfactory fossa. Lateral lamella is vertical on left and oblique on right side. LT concha bullosa (asterisk) and asymmetric aeration of ethmoid sinuses; (D) Bilateral concha bullosa with mucosal thickening left side (arrow). LT Haller cells with mucosal thickening (asterisk); (E) Pneumatized anterior clinoid processes (thin arrows) and lateral recess of sphenoid sinus (thick arrow) with foramen rotundum (arrowhead) projecting into the roof of the aerated lateral recess; and (F) Laterally deviated sphenoid sinus septum (arrow) going toward carotid canal.

Table 9.4: Anatomic variants associated with residual/recurrent disease.	
Anatomic variants	Residual/recurrent disease
Accessory maxillary ostium (behind the natural ostium)	Recurrent sinusitis if both the ostia are not joined during surgery
Hyperpneumatization of maxillary sinus	Dental caries and resultant procedures can cause recurrent infections High rest of oroantral fistula
Anterior and posterior components of maxillary sinus	Incomplete clearance/residual disease
Anterior → middle meatus Small posterior → superior meatus Basal attaches to maxillary sinus instead of LP (missed basal lamella)	Incomplete clearance/residual disease
Sinusitis in lateral recess of sphenoid sinus lateral part of FS	Recurrence

POST-FUNCTIONAL ENDOSCOPIC SINUS SURGERY (POST-FESS) APPEARANCE

- Post-FESS, an early MDCT may be required if there is suspicion of a surgical complication.
- Contrast administration is needed if orbital or cranial complications are suspected.
- Computed tomography (CT) is performed in the late phase if there is persistence or recurrence of symptoms.
- Familiarity with normal post-FESS appearance is necessary while evaluating for complications/disease recurrence (Figs. 9.3 to 9.6).
- Table 9.5 delineates the explanation of the FESS procedures and the normal expected postoperative appearance.

Specific Conditions

Mucocele

- Entails opening up of the drainage pathways with clearing of the sinus contents.
- Stent/packing material may be visualized postoperatively.
- Post-drainage remineralization of the sinus walls is expected over time.
- CT/MRI also helps to identify residual/recurrent mucocele.

Sinonasal debridement for fungal sinusitis:

- Postoperative imaging is challenging as differentiation of residual fungal disease versus postoperative changes (hemorrhage/packing material) is difficult.
- CT and MRI need to be co-evaluated.

Table 9.5: Post-functional endoscopic sinus surgery (FESS) imaging.

Type of endoscopic surgery/indications	Procedures	Postoperative appearance
Osteomeatal unit ESS for blocked OMU	• Uncinotomy/uncinectomy • Middle meatal antrostomy/fenestration • Middle turbinectomy • Ethmoidectomy • Inferior antrostomy (uncommon)	• Widened "neoinfundibulum" on coronal CT In ethmoidectomy: • Medial bowing of lamina papyracea (1–3 mm) • Globe may appear deviated • Defect in the region of inferior turbinate in inferior antrostomy
Frontal sinusotomy: Done for persistent sinonasal disease in spite of infundibular/anterior ethmoid procedures	*Draf classification:* 1. Resection of anterior ethmoid cells and uncinate process around the frontal recess 2. 1 + resection of part of the floor of frontal sinus (nasal septum to lamina papyracea) 3. Entire frontal sinus floor + superior part of nasal septum (modified) • Lothrop procedure ± stenting (if neo-ostium <5 mm)	• Coronal and sagittal sections need to be seen for evaluation of these structures • Position of stent to be assessed
Sphenoidotomy ± sphenoid marsupialization *(exteriorizing the sinus)* for sphenoid sinus obstruction	• Widening of the natural ostium • Creating new opening through posterior ethmoid ± ethmoidectomy	Axial + sagittal reformats
Inferior turbinate reduction Turbinoplasty or lateralization of the inferior turbinate (out-fracture): Hypertrophy of inferior turbinate (allergic rhinitis)	Mucosal volume reduction (RFA/laser ablation/coblation) Submucosal resection of inferior turbinate	Coronal sections
Septoplasty or septorhinoplasty. Deviated nasal septum worsening the nasal obstruction or cosmetic		• Nasal septum appears "straightened" • Previously seen spurs may be reduced or not seen at all • Silicone stents/tubes in early postoperative period

(ESS: Endoscopic sinus surgery; OMU: Osteomeatal unit; CT: Computed tomography; RFA: Radiofrequency ablation).

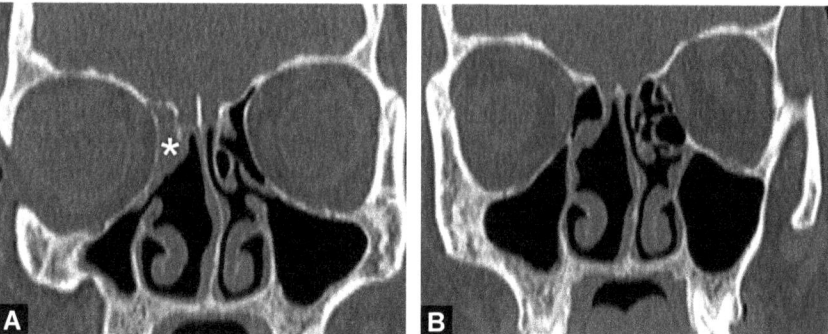

Figs. 9.3A and B: Post-FESS appearance and disease recurrence. Bilateral middle turbinates are not seen and there are no septations in RT ethmoid sinus, suggesting bilateral middle turbinectomies and RT ethmoidectomy; Recurrent mucosal thickening seen in RT frontal drainage pathway (asterisk).

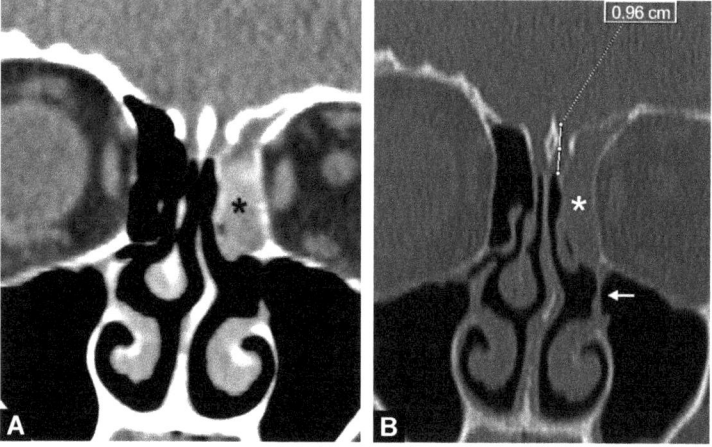

Figs. 9.4A and B: Post-FESS patient with recurrent left sinusitis and anatomic variant posing surgical risk. LT maxillary antrostomy (wide maxillary ostium after uncinectomy and middle turbinectomy). Recurrent LT ethmoid sinusitis (asterisk). Adhesions/fibrotic band at the site of LT uncinate (arrow) may again obstruct the maxillary ostium. Note anatomic variant posing surgical risk—Keros type III (bilateral deep olfactory fossae).

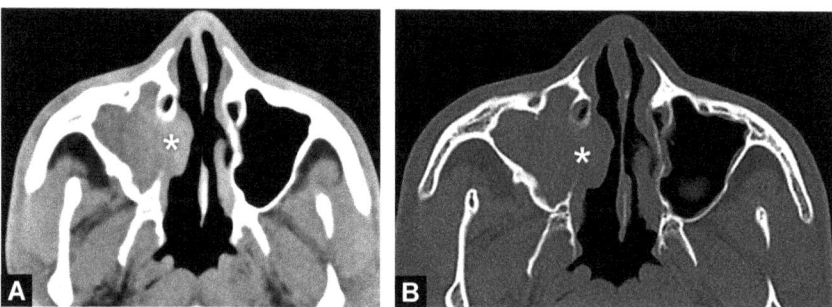

Figs. 9.5A and B: Post-FESS polyp recurrence. Recurrent antrochoanal polyp (asterisk) after RT maxillary antrostomy.

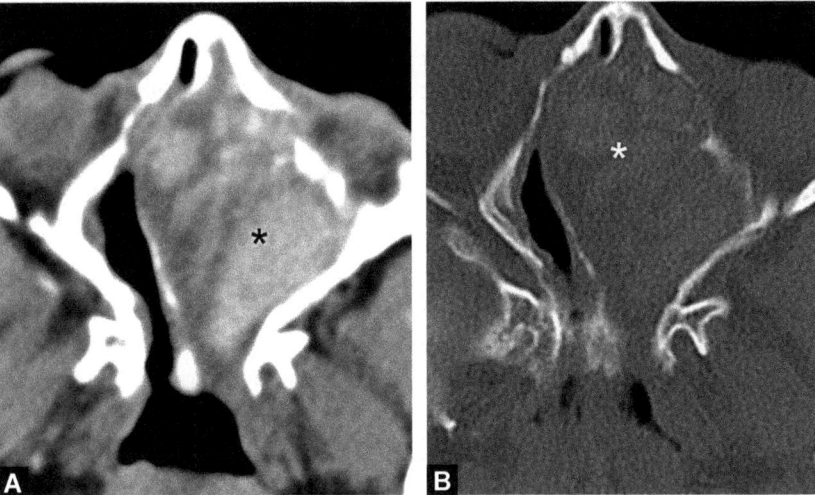

Figs. 9.6A and B: Post-FESS contralateral disease recurrence. RT maxillary antrostomy seen. Contralateral recurrence of allergic fungal sinusitis showing hyperdensity and causing expansion of LT nasal cavity and maxillary sinus (asterisks). Here recurrence is due to nature of disease and affects contralateral side.

COMPLICATIONS OF FESS

Table 9.6 enumerates the complications which may be associated with FESS (Figs. 9.7A to F).

Immediate/Early Complications

These complications often result from direct trauma during surgery due to penetrating injury by surgical instruments.

Cerebrospinal Fluid Rhinorrhea

- Occurs as a consequence of disruption of the ASB.
- It may be associated with intracranial hemorrhage or parenchymal injury, and later with recurrent meningitis/intracranial abscess.
- Anterior skull base defects may even result in formation of cephaloceles.
- A combination of thin section NCCT and contrast-enhanced magnetic resonance (MR) is required for complete delineation of these injuries.

Orbital Complications

- Lamina papyracea (LP) is the most common site of injury. Inferior orbital wall may also be disrupted.
- Resultant orbital hemorrhage appears as fat stranding of the orbital fat.
- Extraocular muscles appear thickened with irregular margins. Associated motility disturbances are seen.
- Optic nerve injury is associated with visual loss. The optic nerve appears thickened with irregular contours. MRI may reveal altered signal intensity within the nerve itself.
- Disruption of the nasolacrimal causes dacryocystitis and epiphora.

Nasal Septum

- Particularly susceptible during septoplasty.
- Hematoma within a closed space (perichondrium) results in ischemic necrosis of the cartilage.
- Patients are usually symptomatic with nasal obstruction, epistaxis, recurrent crushing, secondary infections or "whistling".

Vascular Complications

- Arteries which may be injured include (anterior to posterior): anterior ethmoidal, anterior cerebral, sphenopalatine, and internal carotid arteries.
- Patient presents with epistaxis in the postoperative period.
- Imaging reveals extravasation of contrast/pseudoaneurysm.
- CT angiography delineates the defect and injury. Digital subtraction angiography (DSA) with embolization is the treatment of choice.

Table 9.6: Potential complications of endoscopic sinus surgery.

Skull base complications:
- Cerebrospinal fluid CSF leakage (rhinorrhea) or herniation (encephalocele)
- Infection

Intracranial injuries:
- Cerebral parenchymal injury
- Intracranial hemorrhage
- Infection

Ophthalmic injuries:
- Extraocular muscle injury
- Intraorbital hemorrhage
- Optic nerve injury
- Disruption of lacrimal drainage system
- Periorbital lipogranuloma

Sinonasal complications:
- Recurrent rhinosinusitis and polyposis
- Retained septations
- Neo-osteogenesis
- Adhesions
- Mucus recirculation phenomenon
- Mucocele
- Nasal septal perforation
- Empty nose syndrome

Miscellaneous:
- Gossypiboma
- Vascular injury (pseudoaneurysm)

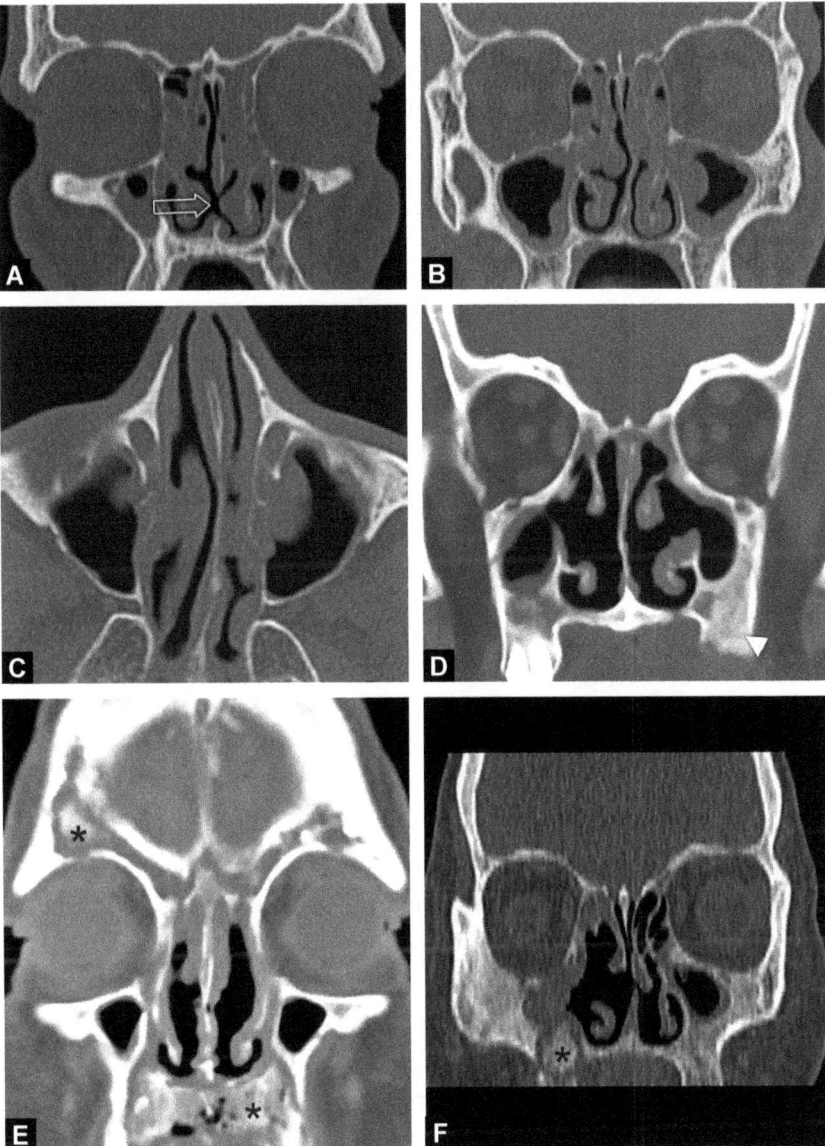

Figs. 9.7A to F: Post-FESS complications. (A to C) Show nasal septal perforation (arrow) in a patient who had undergone LT middle turbinectomy. There is recurrent mucosal thickening in all the visualized sinuses; (D and E) Another patient who had undergone bilateral middle turbinectomy and left uncinectomy showing recurrent mucoperiosteal thickening with neo-osteogenesis (arrowhead). There was also extensive osteomyelitis of frontal and maxillary bones with sequestrum formation (asterisks); and (F) Post RT maxillary antrostomy patient with osteomyelitis of RT maxillary bone in a diabetic patient with sequestrum formation (asterisk). There is bony remodeling of both maxillary sinuses.

Late Complications

Recurrence (Table 9.7 and Figs. 9.8A and B)

- Recurrence of symptoms is a common indication of repeat imaging.
- This may be due to recurrent or residual disease.
- Recurrence of the disease can be due to basic nature of the pathology, e.g. refractory nature of polyps in asthmatics. It is however frequently due to structural causes.
- The role of imaging in this scenario is not only to map the extent of disease but also to identify a structural cause, if any.

Empty Nose Syndrome

- "Empty nose syndrome" refers to a situation wherein a patient experiences symptoms of nasal congestion despite the nasal cavity and sinuses being clear.
- It is a rare complication that follows extensive reaction especially of the inferior turbinate.
- The proposed mechanism is the increase in nasal permeability which effects the functioning of neurosensitive receptors, as also the function of humidification of inhaled air.

Rare Complications

- *Gossypiboma*: Due to retained gauze. May be seen in sinonasal cavity, even intracranial. Simulates a mass lesion.
- CT-MRI low signal intensity of T2-weighted image (T2WI).

Lipogranuloma

- Periorbital fat containing nodules usually located in eyelids. Imaging appearance is of ill-defined and irregular nodules showing heterogenous enhancement.

Table 9.7: Causes of disease recurrence after functional endoscopic sinus surgery (FESS).	
Causes of recurrent disease	CT appearance
Postoperative adhesions and mucosal thickening	Difficult to differentiate, adhesions may appear as linear bands
Residual cells: Haller/agger nasi/ frontal/anterior ethmoidal	
Neo-osteogenesis	Amorphous bony attenuation Can enlarge and increasingly ossify over time
Recirculation	Phenomenon of mucous circulating between the natural ostium and other opening (accessory ostium) that are not connected Ring like appearance on computed tomography (CT)

Chapter 9 Pre- and Post-Functional Endoscopic Sinus Surgery Imaging 133

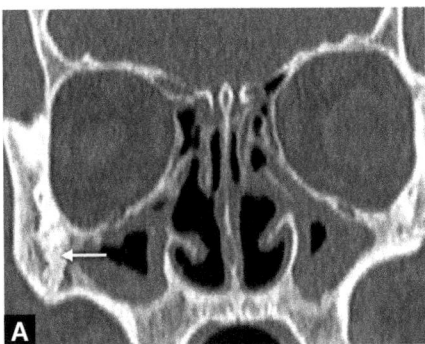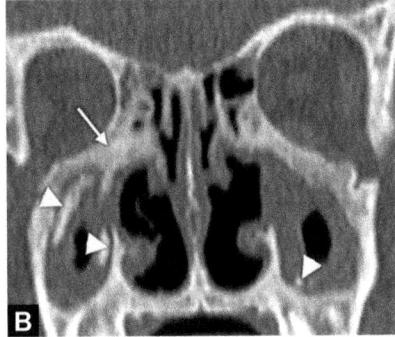

Figs. 9.8A and B: Post-FESS case with calcified mucoperiosteal thickening and neo-osteogenesis. Nonvisualized middle turbinates and RT uncinate process. RT ethmoidectomy had also been done. There are foci of discrete chunky calcification suggesting calcified mucoperiosteal thickening (arrowheads) in all the visualized sinuses, obstructing both osteomeatal complexes (OMCs). Arrows show amorphous new bone formation suggesting neo-osteogenesis.

BIBLIOGRAPHY

1. Figueroa RE. Imaging anatomy in revision sinus surgery. In: Kountakis S, Jacobs J, Gosepath J. (Eds). Revision Sinus Surgery. Berlin, Heidelberg: Springer; 2008.
2. Ginat DT. Posttreatment imaging of the paranasal sinuses following endoscopic sinus surgery. Neuroimaging Clin N Am. 2015;25:653-65.
3. Hoang JK, Eastwood JD, Tebbit CL et al. Multiplanar sinus CT: a systematic approach to imaging before functional endoscopic sinus surgery. AJR Am J oentgenol. 2010;194:W527-36.
4. Vaid S, Vaid N, Rawat S, et al. An imaging checklist for pre-FESS CT: framing a surgically relevant report. Clin Radiol. 2011;66:459-70.

Section 3

Tumor and Tumor-like Conditions

10. Pathology of Sinonasal Lesions
11. Pathology of Bony/Cartilaginous Sinonasal Tumors
12. Benign Tumors of the Nose and Paranasal Sinuses: Imaging
13. Benign Sinonasal Tumors: Surgical Perspective
14. Malignant Tumors of the Sinonasal Cavities: Imaging
15. Malignant Tumors of Nose and Paranasal Sinuses: Surgical Perspective
16. Radiation and Chemotherapy in Management of Malignant Sinonasal Tumors

CHAPTER 10

Pathology of Sinonasal Lesions

Deepali Jain

- Introduction
- Classification of Sinonasal Lesions
- Non-Neoplastic Lesions
  - Infective Rhinosinusitis
  - Allergic Sinusitis
  - Sinonasal Polyps
  - Granulomatosis with Polyangiitis (GPA) (Earlier called as Wegener's Granulomatosis)
- Benign Neoplastic Lesions
  - Sinonasal Papillomas
  - Salivary Gland Tumors
  - Hemangioma
  - Nasopharyngeal Angiofibromas
- Malignant Neoplastic Lesions
  - Carcinomas
    - Keratinizing Squamous Cell Carcinoma and Non-keratinizing Squamous Cell Carcinoma
    - Sarcomatoid (Spindle Cell) Squamous Cell Carcinoma
    - SMARCB1 (INI1)-deficient Sinonasal Carcinoma
    - Intestinala and Non-intestinal Type Adenocarcinomas
  - Malignant
    - Biphenotypic Sinonasal Sarcoma
    - Sinonasal Glomangiopericytoma
  - Teratocarcinosarcoma
  - Hematolymphoid Tumors
  - Olfactory Neuroblastoma

INTRODUCTION

The sinonasal tract may be involved by wide variety of infections, autoimmune disorders and neoplastic lesions. Among non-neoplastic lesions, histopathology laboratories commonly receive specimens of inflammatory nasal polyps, allergic, and fungal sinusitis. In neoplastic lesions, the fourth edition of the *World Health Organization (WHO) Classification of Head and Neck Tumours*[1] includes few new benign and malignant entities which include seromucinous hamartoma, NUT (nuclear protein in testis) carcinoma, biphenotypic sinonasal sarcoma and human papilloma virus (HPV)-related carcinoma with adenoid cystic features. In this chapter, a brief overview of commonly encountered sinonasal lesions in routine pathology practice is given.

CLASSIFICATION OF SINONASAL LESIONS

- Non-neoplastic sinonasal lesions have been described in Table 10.1.

Table 10.1: Non-neoplastic sinonasal lesions.	
Infective	Noninfective
Rhinosinusitis	Sinonasal polyps
Rhinoscleroma	Nasal glial heterotopia
Rhinosporidiosis	Allergic sinusitis
	Wegener's granulomatosis (granulomatosis with polyangiitis)
	Respiratory epithelial adenomatoid hamartoma
	Myospherulosis

Neoplastic: WHO Classification of Head and Neck Tumors classifies nasal cavity and paranasal sinus tumors into different categories according to their cell lineage and clinical behavior[1] (Table 10.2).

Table 10.2: World Health Organization (WHO) classification of sinonasal tumors	
Carcinomas	• Keratinizing squamous cell carcinomas • Non-keratinizing squamous cell carcinomas • Spindle cell (sarcomatoid) squamous cell carcinoma • Lymphoepithelial carcinoma • Sinonasal undifferentiated carcinoma • NUT (nuclear protein in testis) carcinoma • Neuroendocrine carcinoma • Adenocarcinoma
Salivary gland tumors	Pleomorphic adenoma
Sinonasal papillomas	• Inverted papilloma • Oncocytic type • Exophytic type
Benign soft tissue tumors	• Leiomyoma • Hemangioma • Schwannoma • Neurofibroma • Nasopharyngeal angiofibroma*
Malignant soft tissue tumors	• Fibrosarcoma • Undifferentiated pleomorphic sarcoma • Leiomyosarcoma • Rhabdomyosarcoma • Angiosarcoma • Malignant peripheral nerve sheath tumor • Biphenotypic sinonasal sarcoma • Synovial sarcoma • Borderline/low-grade malignant tumors: Fibromatosis, solitary fibrous tumor, sinonasal glomangiopericytoma, and hemangioendothelioma
Hematolymphoid	• Extranodal natural killer (NK)/T-cell lymphoma • Plasmacytoma
Neuroectodermal/melanocytic	• Ewing sarcoma/primitive neuroectodermal tumor • Olfactory neuroblastoma • Mucosal melanoma

*NPA (nasopharyngeal angiofibroma) is classified under soft tissue tumors of nasopharynx.

NON-NEOPLASTIC LESIONS

Inflammatory lesions: Subdivided into allergic and infective categories.
Infective: It can be bacterial, viral or fungal.

Infective Rhinosinusitis

- Infective lesions of nasal cavity and paranasal sinuses is of varying etiology. Bacterial causes include *Streptococcus pneumoniae*, *Haemophilus influenzae*, and *Moraxella catarrhalis*. Rhinovirus, influenza, and parainfluenza viruses are most frequent causes of viral sinusitis. During acute phase of illness biopsy is not required and diagnosis is primarily made by clinical examination and culture results.
- Fungal sinusitis can be invasive or allergic. Invasive and allergic types can be differentiated by immune status of the patients, causative organisms and histopathology.
- Allergic fungal sinusitis (AFS) develops due to allergic reaction to fungal allergens in immunocompetent hosts.
- Microscopically, pools of mucin with degenerating eosinophils, neutrophils and Charcot–Leyden crystals are seen.
- Fungal hyphae are entangled within mucin, which are highlighted by special histochemical stains for fungi (Figs. 10.1A and B).
- Differential diagnosis is with invasive fungal sinusitis (IFS) where tissue infiltration by fungal hyphae is seen. Most common pathogens of IFS are *Aspergillus* and *Mucor* species.
- Different histochemical stains can be used to diagnose fungal organisms (Table 10.3).
- *Rhinosporidiosis*: *Rhinosporidium seeberi* is a protozoa which is responsible for the disease. *Microscopy*: Large cysts with thick walls filled with numerous endospores (Figs. 10.2A and B).

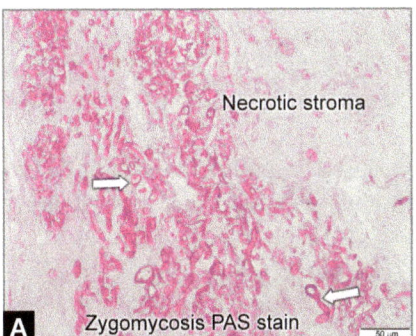 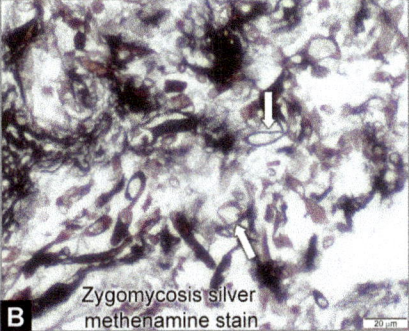

Figs. 10.1A and B: (A) **Zygomycosis:** broad aseptate fungal hyphae (arrow); and (B) Periodic acid-Schiff (PAS) and silver methenamine stains. A is stain. B is sliver methenamine stain. Arrows for A and B are same.

Table 10.3: Commonly used histochemical stains for diagnosis of sinonasal infections.

	Periodic acid-Schiff (PAS)	Silver methenamine	Alcian blue PAS	Mucicarmine	Ziehl–Neelsen	Elastic van Gieson
Fungal sinusitis						
Candida	+	+				
Aspergillus	+	+				
Zygomycosis	+	+				
Cryptococcus	+	+	+	+		
Rhinosporidium	+	+				
Tuberculosis					+	
Leprosy					+	
Vasculitides						
GPA (Granulomatosis with polyangiitis)						+

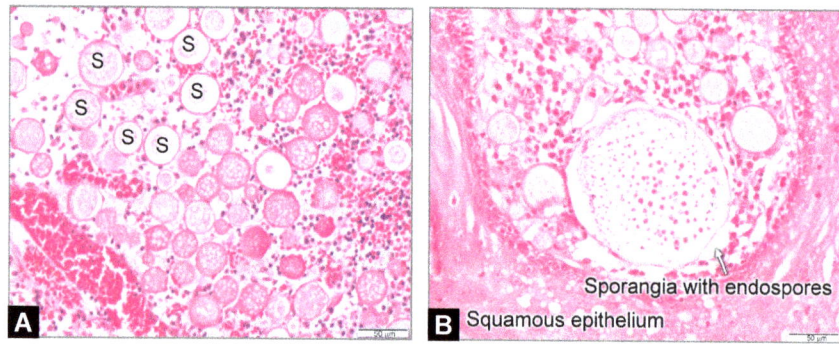

Figs. 10.2A and B: A case of **rhinosporidiosis** which shows subepithelial large sporangia (S) (100–500 μ) filled with small 6–8 μ size endospores (arrow).

Allergic Sinusitis

- *Gross pathology*: Polypoidal sinus mucosa which may be edematous, glistening, and shiny.
- *Histopathology*: Mucosal edema, thickened basement membrane, squamous metaplasia of the epithelium, and eosinophil rich inflammatory infiltrate (Figs. 10.3A and B).

Sinonasal Polyps

Develop due to recurrent chronic sinusitis.
- *Microscopy*: Edematous stroma and chronic inflammation, variable fibrosis usually seen in antrochoanal polyps, and reactive stromal cells in stroma.

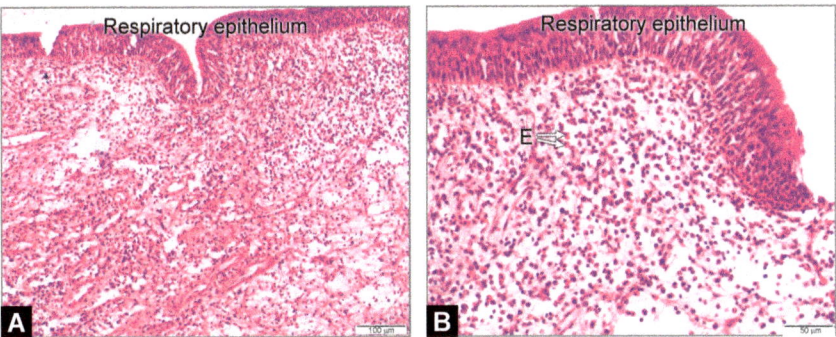

Figs. 10.3A and B: Allergic inflammatory sinusitis which shows subepithelial dense inflammation rich in eosinophils (E).

Granulomatosis with Polyangiitis (GPA) (Earlier called as Wegener's Granulomatosis)

- Type of small vessel vasculitides due to cytoplasmic antineutrophil cytoplasmic antibody (c-ANCA) directed against enzyme proteinase-3.
- Kidneys, lungs and sinonasal tract are most commonly involved.
- *Microscopy*: Necrotizing granulomatous inflammation which includes biocollagenolytic necrosis and giant cells; evidence of vasculitis is difficult to find in extensively involved lesions; elastic stains help in recognition of destruction of elastin layer of the vessel.

BENIGN NEOPLASTIC LESIONS

Sinonasal Papillomas

- Inverted type is the most frequent papilloma. Although a benign entity; malignant transformation is noted in 2–27% cases and recurrences are common.
  On histopathology: Inverted proliferation of epithelium into the stroma (Figs. 10.4A and B).
- *Oncocytic type*: Exophytic and endophytic proliferation of sinonasal epithelium with oncocytic features. The clinical behavior is same as inverted type in terms of recurrences and malignant transformation. Human papilloma virus has not been identified as a causative agent
- *Exophytic type*: Associated with HPV in around 60% of cases. Recurrences are common due to inadequate excision but malignant transformation rare.

Salivary Gland Tumors

- *Pleomorphic adenoma*: Most common benign tumor of salivary glands. Biphasic tumor of epithelial and mesenchymal cells (Figs. 10.5A and B).

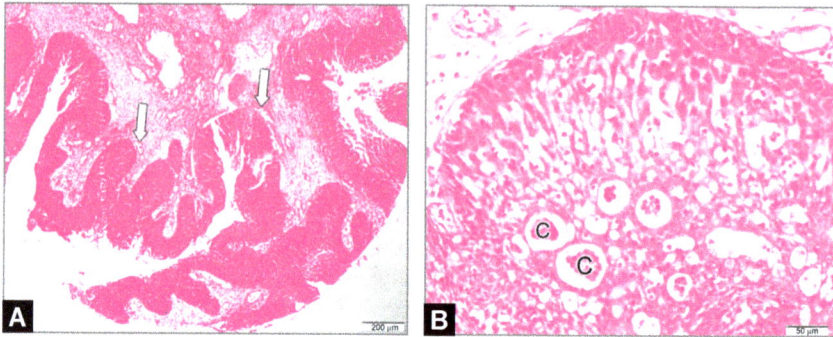

Figs. 10.4A and B: (A) **Inverted papilloma:** islands of sinonasal epithelium inverted into the stroma (arrows); (B) Higher magnification of an inverted frond which shows sinonasal epithelium and cysts (C) filled with inflammatory cells.

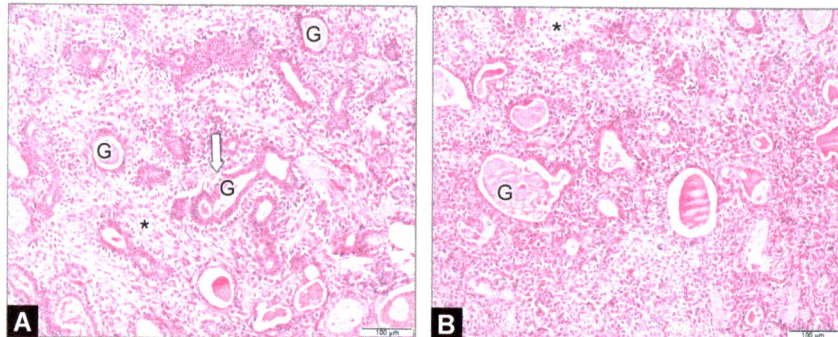

Figs. 10.5A and B: Pleomorphic adenoma: (A) admixture of glands (G) lined by epithelial and myoepithelial cell layer (arrow); (B) Embedded in cellular stroma (asterisk in A and B).

- *Adenoid cystic carcinoma*: Malignant salivary gland tumor arises from nose, sinuses, and upper airways, which is arranged in cribriform, tubular, and solid patterns. Perineural invasion is most frequent (Figs. 10.6A and B).

Hemangioma

- Also called as lobular capillary hemangioma/pyogenic granuloma/capillary hemangioma/cavernous hemangioma.
- Primarily of two types: (1) Capillary and (2) cavernous.

Nasopharyngeal Angiofibromas

- Arises in the nasopharynx of young men.
- Beta-catenin mutation is frequent event and present in about 75% of tumors.
- Locally aggressive tumors.
- Microscopically shows vascular and stromal components (Figs. 10.7A and B).

Chapter 10 Pathology of Sinonasal Lesions 143

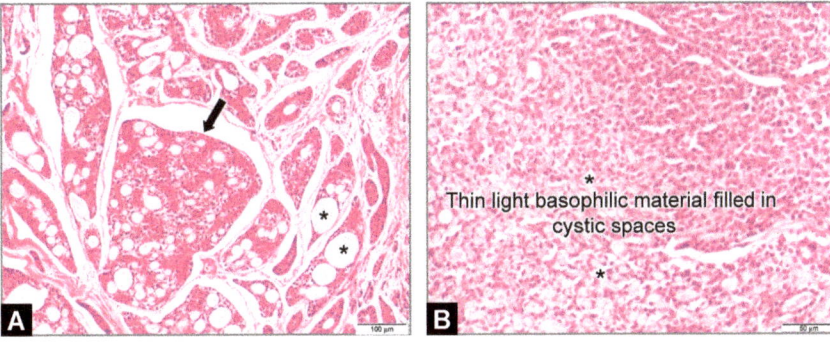

Figs. 10.6A and B: Adenoid cystic carcinoma: (A) Tumor cells are arranged in cribriform pattern (arrow) which means complex tubular pattern with intermittent cystic spaces filled with thin basophilic material (asterisk) (B).

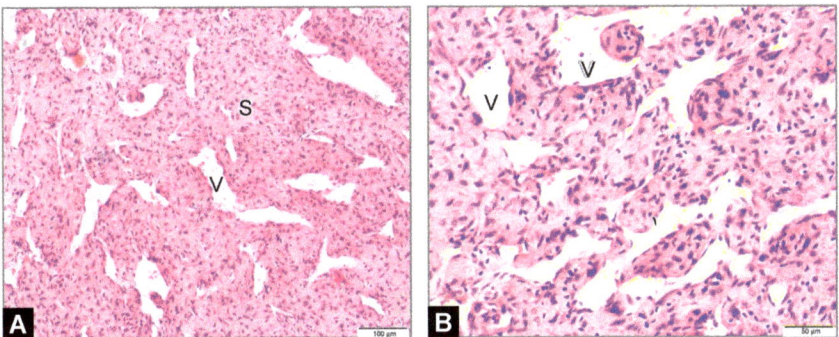

Figs. 10.7A and B: Nasopharyngeal angiofibroma shows an admixture of stellate shaped blood vessels (V) of varying thickness and fibrous to cellular stroma (S).

MALIGNANT NEOPLASTIC LESIONS

Carcinomas

Keratinizing Squamous Cell Carcinoma and Non-keratinizing Squamous Cell Carcinoma (Figs. 10.8 and 10.9)

- These tumors arise from the surface epithelium lining the nasal cavity and paranasal sinuses. In 30–50% cases of non-keratinizing squamous cell carcinoma (NKSCC), high risk HPV association is seen.
- The newly recognized HPV related carcinoma with adenoid cystic-like features shows surface dysplasia and underlying carcinoma with morphology similar to high grade adenoid cystic carcinomas. High risk HPV association is seen.[2,3]

Sarcomatoid (Spindle Cell) Squamous Cell Carcinoma

Variant of squamous cell carcinoma with predominant spindle cell morphology.

Lymphoepithelial carcinoma:
- More than 90% cases harbor Epstein-Barr virus (EBV)
- Mostly seen in Asian countries where EBV is endemic.

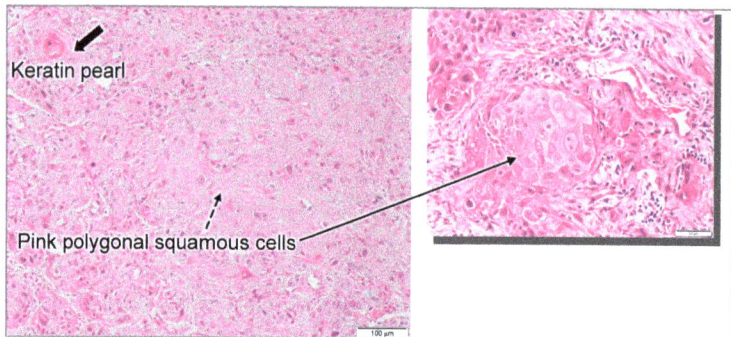

Fig. 10.8: Keratinizing squamous cell carcinoma: infiltrating islands of malignant squamous cells (dashed arrow and inset) with keratin pearls (thick arrow).

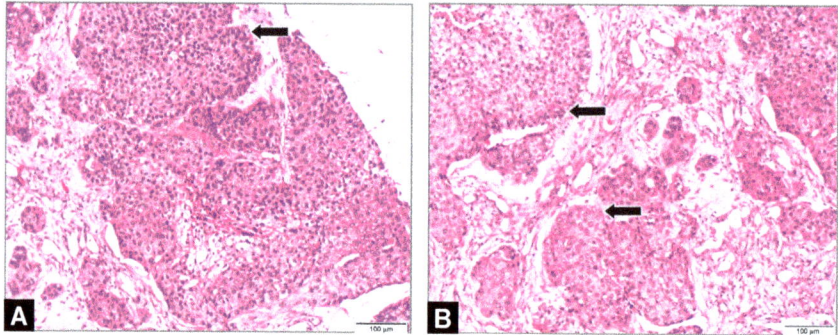

Figs. 10.9A and B: Non-keratinizing squamous cell carcinoma: infiltrating islands of malignant squamous cells (arrows) without intra- or extracellular keratin.

Sinonasal undifferentiated carcinoma (SNUC): No squamous/glandular differentiation
- No viral (EBV/HPV) association

NUT Midline carcinoma:
- Poorly differentiated carcinoma with squamous differentiation.[4]
- Definite diagnosis is made by detection of NUT gene rearrangement t(15;19) by either fluorescence in situ hybridization (FISH) or immunohistochemistry (IHC) (Figs. 10.10A and B).
- No viral association.
- Very poor prognosis.

SMARCB1 (INI1)-deficient Sinonasal Carcinoma

- *SMARCB1 gene is known as* SWI/SNF related, matrix associated, actin-dependent regulator of chromatin, subfamily B, member 1.
- Inactivation of tumor suppressor gene INI1 has been implicated in the pathogenesis of this tumor. Only few cases are available in the literature. It remains unclear if it represents a distinct tumor entity.
- Diagnosis is confirmed by INI1 loss on IHC or *in-situ* hybridization.

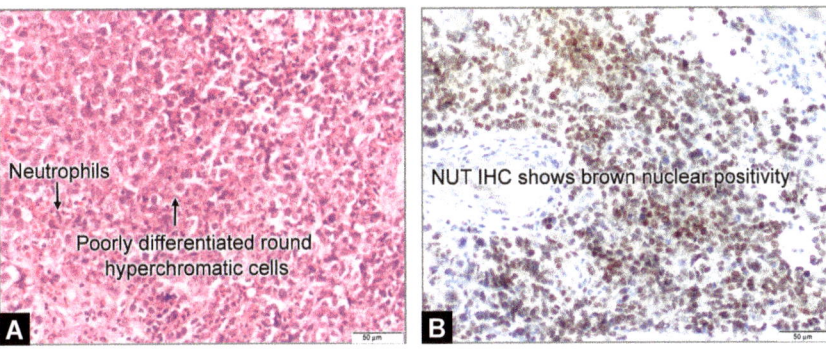

Figs. 10.10A and B: A case of **NUT midline carcinoma** shows poorly differentiated tumor cells admixed with neutrophils. Tumor cells are positive for NUT immunohistochemistry (IHC).

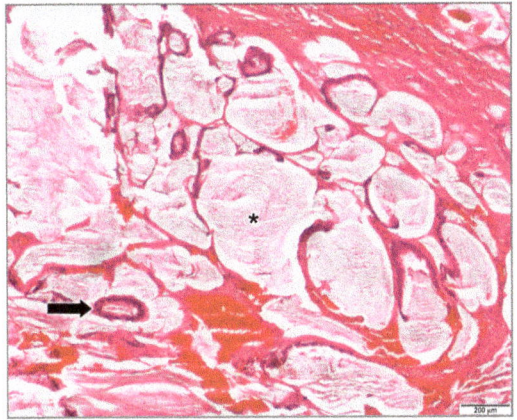

Fig. 10.11: Intestinal adenocarcinoma: malignant glands (arrow) floating in large areas or pools of mucin (asterisk).

Intestinal and Non-intestinal Type Adenocarcinomas (Figs. 10.11 and 10.12)

Intestinal adenocarcinomas are morphologically similar to intestinal tumors (Fig. 10.11) whereas non-intestinal types do not show intestinal phenotypes (Fig. 10.12).

MALIGNANT SOFT TISSUE TUMORS

Biphenotypic Sinonasal Sarcoma

Malignant low-grade spindle cell sarcoma with neural (S100 IHC positive) and myogenic (smooth muscle actin IHC positive) differentiation.

Sinonasal Glomangiopericytoma

- A tumor of perivascular myoid cells.
- Microscopically a patternless architecture with dilated blood vessels (Fig. 10.13).

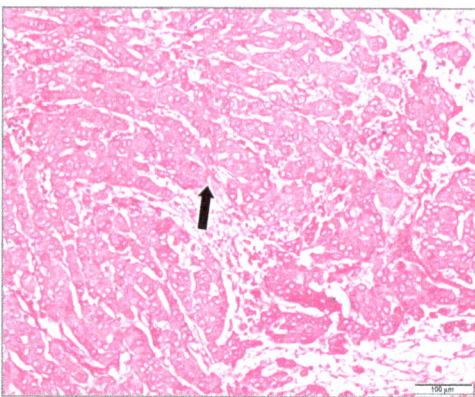

Fig. 10.12: Non-intestinal adenocarcinoma: infiltrating cords and glands of tumor (arrow). The tumor cells show abundant cytoplasm and low-grade nuclei.

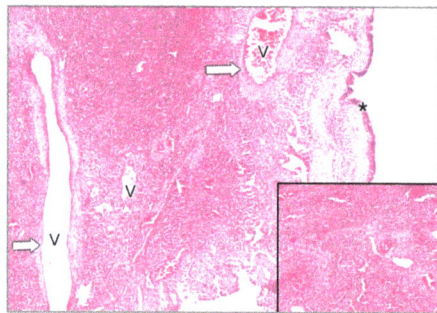

Fig. 10.13: Glomangiopericytoma: a tumor beneath normal respiratory lining epithelium (asterisk). Tumor is composed of large gaping vessels (arrows). Tumor cells are spindle to oval with mild nuclear atypia (Inset).

- Immunohistochemically positive for smooth muscle actin, beta-catenin and cyclin D1.

TERATOCARCINOSARCOMA

Combination of teratoma and admixture of epithelial, mesenchymal and neuroepithelial elements.

HEMATOLYMPHOID TUMORS

- Nearly all hematolymphoid tumors in sinonasal region are non-Hodgkin's lymphomas (NHL) and extramedullary plasmacytomas.
- Sinonasal lymphomas are third most common malignancy after squamous cell carcinoma and adenocarcinoma. Among NHL, extranodal NK/T cell lymphomas (ENKTL) and diffuse large B cell lymphomas are two most common types in nasal cavity and paranasal sinuses.
- ENKTL commonly occurs in East Asians and has a strong association with EBV.

- Histologically, these show angioinvasive growth pattern lead on to geographic areas of necrosis (Fig. 10.14).
- Immunohistochemistry shows positivity for CD3, granzyme, perforin, and CD56.

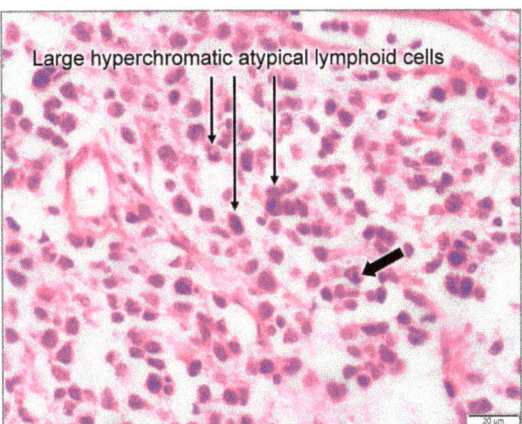

Fig. 10.14: NK-T cell lymphoma: non-Hodgkin's lymphoma shows atypical large lymphoid cells (thin arrows) with high apoptosis (thick arrow).

OLFACTORY NEUROBLASTOMA

- Malignant neuroectodermal tumor with neuroblastic differentiation localized in the superior nasal cavity confined to cribriform plate.
- Histologically low- and high-grade based on tumor architecture, mitotic activity, nuclear pleomorphism, presence of fibrillary matrix, rosettes, and necrosis (Fig. 10.15).
- Immunohistochemistry positive for neuroendocrine markers.
  An algorithmic approach to the malignant sinonasal tumors on IHC is detailed in Flowchart 10.1.

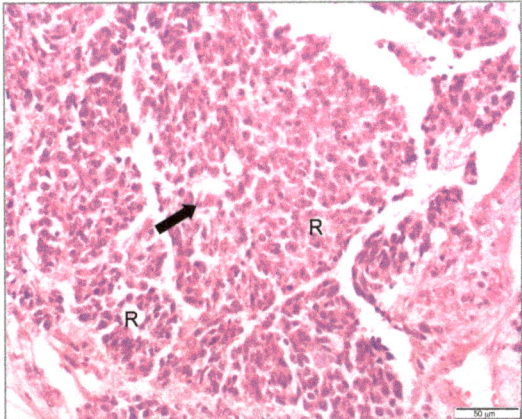

Fig. 10.15: Olfactory neuroblastoma: photomicrograph shows malignant round blue cell tumor with rosettes (R and arrow). The cells are small to intermediate in size, have high nuclear cytoplasmic ratio and hyperchromatic nuclei.

148 Section 3 Tumor and Tumor-like Conditions

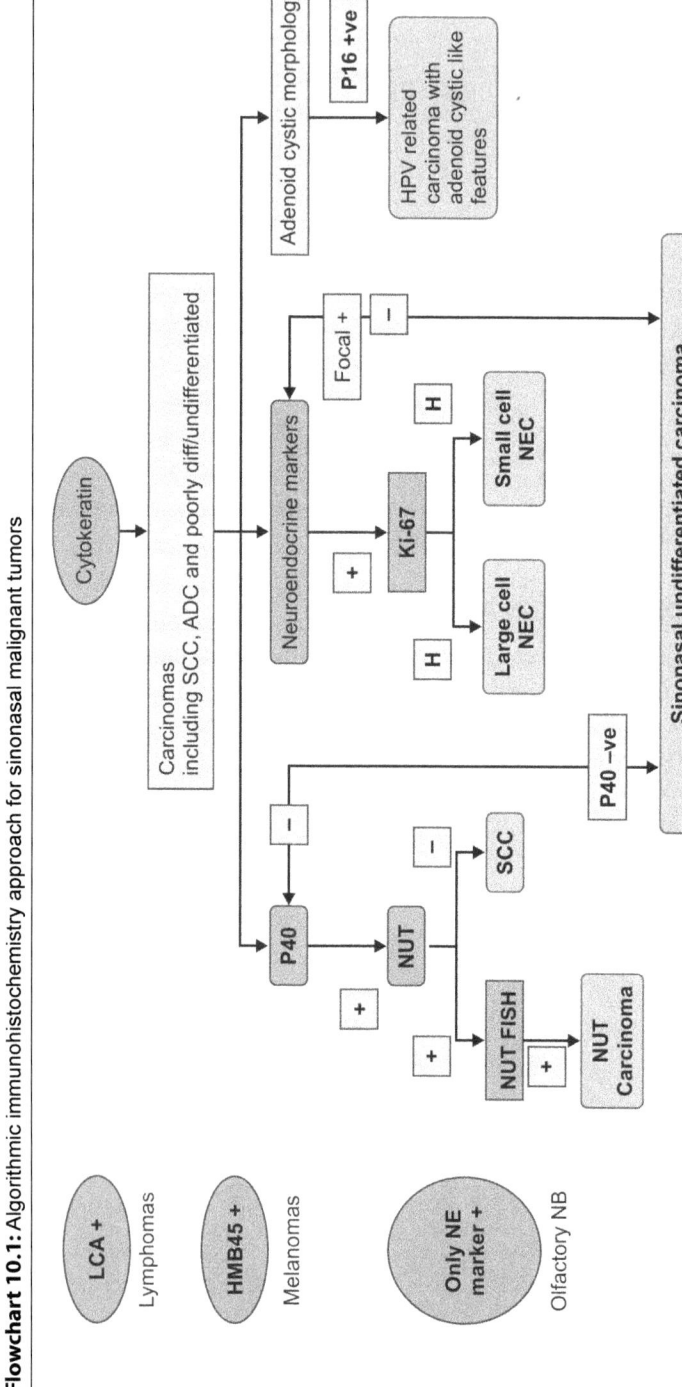

Flowchart 10.1: Algorithmic immunohistochemistry approach for sinonasal malignant tumors

(ADC: Adenocarcinoma; H: High; HPV: Human papilloma virus; NEC: Neuroendocrine carcinoma; NB: Neuroblastoma; SCC: Squamous cell carcinoma).

REFERENCES

1. Slootweg PJ, Chan JKC, Stelow EB, et al. Tumors of the nasal cavity, paranasal sinuses and skull base. In: El-Naggar AK, Chan JKC, Grandis JR, Takata T, Slootweg PJ (Eds). WHO Classification of Head and Neck Tumors, fourth edition. IARC Lyon; 2017. pp. 14-61.
2. Stelow EB, Bishop JA. Update from the 4th Edition of the World Health Organization Classification of Head and Neck Tumours: Tumors of the Nasal Cavity, Paranasal Sinuses and Skull Base. Head Neck Pathol. 2017;1:3-15.
3. Bishop JA, Guo TW, Smith DF, et al. Human papillomavirus-related carcinomas of thesinonasal tract. Am J Surg Pathol. 2013;37:185-92.
4. Bishop JA, Westra WH. NUT midline carcinomas of the sinonasal tract. Am J Surg Pathol. 2012;36:1216-21.

11
CHAPTER

Pathology of Bony/Cartilaginous Sinonasal Tumors

Asit R Mridha, Adarsh W Barwad

- Introduction
- Benign Tumors/Tumor-Like Conditions
  - Central Giant Cell Granuloma
  - Osteoma
  - Ossifying Fibroma
  - Fibrous Dysplasia
- Histopathologic Patterns on Biopsy
  - Aneurysmal Bone Cyst
- Malignant Tumors
  - Chondrosarcoma
  - Plasmacytoma

INTRODUCTION

- World Health Organization (WHO) classification of sinonasal tumors have been discussed in detail in Chapter 11.
- Common benign and malignant bony/cartilaginous tumors will be discussed here (Table 11.1).

Table 11.1: Common osseous/cartilaginous sinonasal tumors.	
Benign tumor/tumor-like lesions	*Malignant*
Central giant cell granuloma	Chondrosarcoma
Chondroma	Plasmacytoma
Osteoma	Osteosarcoma
Ossifying fibroma	Chordoma
Fibrous dysplasia	
Chondroblastoma	
Chondromyxoid fibroma	
Osteochondroma	
Osteoid osteoma	
Osteoblastoma	
Ameloblastoma	
Aneurysmal bone cyst	

BENIGN TUMORS/TUMOR-LIKE CONDITIONS

Central Giant Cell Granuloma (Fig. 11.1)

- Central giant cell granulomas (CGCGs) are intraosseous nonproliferative lesions with obscure etiology and occur almost exclusively in the mandible and maxilla. CGCG is also known as reparative giant cell granuloma.
- There are lot of morphological similarities between giant cell tumor and CGCL and the distinction between jaw bone and extragnathic lesions is difficult on histomorphology. Only comparison between the two is the more number of nuclei present in the giant cells in giant-cell tumor (GCT) of bone. Some authors consider that the GCT and CGCG represent different spectra of same lesion.
- Microscopically, CGCL is characterized by dense proliferation of oval and spindle-shaped mesenchymal cells, a varying number of multinucleated giant cells in small aggregates and dispersed in the fibrous stroma.
- Giant cells are often present in a perivascular location or adjacent areas of hemorrhage and usually contain 4-20 nuclei. These are often small and irregular with few nuclei or large and round containing more nuclei.
- The lesion can also show round macrophages, deposition of hemosiderin, extravasated erythrocytes, foci of osteoid matrix, bony trabeculae and dystrophic calcification.
- The mesenchymal and multinucleated giant cells are strongly immunoreactive to anti-CD68 antibody, which suggesting that they belong to the macrophage lineage.
- An expression of osteoclastogenic nuclear factor of activated T cells (NFATc1) has been seen in giant cells from CGCL, cherubism and brown tumor of hyperparathyroidism.

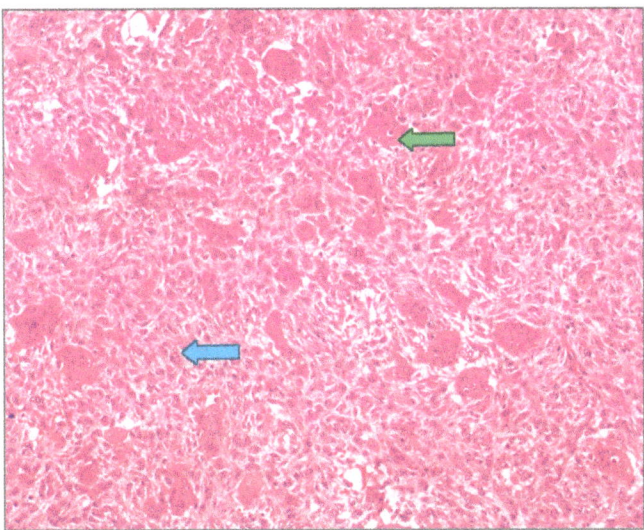

Fig. 11.1: Central giant cell granuloma (CGCG): Histology showing dense proliferation of oval and spindle-shaped mesenchymal cells (blue arrow) along with osteoclastic multinucleated giant cells (green arrow).

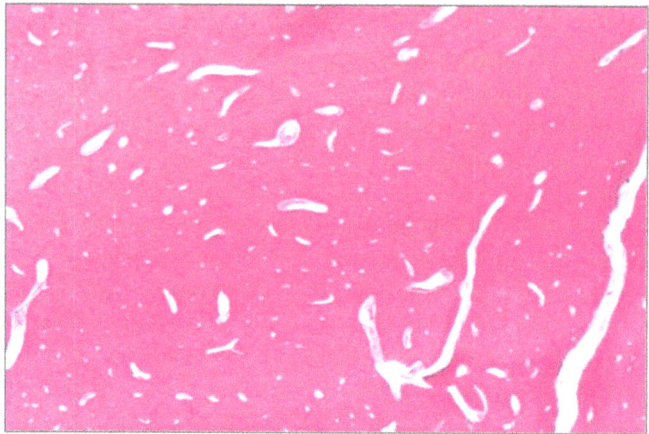

Fig. 11.2: Osteoma: Histological photomicrograph showing dense, compact bone and broad trabeculae of mature bone.

Osteoma (Fig. 11.2)

- Osteoma is characterized by compact cortical bone with scanty intervening fibrovascular stroma. In some cases, there is a peripheral rim of dense sclerotic lamellar bone surrounding trabeculae of lamellar or occasionally woven bone.
- It is usually classified into three histologic types according to bone formation: (1) eburneous type (hard laminated), (2) cancellous type (spongy), and (3) mixed type (combining features of the eburneous and cancellous type).
- Ivory type lesions contain compact, usually lamellar bone, with scant or no intertrabecular spaces.
- In the cancellous type, the ratio of bone volume to intertrabecular space decreases and the morphology becomes similar to normal trabecular bone tissue.
- No significant practical differences are found between these forms of morphology when diagnostic techniques, treatment and prognosis are considered.

Ossifying Fibroma

Depending on the pattern of mineralization, four entities have been described: (1) Juvenile psammomatous ossifying fibroma (JPOF), (2) Juvenile trabecular ossifying fibroma (JTOF), (3) Gigantiform cementoma (GC), and (4) Cemento-ossifying fibroma (COF) and ossifying fibroma-not otherwise specified (NOS).

Histopathologic Patterns on Biopsy

Ossifying fibroma NOS—shows three histologic or a mixture of these patterns (Table 11.2; Figs. 11.3 and 11.4).

Chapter 11 Pathology of Bony/Cartilaginous Sinonasal Tumors

Table 11.2: Ossifying fibroma not otherwise specified (NOS).

Ossifying form (most common) (Fig. 11.3)	Cementifying form (Fig. 11.4)	Storiform form
• Small irregular osteoid trabeculae typically rimmed by osteoblasts (similar to fibrous dysplasia) • Hypercellular stromal element • Fbroblastic cells devoid of any atypical cytologic features • Mature lesions: osteoblastic rimming is minimal, lamellar irregular trabeculae	• Osseous trabeculae and cemental structures (ovoid or droplet in shape) • Resemble normal cementicles present in periodontal ligament • Ovoid lesions are often referred to as cementifying fibromas • Those with both osseous and cementoid calcifications are labeled as cemento-ossifying fibromas	• Streaming of the fibroblastic stromal elements in a pinwheel configuration similar to benign fibrous histiocytoma • Mimics dystrophic bone

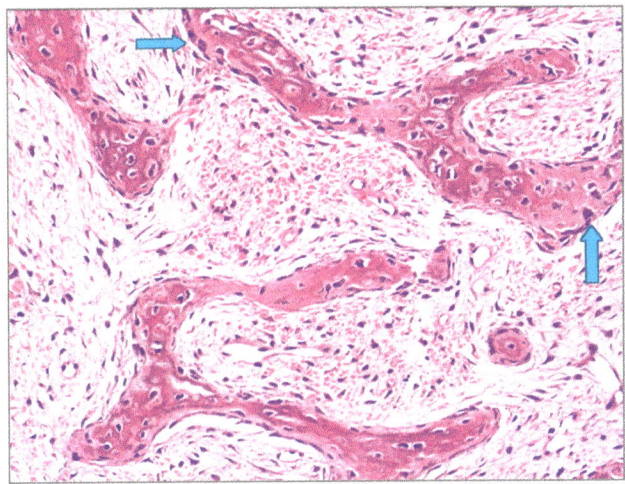

Fig. 11.3: Ossifying form of ossifying fibroma (OF): Small irregular osteoid trabeculae that are typically rimmed by osteoblasts (arrows) and are suspended in mildly cellular stroma.

Juvenile ossifying fibromas: Two distinct clinic-pathologic entities are known:

Trabecular juvenile ossifying fibroma:
- Cell-rich fibrous stroma containing bundles of cellular osteoid and bone trabeculae without osteoblastic rimming, and aggregates of giant cells.
- Stromal cells are spindle or polyhedral and produce little collagen and the fibrillary osteoid matrix gives the tumor a characteristic loose structure.
- Cellular, immature osteoid, with plump eosinophilic osteoblastic cells, forms strands that may be long and slender or plump (paint brush strokes).

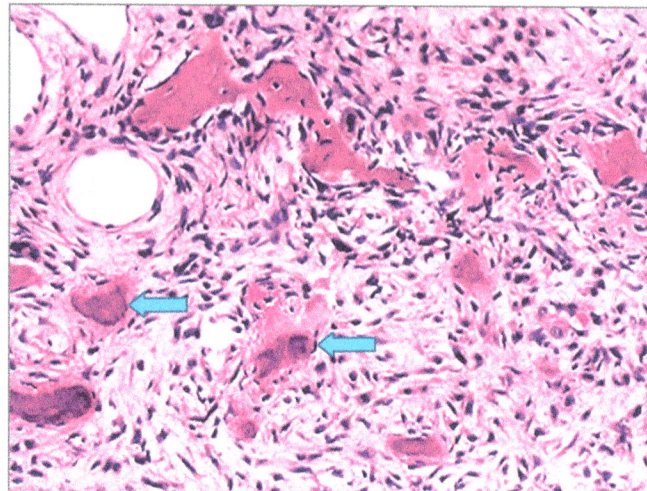

Fig. 11.4: Cementifying form of ossifying fibroma (OF): Typical osseous trabeculae in addition to the cemental structures (arrows).

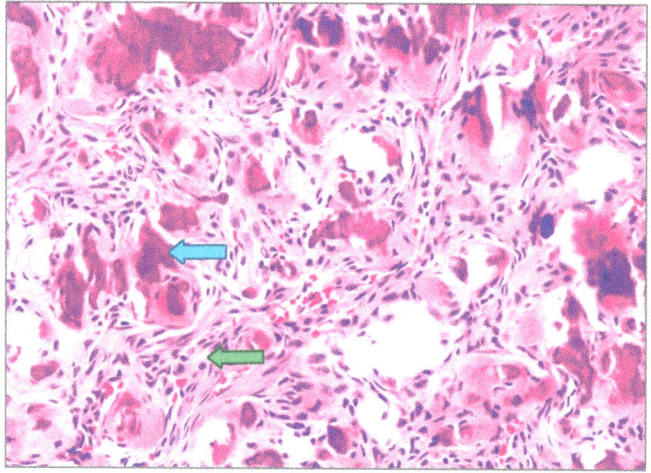

Fig. 11.5: Juvenile psammomatoid ossifying fibroma (OF): Multiple small acellular calcified structures—psammomatoid bodies (blue arrow); suspended in cellular stroma (green arrow), composed of uniform, stellate, and spindle-shaped cells.

- Irregular mineralization takes place at the center of the osteoid strands, and progressive calcification results in anastomosing trabeculae of immature woven bone.

Juvenile psammomatoid ossifying fibroma:
- Multiple small acellular calcified structures, round and uniform and with concentric lamellar calcification, called ossicles/psammomatoid bodies—homogenously distributed (Fig. 11.5).
- Relatively cellular stroma that may have whorled appearance, composed of uniform, stellate, and spindle-shaped cells.

Fibrous Dysplasia (Fig. 11.6)

- Fibrous dysplasia is a benign intramedullary fibro-osseous lesion originally described by Lichtenstein in 1938 and by Lichtenstein and Jaffe in 1942.
- Fibrous dysplasia can present in one bone (monostotic) or multiple bones (polyostotic) and can be associated with other conditions.
- The lesions of fibrous dysplasia develop during skeletal formation and growth and have a variable natural evolution.
- The etiology has been linked with a mutation in the Gs α gene that occurs after fertilization in somatic cells and is located at chromosome 20q13.2-13.3.
- Gs α mutation was first identified in patients with McCune-Albright syndrome, a rare disorder that combines polyostotic fibrous dysplasia, skin pigmentation, and one of several endocrinopathies.
- Biopsy from the lesion is mandatory for confirmation of diagnosis.

Histologic Features

Gross examination
- A yellowish white tissue with a distinctive gritty feel, imparted by the small trabeculae of bone.
- Can be cut with a scalpel and may bleed briskly when cut, as a result of its concentration of small vessels.

Histologic Features

- Key histologic feature—delicate trabeculae of immature bone, with no osteoblastic rimming, enmeshed within a bland fibrous stroma

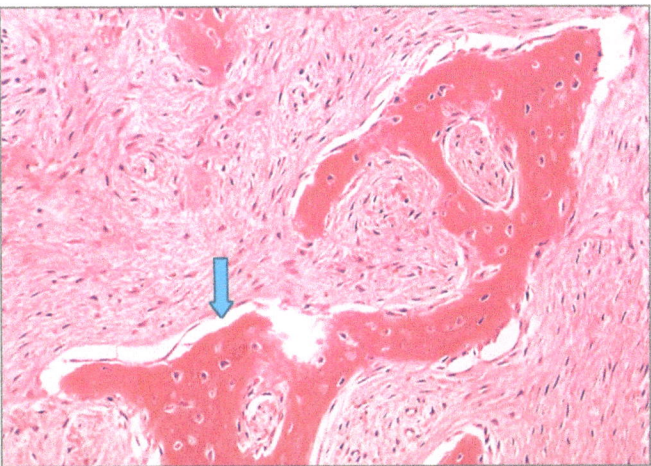

Fig. 11.6: Fibrous dysplasia: High power view showing irregular bony trabeculae lacking osteoblastic rimming (arrow) and are suspended in mildly cellular stromal mesenchyme.

of dysplastic spindle-shaped cells without any cellular features of malignancy.
- Margins of the lesion to be separated from surrounding bone by a thin shell of mature lamellar reactive bone.
- Variable number of immature, non-stress oriented, disconnected dysplastic trabeculae floating in a sea of immature mesenchymal cells that have little or no collagen—"alphabet soup."
- Characteristic absence of plump osteoblasts rimming the isolated immature trabeculae.
- Bland fibrous stroma of monomorphic spindle-shaped cells without any cellular features of malignancy.
- Multiple delicate capillaries are found throughout the lesion.
- Lobules of cartilage are infrequently seen composed of mature hyaline cartilage.

Aneurysmal Bone Cyst

- The morphologic characteristics of aneurysmal bone cyst (ABC) include the most conspicuous pattern of presence of cavernous spaces separated by fibrous tissue walls which contains osteoclastic giant cells, and strands of bone.
- Solid ABC has been mentioned as giant cell reparative granuloma in extragnathic location by some authors.

Histopathology (Fig. 11.7)

- *Microscopically* it shows cavernous spaces with fibrous walls which contain scattered or small aggregates of osteoclastic giant cells, and strands of woven or mature bone.

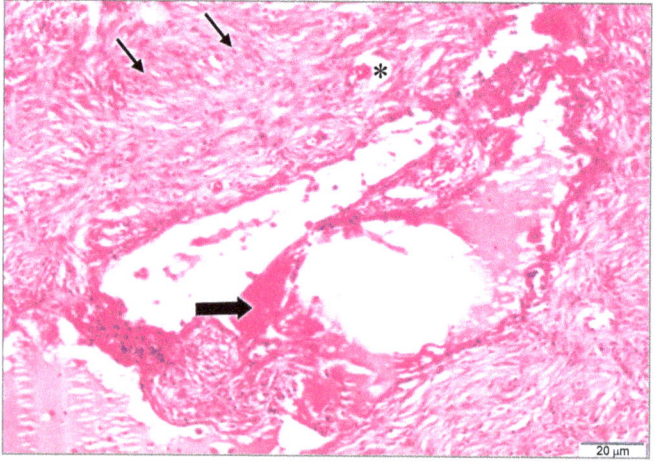

Fig. 11.7: Aneurysmal bone cyst: Histological photomicrograph showing blood-filled cavernous spaces (asterisk) with fibrous septae (thin arrows) and a fibrous osteoblastic solid component (thick arrow) with giant cell.

- Spindle fibroblastic/fibrohistiocytic cells.
- Calcifying fibromyxoid foci, if present represent one of characteristic features.
- Mitosis usually present and may be high, but atypical mitosis is never seen.

MALIGNANT TUMORS

Chondrosarcoma (Fig. 11.8)

- Chondrosarcoma of the head and neck region is a rare disease, representing approximately 0.1% of all head and neck neoplasms and constituting only 4% of nonepithelial tumors of the nasal cavity, paranasal sinuses and nasopharynx.

Histological Features

- Chondrosarcomas show various histological patterns ranging from benign chondroid tumor to undifferentiated neoplasm, which make them difficult to diagnose pathologically.
- Histologic examination reveals lobules of hyaline cartilage with variable degrees of cellularity, myxoid change, and calcification. The chondrocytes usually have enlarged hyperchromatic nuclei with binucleation. Necrosis and mitoses are mostly seen in high-grade lesions.
- Evans et al.[5] classified chondrosarcomas into three grades, from grade I to grade III, according to cellular density, nuclear differentiation, and the size of nucleus.

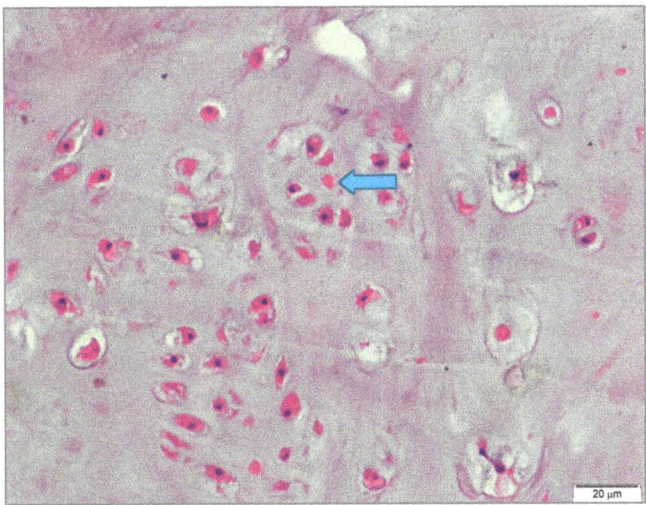

Fig. 11.8: Well-differentiated chondrosarcoma: Photomicrograph showing lobulated appearance of hyaline cartilage and mild increase in cellularity (arrow).

Immunohistochemical characteristics of common bony/cartilaginous tumors are listed in Table 11.3.

Tumor	Immunohistochemistry
Table 11.3: Immunohistochemical characteristics of common bony/cartilaginous tumors.	
Central giant cell granulomas (CGCG)	Immunoreactive to anti-CD68 antibody
Chondrosarcoma	S 100 IDH1 (isocitrate dehydrogenase)
Plasmacytoma	Immunopositive for CD138, CD38 and vs38c. Variable immunoreactivity is seen with CD45 and CD79a

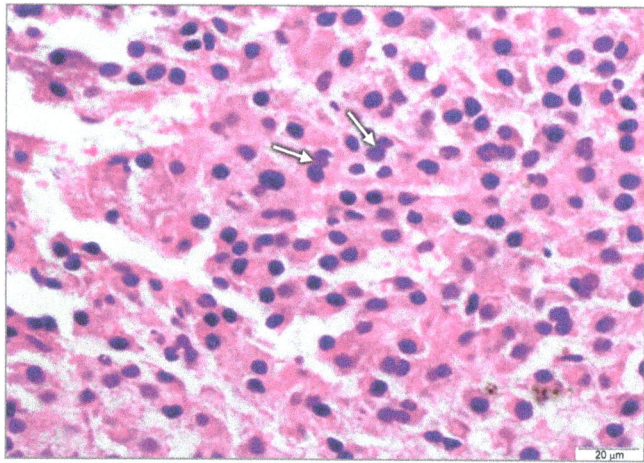

Fig. 11.9: Plasmacytoma: Histological (H&E) section showing sheets of plasma cells (arrows) including few binucleated one in cases of plasmacytoma of nasal bone.

Plasmacytoma (Fig. 11.9)

- Plasma cell neoplasms include multiple myeloma, medullary (solitary plasmacytoma of the bone) and the extramedullary plasmacytoma.
- It accounts for less than 1% of head and neck tumors. In nasal cavity, however, plasmacytoma represents approximately 4% of tumors. About 80–90% of extramedullary plasmacytomas involve the mucosa-associated lymphoid tissue (MALT) of the upper airways, and 75% of these affect the nasal and paranasal regions.

Histopathology

- There is neoplastic proliferation of plasma cells frequently in large nodules or sheets. Binucleated and immature forms are often admixed among mature plasma cells.

- Plasma cells contain abundant rough endoplasmic reticulum which stains red with methyl green-pyronin (MGP). There is usually cytoplasmic accumulation of immunoglobulin, which forms spherical cytoplasmic inclusions that are either clearly within the cytoplasm (Russell bodies) or are overlying the nucleus or invaginated into it (Dutcher body). These inclusions are positive with Periodic acid-Schiff (PAS) reaction and diastase-resistant. Amyloid deposition may be present, which is stained by Congo red and under polarized light it has a characteristic "apple-green" birefringence.

Differential Diagnosis

- The differential diagnoses include reactive plasma cell lesions such as plasma cell granuloma, granulomatous inflammation, rhinoscleroma, and lymphoma.

BIBLIOGRAPHY

1. El-Mofty S. Psammomatoid and trabecular juvenile ossifying fibroma of the craniofacial skeleton: two distinct clinicopathologic entities. Oral Surg Oral Med Oral Pathol Oral Radiol Endod. 2002;93:296-304.
2. Evans HL, Ayala AG, Romsdahl MM. Prognostic factors in chondrosarcoma of bone. A clinicopathologic analysis with emphasis on histologic grading. Cancer. 1977;40(2):818-31.
3. Eversole R, Su L, ElMofty S. Benign fibro-osseous lesions of the craniofacial complex a review. Head Neck Pathol. 2008;2:177-202.
4. MacDonald-Jankowski DS. Ossifying fibroma: a systematic review. Dentomaxillofac Radiol. 2009;38:495-513.
5. Soyele OO, Braimah RO, Taiwo AO, et al. Fibrous dysplasia of the maxillofacial region, a review of 134 cases at Lagos University Teaching Hospital, Lagos, Nigeria; 2017.

12 CHAPTER

Benign Tumors of the Nose and Paranasal Sinuses: Imaging

Smita Manchanda, Ashu Seith Bhalla

- Introduction
- Benign Epithelial Tumors
  - Sinonasal Papillomas
    - Inverted Papilloma
    - Fungiform Papilloma
    - Oncocytic Papilloma
  - Salivary Gland Type Adenomas
    - Pleomorphic Adenoma
- Borderline/Low Malignant Potential Soft Tissue Tumors
  - Inflammatory Myofibroblastic Tumor
  - Glomangiopericytoma
- Benign Soft Tissue Tumors
  - Hemangioma
  - Peripheral Nerve Sheath Tumors
    - Schwannoma
    - Neurofibromas
- Benign Tumors of Bone and Cartilage
  - Giant Cell Lesions
    - Giant Cell Reparative Granuloma
    - Giant Cell Tumor
    - Aneurysmal Bone Cyst (ABC)
  - Osteoma
  - Osteoblastoma
- Benign Germ Cell Tumors
  - Mature Teratoma
- Miscellaneous Entities
  - Juvenile Nasopharyngeal Agiofibroma (JNA)
  - Hemophilic Pseudotumor
  - Fibro-osseous Lesions
  - Fibrous Dysplasia (FD)
  - Ossifying Fibroma

INTRODUCTION

- Amongst the head and neck tumors, sinonasal (SN) tumors are relatively rare.
- Malignant lesions are encountered more frequently than the benign entities.
- Besides sinonasal masses may also originate in the cranium/skull base (*see* Chapter 23) or arise from the maxillary alveolus (*see* Chapter 24).
- The recent WHO classification of these tumors is detailed in Chapter 10. This classification divides the tumors into broad categories of epithelial tumors, soft tissue tumors, tumors of bone and cartilage, germ cell tumors, hematolymphoid tumors, neuroectodermal tumors and secondary tumors. These are further subdivided into benign and malignant in the

first four groups. The hematolymphoid tumors, neuroectodermal tumors and secondary tumors include only malignant lesions.
- SN tumors need to be differentiated from other masses like inflammatory/infective lesions, such as polyps and mycetoma.

BENIGN EPITHELIAL TUMORS

Sinonasal Papillomas

- Papillomas arise from the Schneiderian mucosa of the sinonasal tract (which is of ectodermal origin).
- Papillomas are of three types: Inverted, Fungiform or Oncocytic.
- These are uncommon lesions comprising about 0.4 to 4.7 percent of all SN tumors[1] Inverted papilloma and fungiform forms comprise the majority (about 50% each) and the oncocytic form is rare.

Inverted Papilloma (IP)

- Synonym: Inverting papilloma.
- Occurs more frequently in middle aged men (40–70 years).
- IP characteristically originates from the lateral wall of the nasal cavity near the maxillary ostium and also extends into the maxillary sinus. Other sites of origin include the other paranasal sinuses.
- IP can also show malignant transformation (synchronous or metachronous).
- Numerous staging systems are used, *Krouse system* being most commonly followed. Four stages[2] are described in it:
  - Stage 1: Confined to nasal cavity.
  - Stage 2: Ethmoid sinuses, maxillary sinus (medial and superior region involved).
  - Stage 3: All paranasal sinuses but confined to nose/sinuses.
  - Stage 4: Not confined to sinuses/malignant.
- Tumor has high recurrence rates of 4 to 22%.[3]
- Imaging Findings:
  - Variable size from small polypoidal lesions to large expansile masses.
  - Larger lesions expand the nasal cavity with thinning and remodeling of the bony walls.
  - CT (Figs. 12.1A to D):
    - Soft tissue attenuation lesions.
    - *A focal area of hyperostosis at the site of origin is characteristic.*
    - Resection of this involved area is critical to reduce recurrence rates.
    - Bony fragments may be seen within the soft tissue mass. The calcific foci are thought to represent "entrapped bone" and true tumoral calcification is in fact uncommon.
    - Calcific foci are seen in up to 40% tumors.[4]
    - The convoluted cerebriform pattern of enhancement characteristically described on MRI may occasionally be seen on CT.

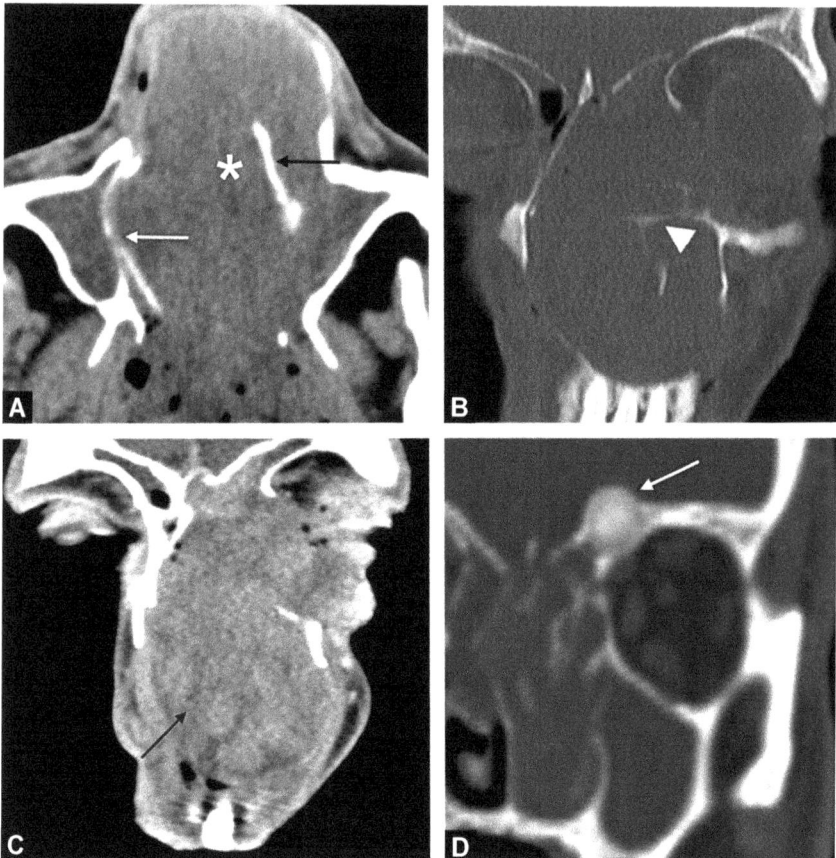

Figs. 12.1A to D: Inverted papilloma (CT).
- Large expansile soft tissue density lesion (on NCCT) left nasal cavity (asterisk in A) and sclerosis along lateral nasal wall (black arrow in A)
- Nasal septum deviated to right (arrow in A)
- Thinning and remodeling of the bony walls with bone erosion (arrowhead in B)
- Characteristic "convoluted cerebriform" pattern of enhancement (black arrow in C)
- Focal hyperostosis (arrow in D) in another case of IP.

- MRI (Figs. 12.2A to C):
  ▶ A typical "cerebriform" appearance is seen on the T_2 weighted images and postcontrast T_1 weighted images. It is also referred to as a convoluted pattern and may be diffuse or partial.[1]
- Malignant transformation is suspected in IP, if there is bone erosion/destruction with extension outside the sinonasal cavity. Presence of necrosis and the partial form of cerebriform pattern should also alert to possibility of malignant change.

Fungiform Papilloma

- Seen at a younger age than IP (20–50 years). Also more frequent in males.
- Site of origin is the nasal septum.

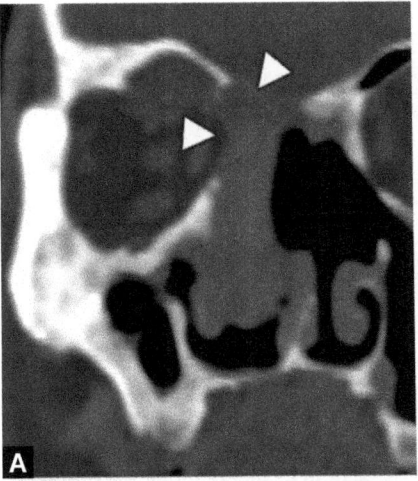
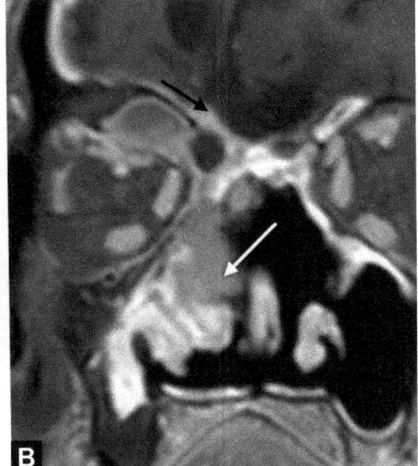
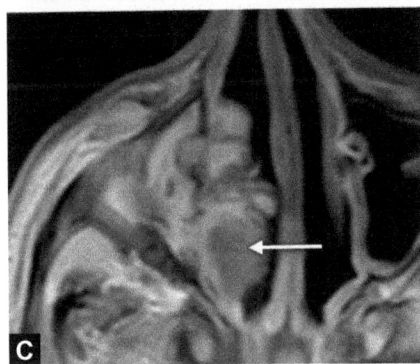

Figs. 12.2A to C: Recurrent inverted papilloma (post open surgical reduction). (A) NCCT: Soft tissue density mass along lateral nasal wall with erosion of cribriform plate and lamina papyracea (arrowheads) (B) Post gad T1WI: Cerebriform pattern of enhancement (white arrow). Intracranial extension in the form of dural enhancement right basifrontal lobe (black arrow). Gliotic changes also seen. (C) T2WI: T2 intermediate signal intensity mass with convoluted appearance (white arrow).

- This form of papilloma has no malignant potential.
- Imaging findings are nonspecific of an expansile nasal mass.

Oncocytic Papilloma

- Rare form that occurs in middle aged men.
- It arises from the lateral nasal wall, and similar to IP has malignant potential.
- Imaging findings are of a polypoidal lesions similar to the other two forms.

Salivary Gland Type Adenomas

Pleomorphic Adenoma

- Benign salivary gland tumor, rarely seen in the nasal cavity.[1]
- Well-defined soft tissue mass (Figs. 12.3A to C).
- CT: Punctate calcification, if seen is characteristic.
- MRI: T_2 weighted images: Hyperintense with hypointense capsule. Heterogeneous contrast enhancement, free diffusion.

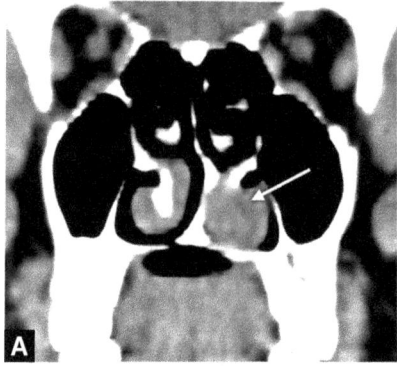
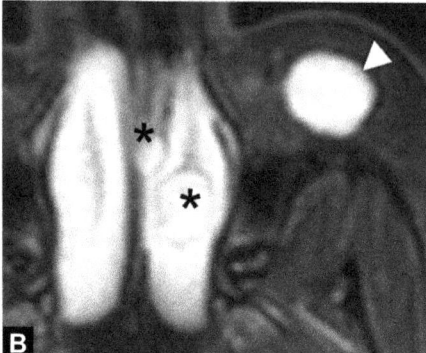
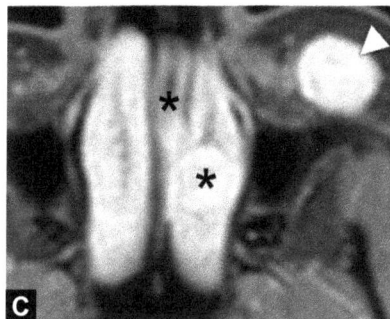

Figs. 12.3A to C: Pleomorphic adenoma. (A) NCCT. Well-defined soft tissue density mass in left inferior meatus (arrow). (B) Fat suppressed T2WI. Multiple, T2 hyperintense masses with hypointense rim; in inferior meatus (asterisks) and left premaxillary space (arrowhead). (C) Post gad T1WI. These lesions in the inferior meatus (asterisks) and left premaxillary space (arrowhead) are intensely enhancing.

BORDERLINE/ LOW MALIGNANT POTENTIAL SOFT TISSUE TUMORS

Inflammatory Myofibroblastic Tumor

- Inflammatory pseudotumor.
- Rare in head and neck region, with commonest site here being the orbit.
- Sinonasal—rare, reported in sphenoid.[5]
- Imaging findings (Figs. 12.4A and B) mimic a malignant lesion.
- CT: May appear hyperdense, bone erosion seen.
- MRI: T_1WI isointense to grey matter. T_2WI hypointense. Enhancement homogenous.

Glomangiopericytoma

- Synonym: Sinonasal-type hemangiopericytoma.[6]
- Rare tumor with perivascular myxoid phenotype.
- Clinical presentation: Nasal obstruction, recurrent epistaxis. Is a cause of oncogenic osteomalacia.
- CT: Noncalcified soft tissue density mass in nasal fossa or paranasal sinus with intense homogenous enhancement.
- MRI: T_1WI isointense; T_2WI hyperintense. Enhancement is homogenous.
- Somatostatin receptor expressing tumor on ^{68}Ga DOTANOC PET CT (Figs. 12.5A to C).

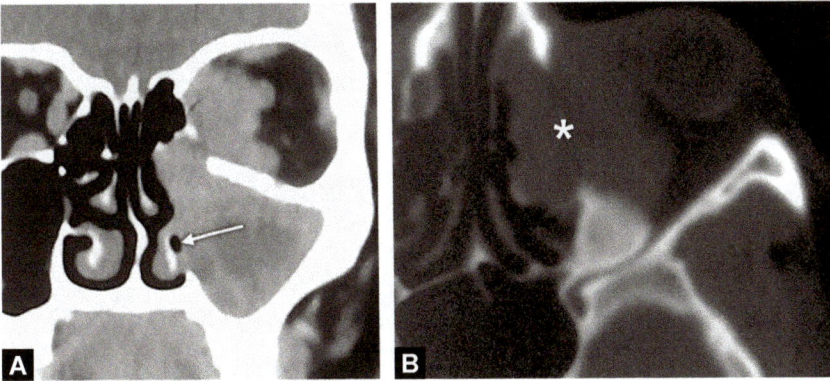

Figs. 12.4A and B: Inflammatory myofibroblastic tumor/inflammatory pseudotumor. NCCT.
- Heterogeneous, hyperdense mass in left maxillary and ethmoid sinuses, nasal cavity and orbit
- Erosion of lateral nasal wall (arrow) and lamina papyracea (asterisk).

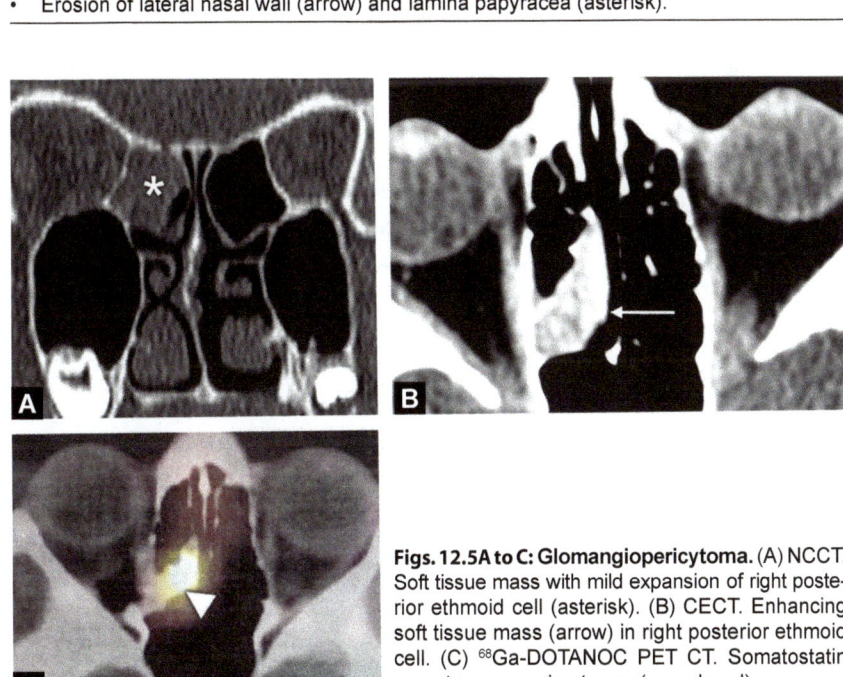

Figs. 12.5A to C: Glomangiopericytoma. (A) NCCT. Soft tissue mass with mild expansion of right posterior ethmoid cell (asterisk). (B) CECT. Enhancing soft tissue mass (arrow) in right posterior ethmoid cell. (C) ^{68}Ga-DOTANOC PET CT. Somatostatin receptor expressing tumor (arrowhead).

- Biopsy: Characteristic perivascular hyalinization, no or minimal atypia seen.

BENIGN SOFT TISSUE TUMORS

Hemangioma
- Benign vascular tumors. Unlike soft tissue hemangioma elsewhere in the head and neck region, SN hemangiomas are uncommon lesions.

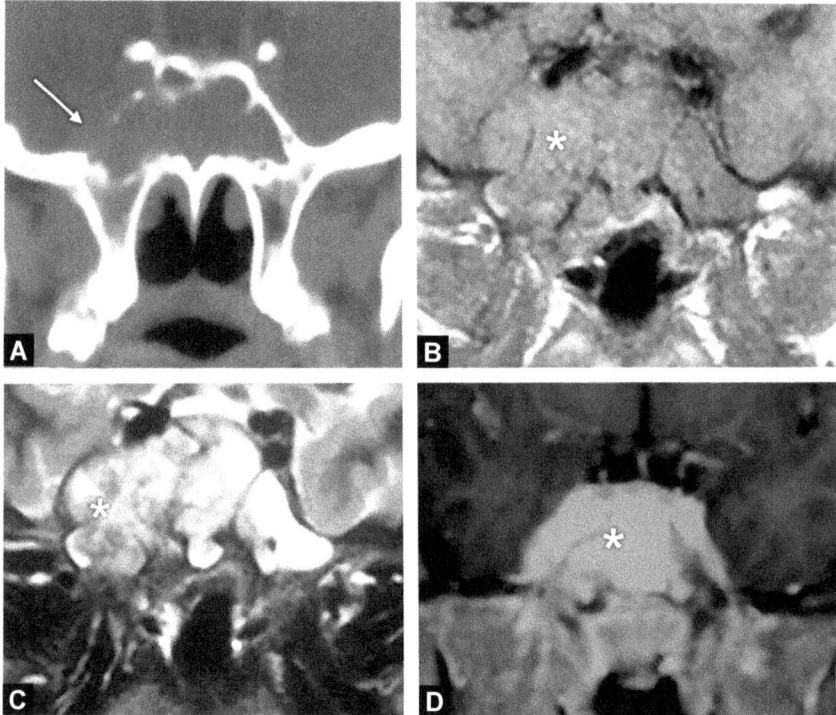

Figs. 12.6A to D: Hemangioma sphenoid sinus. (A) CECT (bone window). Large expansile lesion sphenoid sinus with focal bone erosion (arrow). (B) T1WI and (C) T2WI. Intermediate signal on T1WI and T2WI (asterisk in B and C). (D) Post gad T1WI. Intense postcontrast enhancement (asterisk).

- Most of these are in nasal cavity, and less frequently in sinuses.
- Seen in young patients.
- Imaging:
  - Expansile lesions with bone remodeling/focal erosions. Sclerosis may also be seen. However, lesions can be aggressive with significant bone destruction.[7]
  - Contrast enhancement can be variable—Intense or scattered nodular with gradual fill-in, depending on the amount of fibrosis/hemorrhage vs the vascular proliferation (Figs. 12.6A to D).
  - Calcification may be seen.
  - MRI is nonspecific. It appears hyperintense on T2WI and hypointense on T1WI.
  - Intraosseous hemangioma (Figs. 12.7A and B) reveal an expansile lesion (sun-burst appearance) which is of mixed density but well-defined. The nonossified component shows enhancement.

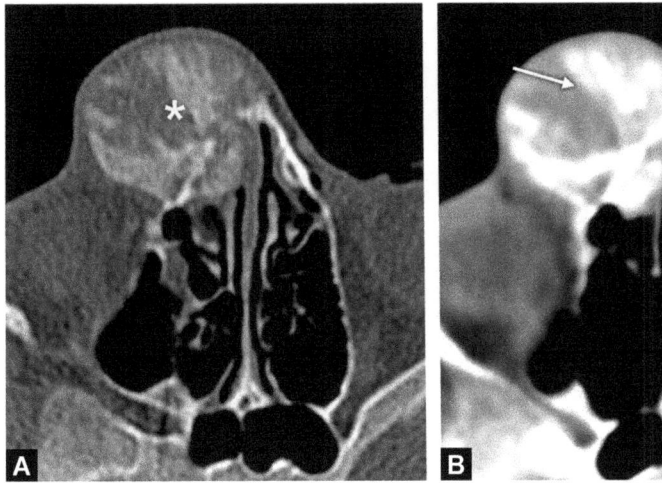

Figs. 12.7A and B: Nasal bone hemangioma. (A) NCCT. Expansile lytic sclerotic lesion of right nasal bone with sun-burst appearance (asterisk). (B) CECT. Heterogeneous contrast enhancement (arrow).

- Also *see* Chapter 20 for imaging features of hemangiomas in the pediatric age group.
- Differential Diagnosis:
  - Should be suspected in any young patient presenting with enhancing nasal cavity mass. However, in the sinuses the differential is more wide depending on the location, especially in those forms with more fibrous component or more with aggressive behavior.

Peripheral Nerve Sheath Tumors

- The benign tumors (Figs. 12.8A to C) include schwannomas (from the Schwann cells) and neurofibroma.[1]

Schwannoma

- Rare SN tumors; arise in relation to trigeminal nerve branches.
- Soft tissue masses which are often heterogeneous with areas of necrosis.
- Bone expansion and remodeling is seen, while presence of bone erosion alerts to possible malignant change.
- MRI: These appear hypertense on T2WI.

Neurofibromas

- More well-defined, homogenous lesions which may cause expansion (Figs. 12.9A to C).
- Plexiform types seen in patients of neurofibromatosis.

For those lesions occuring in the root of nose/ethmoids please *see* Chapters 20 and 23.

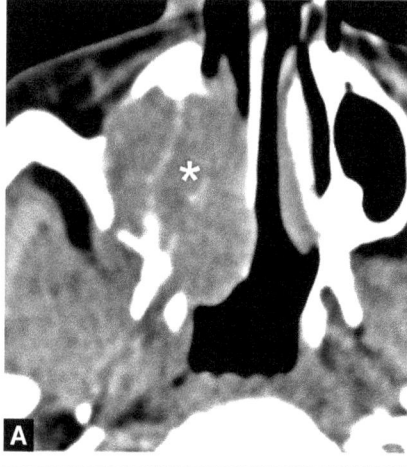
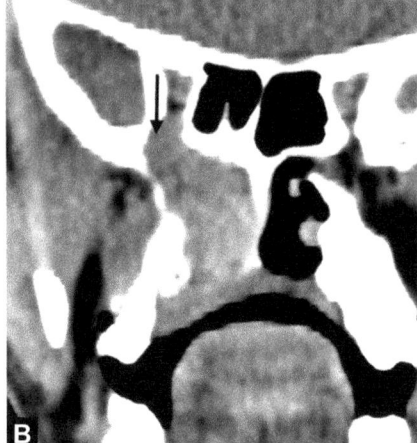
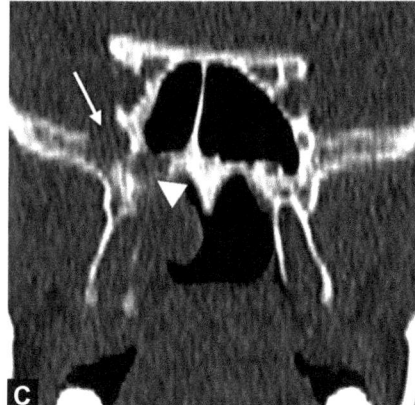

Figs. 12.8A to C: Nerve sheath tumor. NCCT.
- Large expansile soft tissue density mass (asterisk) right maxillary sinus, nasal cavity
- Widening of inferior orbital fissure (black arrow)
- Widening of right foramen rotundum (arrow) and canal for vidian nerve (arrowhead).

BENIGN TUMORS OF BONE AND CARTILAGE
Giant Cell Lesions

- Include giant cell tumors (GCT), Giant cell reparative granuloma (GCRG), Brown tumors, Aneurysmal bone cyst (ABC).
- Have hemosiderin content which shows blooming on the gradient sequences.
- Parathormone (PTH) levels should be ascertained in giant cell lesions.

Giant Cell Reparative Granuloma

- Common sites are mandible/maxilla, infrequently seen involving sinonasal cavity.
- Hypothesis of origin: It is a reactive response to hemorrhage which occurs within the bone consequent to trauma/chronic inflammation.
- Age: Young adults, females > males.
- Imaging findings (Figs. 12.10A to C): Nonspecific.
- CT Scan:

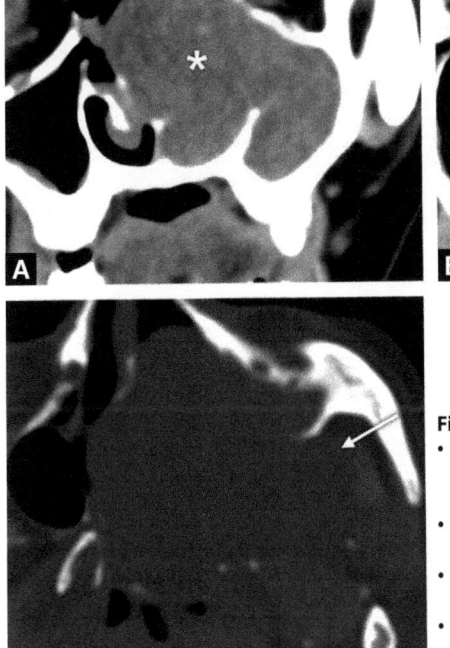
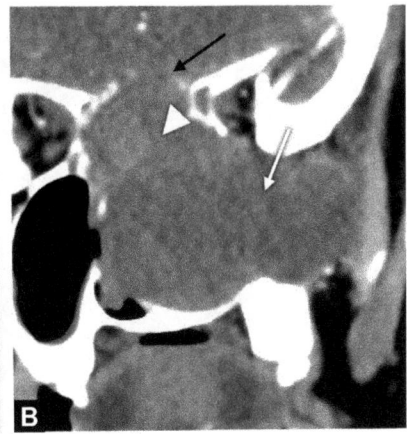

Figs. 12.9A to C: Neurofibroma. CECT.
- Large expansile soft tissue density mass (asterisk) left maxillary sinus, nasal cavity and sphenoid sinus
- Erosion of roof of sphenoid sinus (black arrow)
- Homogenous mass with mild post contrast enhancement (arrowhead)
- Widening of pterygomaxillary fissure and extension into pterygopalatine fossa and infratemporal fossa (arrow in B and C).

- Soft tissue masses with bone erosion.
- Cystic/hemorrhagic foci may be seen within. Expansile but can be aggressive.
- Erosion of nasal septum, ethmoid bones, sphenoid bones and even cribriform plate/clivus may be seen.
- MRI:
  - Both T1WI, T2WI reveal a heterogeneous signal intensity.
  - Contrast enhancement is also heterogeneous.
- Treatment: Intralesional steroids or calcitonin are used. Occasionally surgery is required.

Giant Cell Tumor

- These are also rare tumors in the sinonasal cavity and are usually benign.[8]
- GCT can occasionally show aggressive behavior and metastasize.
- Imaging (Figs. 12.11A and B):
  - CT: Appear as multilocular lesions with fluid levels.
  - MRI: Low signal intensity on all sequences with moderate degree of post contrast enhancement.

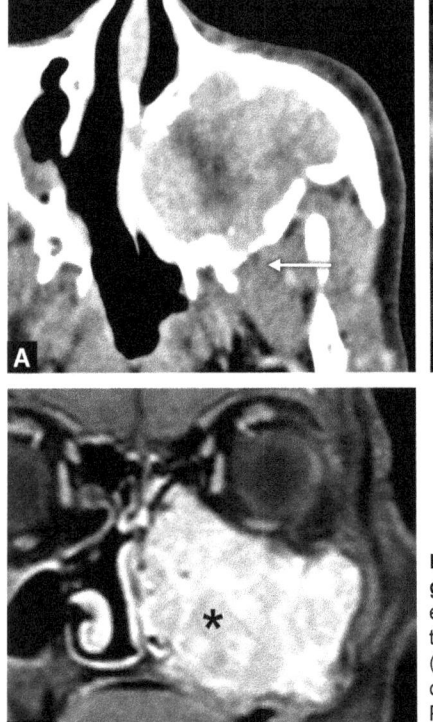
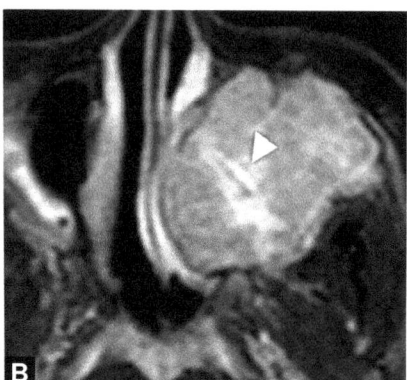
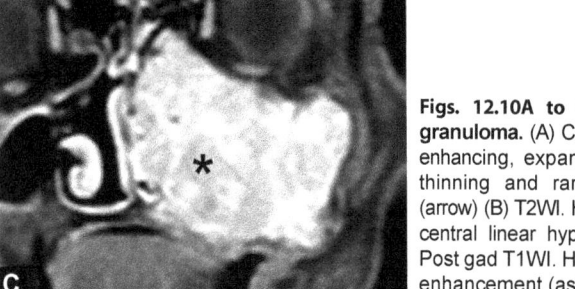

Figs. 12.10A to C: Giant cell reparative granuloma. (A) CECT. Large, heterogeneously enhancing, expansile mass left maxilla with thinning and rarefaction of posterior wall (arrow) (B) T2WI. Heterogeneous T2 signal with central linear hyperintensity (arrowhead) (C) Post gad T1WI. Heterogeneous post contrast enhancement (asterisk).

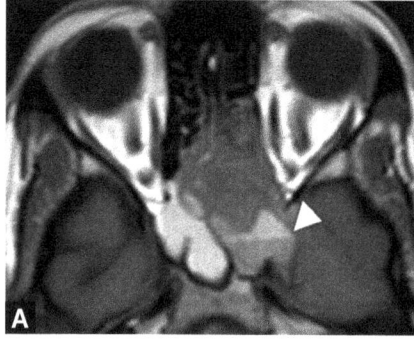
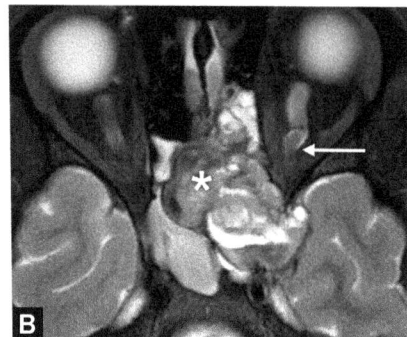

Figs. 12.11A and B: Giant cell tumor. (A) T1WI and (B) T2WI.
- Blood-fluid levels within the lesion (arrowhead)
- Expansile mixed intensity lesion left sphenoid and posterior ethmoid cells (asterisk)
- Mass effect over left optic canal with buckling of the left optic nerve (arrow)
- Retained secretions in the right sphenoid sinus.

Aneurysmal Bone Cyst (ABC)

- ABC usually develops secondarily within another tumor. Primary ABC in sinonasal masses is far less common than secondary ABC.
- Appear as expansile mixed density/lytic lesions on CT.

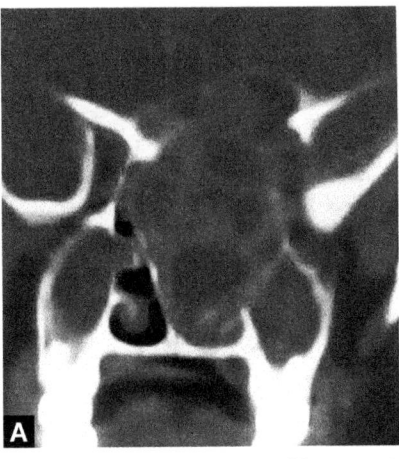
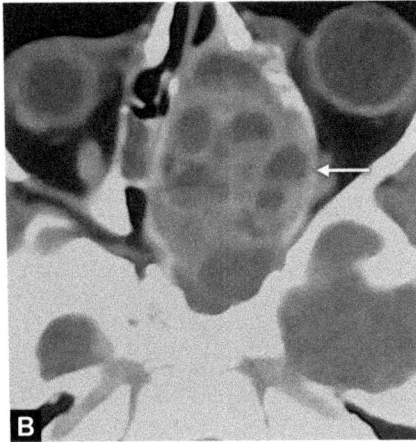

Figs. 12.12A and B: Aneurysmal bone cyst. CECT.
- Expansile mixed density lesion left nasal cavity and ethmoid sinuses
- Multiple fluid-fluid levels (arrow).

- As elsewhere, blood-fluid levels are characteristic of ABC (Figs. 12.12A and B).
- Gradient sequences maybe used to demonstrate hemosiderin content within the lesion.

Osteoma
- Common benign SN tumor.
- Often incidentally detected lesions.[1]
- However depending on location, may cause obstruction of sinus drainage pathways resulting in accumulation of secretions.
- There are reported cases of large lesions with skull base erosions and resultant CSF leak.
- Common sites: Ethmoid or frontal sinuses.
- CT: Well-defined high density lesions (Figs. 12.13A to C). The density will depend upon whether the composition of the lesion is predominantly fibrous tissue, spongy bone or compact bone, with respectively increasing density.
- MRI: Hypo/isointense on T2 weighted sequences.

Osteoblastoma
- Osteoblastoma is rare in the craniofacial region, being more frequent in the vertebral column and long bones.
- In the paranasal sinuses, its description in literature is confined to case reports.
- It occurs in young patients (<30 years of age), with no sex predilection.
- Imaging:[9]
  - Plain radiographs and CT scan: Expansile masses with mixed appearance of dense sclerotic component, and a nonossified component (fibrous on histopathology). Causes bone remodeling.

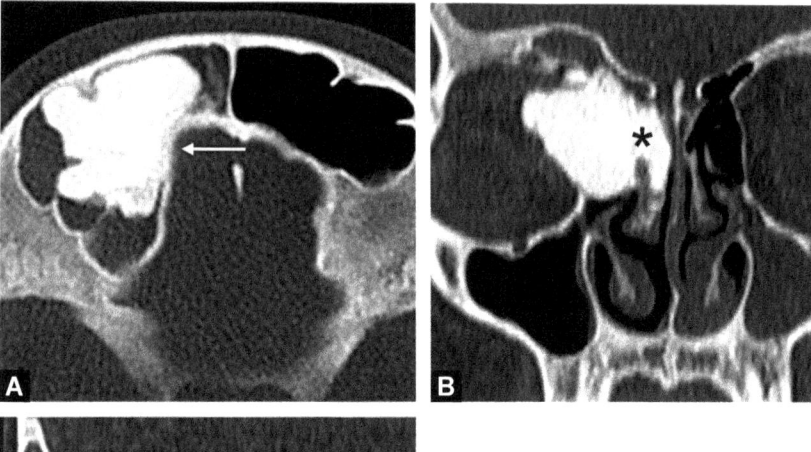
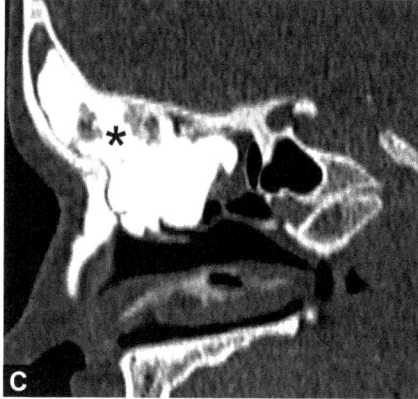

Figs. 12.13A to C: Frontoethmoidal osteoma. NCCT.
- Large, lobulated dense bony mass (arrow)
- Expansion of right frontal and ethmoid sinuses
- Obstruction of frontonasal drainage pathway (asterisks in B and C).

- On MRI, while the sclerotic component is a signal void, the fibrotic component can show intermediate signal intensity on T1 and T2WI with intense enhancement.
- Differential Diagnosis: Osteogenesis imperfecta, GCT, osteoid osteoma, fibrous dysplasia:
  - Fibrous dysplasia: In FD, the sclerotic component is more homogenous, while it is more nodular in osteoblastoma.
  - On CEMR: FD shows marginal enhancement. Osteoblastoma shows more uniform enhancement.
- On HPE, osteoblastoma is similar to an osteoid osteoma with only differentiating point being size (1.5 cm cut-off).

BENIGN GERM CELL TUMORS

Mature Teratoma
- Uncommon benign germ cell tumor of the nasal cavity and paranasal sinuses.
- Shows the typical imaging morphology of teratomas elsewhere in the body.
- Characteristic presence of soft tissue density lesion with internal fat, fluid and calcification.

MISCELLANEOUS ENTITIES

There are several tumors which are not classified in the WHO classification of Sinonasal tumors but they are frequently encountered clinicoradiological entities. These common entities are covered in this section.

Juvenile Nasopharyngeal Angiofibroma (JNA)

- JNA for instance is classified under **Benign nasopharyngeal tumors** in the WHO classification system.
- It is characterized by high vascularity, locally aggressive behavior and high recurrence rates.
- Almost exclusively seen in males.
- Age: Adolescence.
- Site of origin: Sphenopalatine foramen with extension into sinonasal cavity, pterygomaxillary fossa and intracranially with characteristic pattern of spread (Flowchart 12.1).
- The combination of clinical profile, radiological findings and risk of bleeding obviate the need for biopsy in majority of patients. However, tumors with aggressive behavior and atypical patterns of spread mimic malignant lesions and may require sampling.[1]
- Radkowski's classification: This is used for staging of tumors and is detailed in Chapter 13.

Flowchart 12.1: Pathways of spread of Juvenile nasopharyngeal angiofibroma.

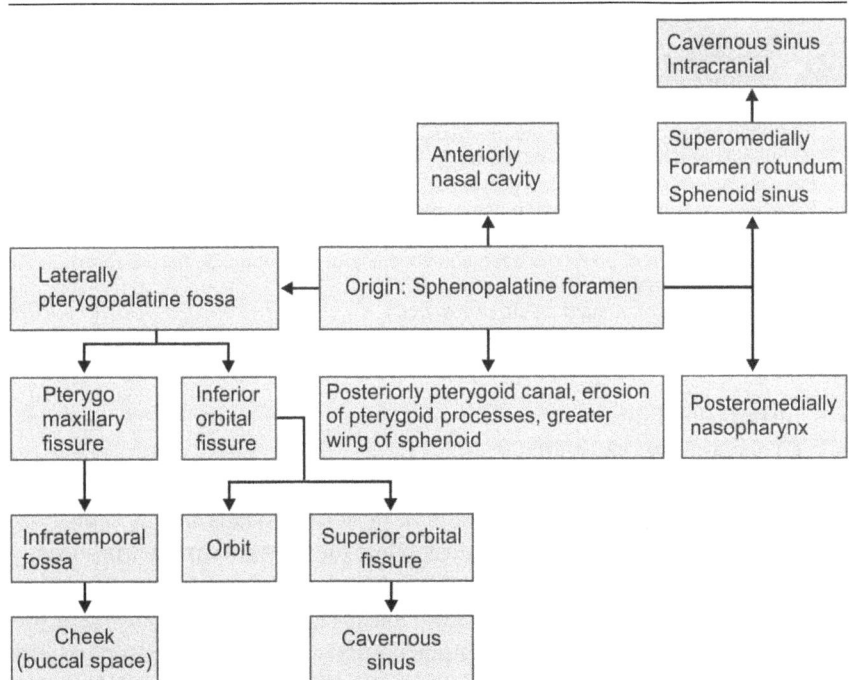

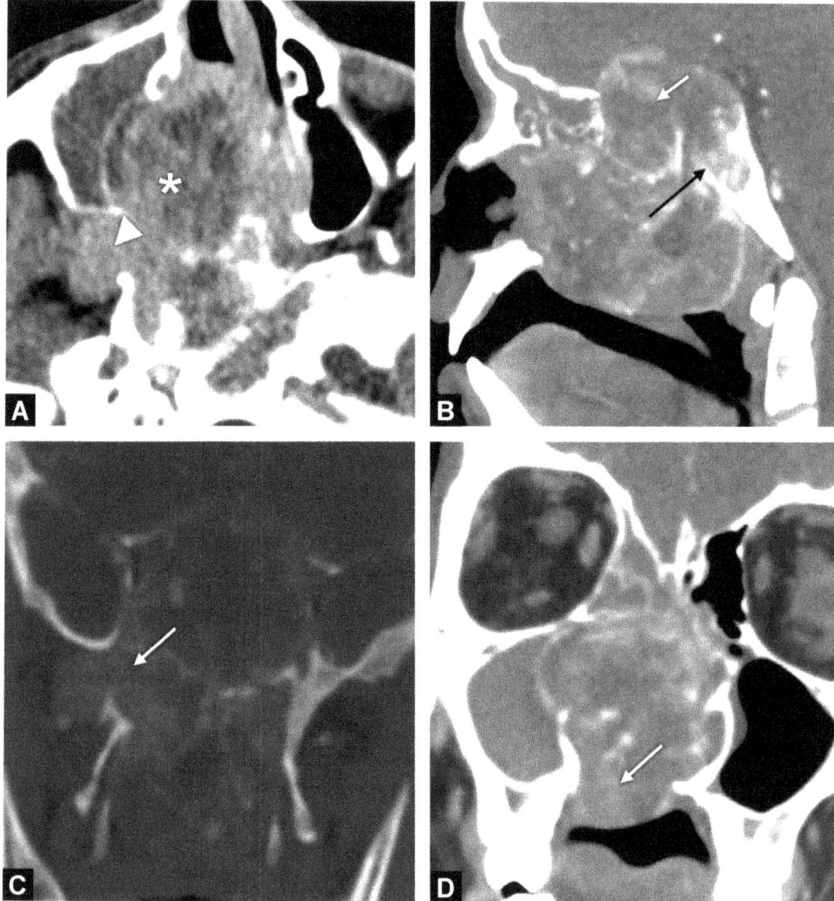

Figs. 12.14A to D: Juvenile nasopharyngeal angiofibroma CECT (Stage III B).
- Intensely enhancing heterogeneous mass lesion centered near right sphenopalatine foramen extending into, bilateral ethmoids, posterior choana and nasopharynx (asterisk)
- Laterally extension into the pterygomaxillary fissure (arrowhead in A)
- Superiorly, erosion of lesser wing and body of sphenoid and planum sphenoidale (white arrow in B)
- Posteriorly erosion of pterygoid base and widening of inferior orbital fissure (arrow in C) and clivus (black arrow in B).
- Inferiorly destruction of hard palate (arrow in D).

- Imaging Findings.
- CT Scans (Figs. 12.14A to D):
  - Intensely enhancing homogenous/heterogeneous mass lesions centered near the sphenopalatine foramen, posterior choana and nasopharynx with characteristic lateral extension into the pterygomaxillary fissure.
  - Initially tumor causes bone expansion and remodeling with typical mass effect on the posterior wall of the maxillary sinus (antral bowing or the Holman-Miller sign). The tumor demonstrates characteristic pattern of spread through fissures and foramina. (Figs. 12.15A to D). However,

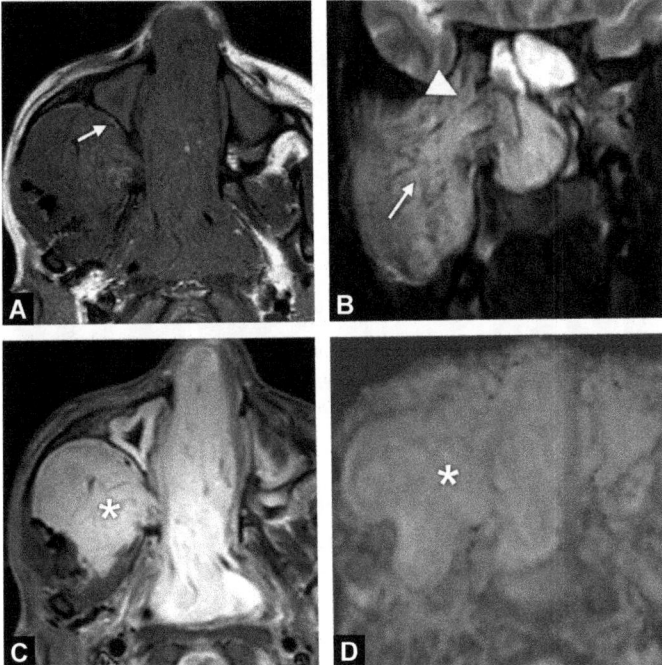

Figs. 12.15A to D: Juvenile nasopharyngeal angiofibroma MRI (Stage II C).
- Bowing of posterior antral wall (arrow in A)
- Widening of inferior orbital fissure (arrowhead in B)
- Intermediate SI with prominent flow voids on T2WI (arrow in B) and hypointense on T1WI
- Free diffusion (bright on ADC map-asterisk in D) with intense postcontrast enhancement (asterisk in C)
- Large, heterogeneous mass in nasal cavity, pterygopalatine fossa and infratemporal fossa.

it is a locally invasive tumor and can display aggressive behavior with bone erosion.
- Bone expansion is however seen far more frequently than erosive destruction.
- Intracranial extension is usually extradural.
- MRI (Figs. 12.15A to D):
    - The tumor shows heterogeneous signal on T_1 and T_2 weighted images. It is however predominantly T_2 hyperintense.
    - Flow voids are often seen within the lesion.
    - There is intense enhancement with contrast.
    - On diffusion weighted imaging, the lesion shows free diffusion with high ADC values ($2.168 \pm 0.270 \times 10^{-3}$ mm^2/s).[10] This feature aids in differentiating the aggressive JNAs from other malignant entities.

Hemophilic Pseudotumor

- Uncommon complication in patients of hemophilia A and B; and rarely seen in those without hemophilia (in other bleeding diathesis).
- Trauma may incite the lesion.
- Consequence of recurrent hemorrhage into soft tissue/ bones resulting in mass lesions.

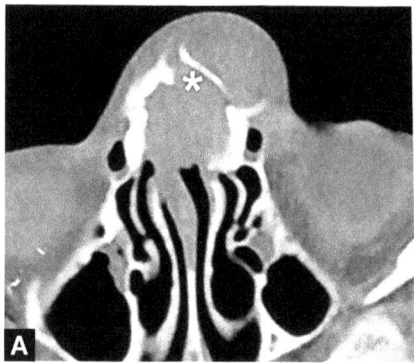 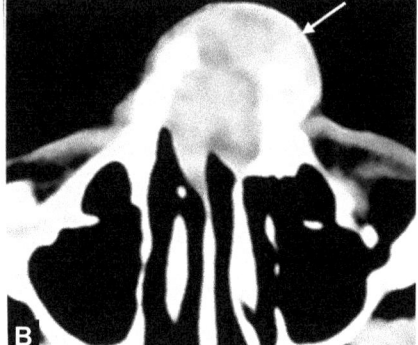

Figs. 12.16A and B: Hemophilic pseudotumor.
- Large soft tissue mass with erosion of anterior nasal septum (asterix in A)
- Mass is predominantly hyperdense on NCCT (arrow in B)

- Due to their tendency to enlarge and cause bone erosions due to increasing pressure, these can mimic a malignancy.
- Osseous forms reported in pelvis, femur, tibia and soft tissue forms in muscles. Rare in sinonasal cavity.
- Appearance is of a lytic lesion with irregular contour, bone erosion or sclerosis. May appear hyperdense on CT (Figs. 12.16A and B).
- Soft tissue component on MRI reveals hemorrhage in various stages and surrounding fibrous capsule.
- Heterogeneous enhancement may be seen.
- High index of suspicion required for diagnosis.

Fibro-osseous Lesions

- Although not classified as a category in WHO classification, due to variable genetic and etiological basis, these are frequently encountered lesions in practice.
- These lesions are clubbed together due to several common clinical, radiological and histological features.
- Tumors of osseous origin that involve the SN cavity may arise from the bony structures within the SN cavity or from adjacent structures, such as the anterior or central skull base, and maxillary alveolus.
- Included in this group are ossifying fibroma and fibrous dysplasia.
- Common points: Lesions characterized by normal bone being replaced by a cellular, fibroid, stroma which over time shows variable amount of ossification/mineralization.
- Seen in young patients.
- Radiologically this is reflected as mixed density lesions which are expansile with variable amounts of fibrous stroma vs ossified components.

Fibrous Dysplasia (FD) (Figs. 17A and B)

- Fibrous dysplasia is not a neoplastic disorder, but a benign disorder involving multiple bones wherein the medulla is replaced by immature fibrous tissue and eventually osseous tissue.[1]

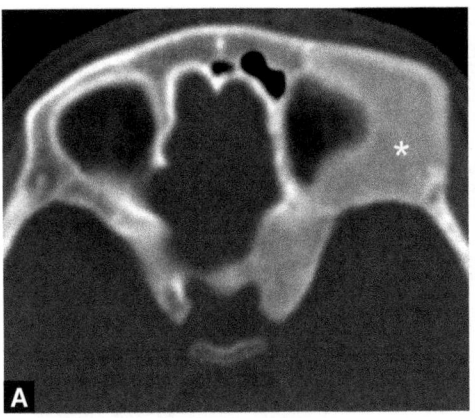 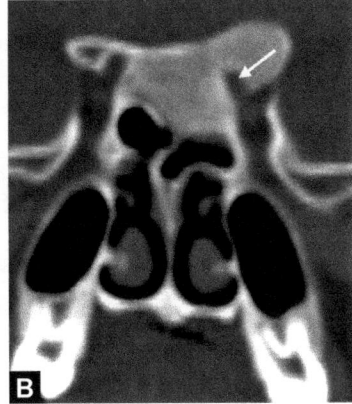

Figs. 12.17A and B: Fibrous dysplasia.
- Expanded left frontal and sphenoid bones with intact contour
- Ground glass density (asterisk)
- Narrowing of left optic canal (arrow).

- Craniofacial bones are a frequent site of involvement, may be part of the polyostotic form.
- Facial appearance referred to as 'Leontiasis Ossea'.
- Imaging Findings:
  - Involved bone is expanded. Its margins with the adjoining bone are ill-defined, i.e. it merges imperceptibly.
  - Matrix may initially appear lucent, then assume a "cotton wool" appearance and finally evolves into "ground glass" density.
  - MRI: Intermediate signal on T1 weighted images, intermediate or low signal intensity on T2 weighted images with significant contrast enhancement in fibrous tissues.
- Critical Issues:
  - Expansion of bone causes narrowing of drainage pathways and skull base foramina.
  - Complications, such as secondary infection and malignancies.

Ossifying Fibroma

- Based on histology ossifying fibroma[1] is divided into two major subtypes (conventional OF and juvenile OF).
- Juvenile type has a more aggressive behavior, are seen in younger patients, are larger at presentation, have less mineralization and show more bone erosion. The juvenile type also has a higher recurrence rate.
- Imaging Findings:
  - CT (Figs. 12.18A and B): Well-defined mixed density lesion with soft tissue component, matrix mineralization and calcification along the periphery. The amount of soft tissue vs mineralized matrix is variable.
  - Expansile lesion, occasionally bone erosion seen.

- MRI (Figs. 12.19A to C): The soft tissue component of the lesion shows heterogeneous enhancement, while the mineralized matrix/rim appear as signal voids.

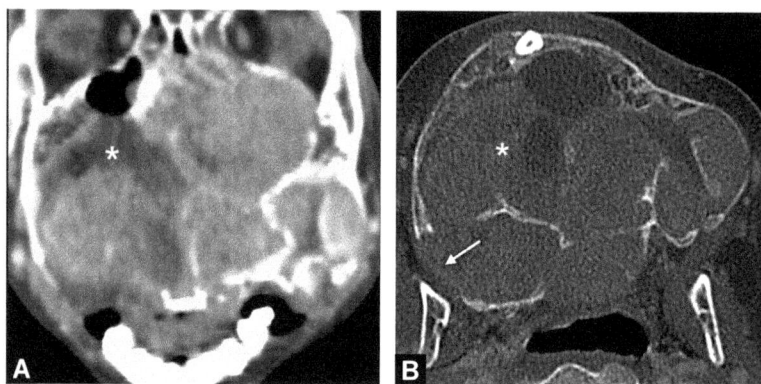

Figs. 12.18A and B: Ossifying fibroma CT.
- Large well-defined heterogeneously enhancing expansile mass lesion nasal cavity and bilateral maxilla
- Mixed density lesion with few internal bony trabeculae (asterisks in A and B)
- Thinning of bony margins with erosion at places (arrow in B).

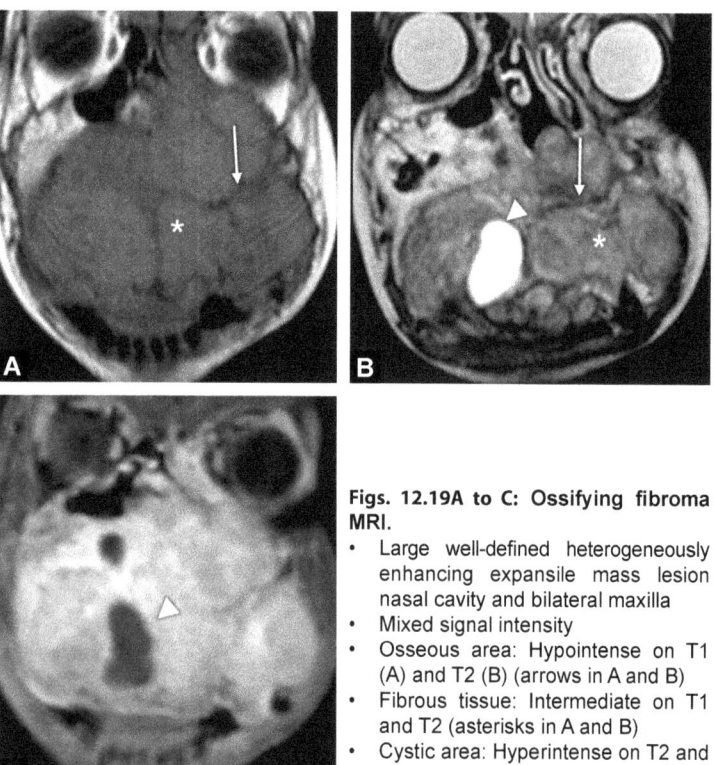

Figs. 12.19A to C: Ossifying fibroma MRI.
- Large well-defined heterogeneously enhancing expansile mass lesion nasal cavity and bilateral maxilla
- Mixed signal intensity
- Osseous area: Hypointense on T1 (A) and T2 (B) (arrows in A and B)
- Fibrous tissue: Intermediate on T1 and T2 (asterisks in A and B)
- Cystic area: Hyperintense on T2 and non enhancing (arrowhead in C).

- The ethmoidal OFs can result in secondary mucocele of the frontal sinuses (also *see* Chapter 5).

Fibrous dysplasia and ossifying fibroma are fibro-osseous lesions with similar presentation. The key differentiating features between these two entities are described in Table 12.1 and illustrated in Figures 12.20A to D.

Table 12.1. Key differentiating features between ossifying fibroma and fibrous dysplasia.	
Ossifying fibroma	*Fibrous dysplasia*
• Classified as a benign tumor	• Classified as a dysplasia, hence not a neoplasm
• Increases in size	• Growth stops after puberty
• Complete removal advocated • High recurrence rate in case of complete removal	• "Wait and watch" policy adopted with surgery only for relief of specific pressure symptoms
• Biopsy required	• Imaging sufficient for diagnosis
CT: • Expansile mass with loss of normal shape/contour of bone often seen as a soft tissue mass • Mixed soft tissue with bone density, thick bony walls may be seen • Sharply defined margins (vs osteosarcoma/chondrosarcoma) • Contrast: Mild enhancement	CT: • Bone expanded but basic shape and contour intact • Characteristic ground glass appearance • May be defined/merge into surrounding tissue
MRI: • T1WI • Osseous area: Hypointense • Fibrous area: Intermediate intense • T2WI: Osseous area—Hypointense (profound) • Fibrous tissue: Hypointense • CEMR: Fibrous area enhance • Fluid-fluid levels may be seen, suggest a secondary ABC	MRI: • Similar signal characteristics depending on degree of ossification
HPE: • COF: Fibrous + Mineralized tissue • Sharp margin from healthy tissue • Mineralization pattern variable	HPE: • Ill-defined • Homogenous

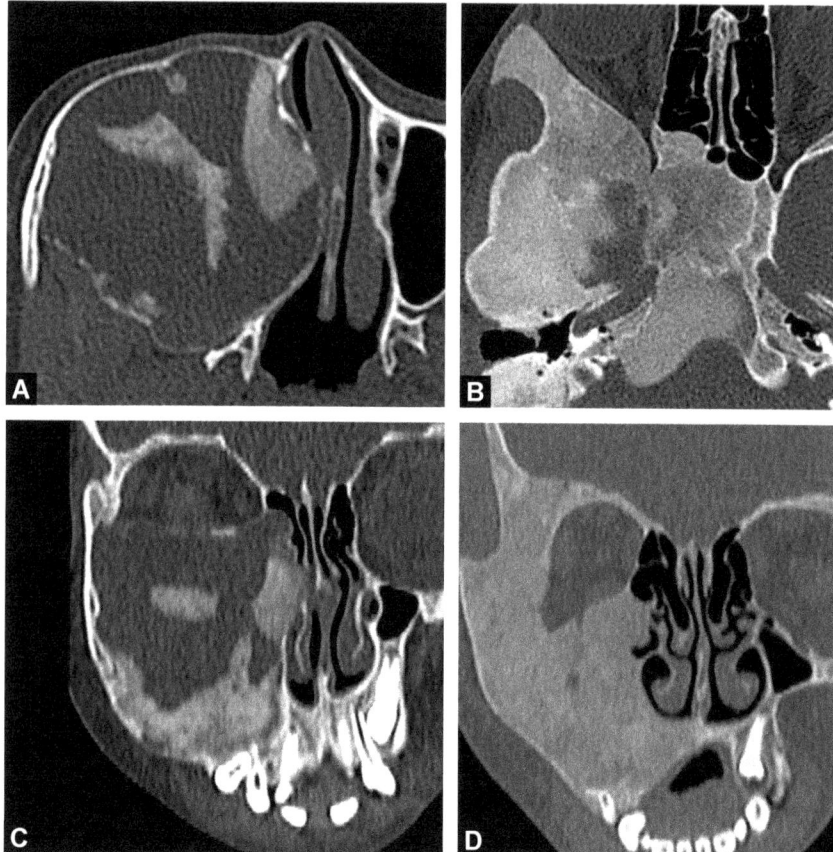

Figs. 12.20A to D: Ossifying fibroma (OF) (A and C) versus fibrous dysplasia (FD) (B and D).
- Expansile mass in OF; Bone expanded with intact contour in FD
- Mixed soft tissue with bone density in OF; Ground glass appearance in FD
- Bony margin in OF; Margin merging with surrounding tissue in FD.

CONCLUSION

Most benign sinonasal tumors show bone expansion and remodelling, several can show aggressive behaviour simulating malignant masses. The approach to sinonasal masses is detailed in Chapter 28.

REFERENCES

1. Sen S, Chandra A, Mukhopadhyay S, et al. Sinonasal tumors computed tomography and MR imaging features. Neuroimag Clin N Am. 2015;25: 595-618.
2. Krouse JH. Development of a staging system for inverted papilloma. Laryngoscope. 2000;110(6): 965-8.

3. Lombardi D, Tomenzoli D, Butta L, et al. Limitations and complications of endoscopic surgery for treatment for sinonasal inverted papilloma: a reassessment after 212 cases. Head Neck. 2011;33(8):1154-61.
4. Whyte A, Chapeikin G. Opaque maxillary antrum: a pictorial review. Australasian Radiology. 2005:49;203-13.
5. Desai SV, Spinazzi EF, Fang CH, et al. Sinonasal and ventral skull base inflammatory pseudotumor: a systematic review. Laryngoscope. 2015;125(4):813-21.
6. Chihani M, Aljalil A, Touati M, et al. Glomangiopericytoma: an uncommon sinonasal perivascular tumor with particular characteristics. Egyptian J Ear, Nose, Throat, Allied Sciences. 2011;12(3):167-70.
7. Jung WS, Yoo CY, Park Y-J, et al. Hemangioma of the maxillary sinus presenting as a mass: CT and MR features. Iran J Radiol. 2015;12(2):e6923.
8. Dubey RB, Tara NP, Desai SM. Giant cell tumor of sinonasal cavity an uncommon location for a common bone tumor. Indian J Radiol Imaging. 2003;13:13-14.
9. Sidani CA, Karam AR, Bruce JH, et al. Osteoblastoma of the frontal sinuses presenting with headache and blurred vision: case report and review of the literature. Radiology Case. 2010;4(6):1-7.
10. Das A, Bhalla As, sharma R, et al. Can diffusion weighted imaging aid in differentiating benign from malignant sinonasal masses: a useful adjunct. Pol J Radiol. 2017;82:345-55.

13
CHAPTER

Benign Sinonasal Tumors: Surgical Perspective

Chirom Amit Singh, Suresh C Sharma

- Introduction
- Clinical Presentation
- Investigations
  - Radiology
  - Biopsy
- Preoperative Workup
  - Workup for Fitness for General Anesthesia
  - Ophthalmology Evaluation
- Treatment
  - Surgery
  - Medical Treatment
  - Wait and Watch Policy
- Approaches for Surgery
  - Open Approach
    - Lateral Rhinotomy Incision
    - Weber-Fergusson Incision
    - Lynch Incision
  - Midfacial Degloving Approach
  - Transpalatal Approach
  - Endoscopic Sinus Surgery
- Specific Tumor Management Considerations
  - Inverted Papilloma
  - Fibro-osseous Tumors
  - Juvenile Nasopharyngeal Angiofibroma

INTRODUCTION

World Health Organization classifies the sinonasal tumors into benign and malignant epithelial tumors, soft tissue tumors, tumors of bone and cartilage, hematolymphoid tumors, neuroectodermal and germ cell tumors. Out of these, hematolymphoid and neuroectodermal tumors do not have any benign entity. Mature teratomas of the sinonasal cavity are rare. This chapter will discuss the commoner benign tumors of sinonasal cavity namely inverted papilloma, fibro-osseous tumors and juvenile nasopharyngeal angiofibroma.

CLINICAL PRESENTATION

Initially, when the tumors are confined to the nose and paranasal sinuses, the patients may present with:
- Nasal obstruction
- Nasal discharge which may be blood stained

- Hyposmia or anosmia
- Headache.

Subsequently, these tumors may progress and extend to the surrounding structures:
- Extension to orbit or compression of optic nerve causing proptosis, diplopia and decrease in vision.
- Extension to pterygopalatine fossa or infratemporal fossa causing cheek swelling and rarely trismus.
- Extension to palate causing palatal swelling.
- Often extension to anterior cranial fossa and cavernous sinus remain asymptomatic.

INVESTIGATIONS

Radiology

Once clinical examination reveals a mass in the nasal cavity or suspicious to have a mass lesion in paranasal sinus, these patients are subjected to imaging to evaluate the characteristic of the tumor and extent of the tumor. Radiological characteristics of different sinonasal tumors are discussed separately in the radiology chapter.

Biopsy

Definitive diagnosis is made from histopathological examination of the biopsy specimen of the tumor. Imaging helps in guiding about decision of biopsy and the site from which the biopsy has to be taken. As for example biopsy is contraindicated in vascular lesion like juvenile nasopharyngeal angiofibroma where the diagnosis is mainly based on clinico-radiological findings.

PREOPERATIVE WORKUP

Workup for Fitness for General Anesthesia

These include routine hemogram, blood sugar level, liver function test, kidney function test, electrocardiography and chest X-ray.

Ophthalmology Evaluation

This is important for:
- Patients who have visual complaints
- Patients with tumors extending into orbit or optic canal without visual complaints.

Ophthalmology evaluation should include:
- Visual acuity
- Field of vision
- Fundus.

TREATMENT

Surgery

- Surgery is the mainstay of treatment for all benign sinonasal tumors.
- Goal of surgery is complete excision of the tumor.

Medical Treatment

This will be discussed later under specific tumors.

Wait and Watch Policy

This is suitable for only those asymptomatic, very slow-growing benign tumors, e.g. asymptomatic frontal osteoma.

APPROACHES FOR SURGERY

Open Approach

Lateral Rhinotomy Incision (Fig. 13.1a)

- Provides wide exposure of the nasal cavity, maxillary antrum, ethmoid sinuses and sphenoid sinus.
- Can be used for excision of benign tumors involving nasal cavity, medial aspect of maxillary sinus, ethmoid sinus and sphenoid sinus.
- This incision has also been used as an approach for *medial maxillectomy* which is the main surgery for inverted papilloma. Medial maxillectomy requires removal of medial part of maxilla medial to inferior orbital foramen, inferior turbinate and infero-medial wall of orbit.

Weber-Ferguson Incision (Fig. 13.1b)

- Provides complete exposure of the maxilla from inferior orbit to superior alveolus.
- This incision has been classically used for *total maxillectomy*.

Lynch Incision (Fig. 13.1c)

- Provides good exposure for frontal sinus and ethmoid sinus.
- This incision is mainly used for *frontoethmoidectomy*.

Midfacial Degloving Approach

- Main advantage of this approach is avoidance of facial incision.
- Approach is from bilateral sublabial area and requires sublabial incision from 1st molar of one side to 1st molar of other side and intranasal incisions.
- Provides good exposure to nasal cavity, inferior part of maxillary sinuses, ethmoid and sphenoid sinuses.

Transpalatal Approach (Fig. 13.2)

- Provides adequate exposure for posterior part of nasal cavity and to some extent pterygopalatine fossa.

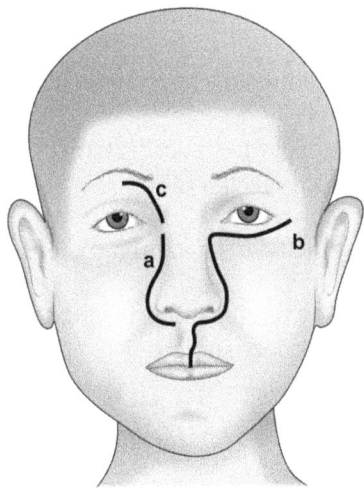
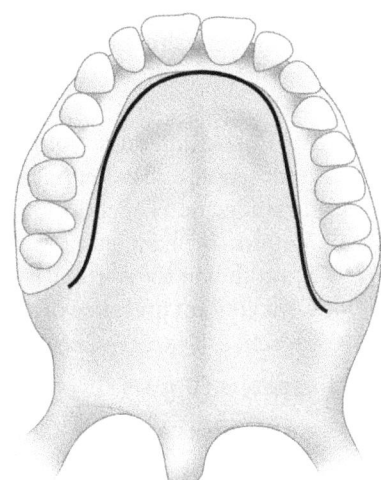

Fig. 13.1: (a) Lateral rhinotomy incision; (b) Weber-Ferguson incision; (c) Lynch incision.

Fig. 13.2: Incision for transpalatine approach.

- This approach has been mainly used for juvenile nasopharyngeal angiofibroma confined to nasal cavity, sphenoid sinus and pterygopalatine fossa.
- Main advantage here also is avoidance of facial scar.

Endoscopic Sinus Surgery

- Endonasal endoscopic approach can provide excellent exposure essentially to all parts of nasal cavity and paranasal sinuses with good magnified view except lateral part of frontal sinus and anterior maxillary sinus.
- It can also be used to approach pterygopalatine fossa and infratemporal fossa.

SPECIFIC TUMOR MANAGEMENT CONSIDERATIONS

Inverted Papilloma

- Site of origin of inverted papilloma is important as it helps in deciding the approach of surgery. The following are the sites of origin of inverted papilloma:[1]
  - Lateral nasal wall (82%)
  - Maxillary sinus (53.9%)
  - Ethmoid sinus (31.6%)
  - Nasal septum (9.9%)
  - Frontal sinus (6.5%)
  - Sphenoid sinus (3.9%).

- Recurrence rate as per different approaches are as follows:[1]
  - Intranasal (without endoscopy): 67.3%
  - Conservative (Caldwell-Luc, external ethmoidectomy procedures): 44%
  - Aggressive (lateral rhinotomy, midface degloving, maxillectomy): 18%
  - Endoscopic and extended endoscopic approach: 11.8%.
- Contraindications of endoscopic approach are:
  - Massive involvement of frontal sinus mucosa or supraorbital cells
  - Intradural or transorbital extension
  - Concomitant presence of malignancy
  - Presence of excessive scar tissue from previous surgery.

Fibro-osseous Tumors

- Fibrous dysplasia usually stabilizes over time and has low malignancy potential.
- Management of fibrous dysplasia is mainly conservative and surgery is indicated for:
  - Symptomatic disease: Optic nerve decompression for tumors compressing the optic nerve, partial excision of intranasal mass to restore nasal patency.
  - Cosmetic recontouring surgery, which can be achieved by partial excision of the tumor.
- Bisphosphonate, e.g. pamidronate has been used in fibrous dysplasia and found to decrease bone pain and stimulate remineralization of osteolytic area.
- Out of total, 95% of sinonasal osteoma is found in frontoethmoidal region[2]
- Indication for surgery in osteomas are:[3]
  - Rapid growth
  - Obstructive sinusitis or mucocele
  - Compression of vital structures
  - Severe pain or headache
  - Facial deformity.
- Ossifying fibroma is the most aggressive form of fibro-osseous lesion with high recurrence rate and treatment should be complete excision of the tumor.

Juvenile Nasopharyngeal Angiofibroma

- Radkowski staging (Table 13.1).[4]
- Preoperative angiography helps in providing the information of blood supply to the tumor, i.e. whether the tumor is receiving blood supply only from external carotid artery branches or from both internal and external carotid artery systems. Preoperative embolization significantly decreases blood loss during tumor resection.
- Surgery is the mainstay of treatment.

Table 13.1: Radkowski staging.	
Stage	Tumor extent
IA	Limited to nose and nasopharyngeal area
IB	Extension into one or more sinuses
IIA	Extension into one or more sinuses
IIB	Full occupation of the pterygopalatine fossa with or without orbital erosion
IIC	Infratemporal fossa extension with or without cheek or pterygoid plate involvement
IIIA	Erosion of the skull base (middle cranial fossa or pterygoids)
IIIB	Erosion of skull base with intracranial extension with or without cavernous sinus involvement

- Endoscopic approaches are more suitable for early stage tumors (IA, IB, IIA, IIB, and some types of IIC).
- External approaches are more preferable for larger tumors (IIC, IIIA, IIIB).
- Radiation therapy is mainly reserved for unresectable tumor. For example, tumor encasing internal carotid artery and massive intracranial extension. It can provide local control rate of 85-91%.[5]
- Preoperative antiandrogen treatment with flutamide have been shown to provide partial tumor regression especially in postpubertal patient.[6]

REFERENCES

1. Krouse JH. Endoscopic treatment of inverted papilloma: safety and efficacy. Am J Otolaryngol. 2001;22(2):87-99.
2. Sayan NB, Ucok C, Karasu HA, et al. Peripheral osteoma of the oral and maxillofacial region: a study of 35 new cases. J Oral Maxillofac Surg. 2002;60(11):1299-301.
3. Eller R, Sillers M. Common fibro-osseous lesions of the paranasal sinuses. Otolaryngol Clin North Am. 2006;39(3):585-600.
4. Radkowski D, McGill T, Healy GB, et al. Angiofibroma. Changes in staging and treatment. Arch Otolaryngol Head Neck Surg. 1996;122:122-9.
5. Blount A, Riley KO, Woodworth BA. Juvenile nasopharyngeal angiofibroma. Otolaryngol Clin North Am. 2011;44(4):989-1004.
6. Thakar A, Gupta G, Bhalla AS, et al. Adjuvant therapy with flutamide for presurgical volume reduction in juvenile nasopharyngeal angiofibroma. Head Neck. 2011;33(12):1747-53.

14
CHAPTER

Malignant Tumors of Sinonasal Cavities: Imaging

Mukesh Yadav, Devasenathipathy Kandasamy

- Introduction
- Epithelial Malignancies
  - Squamous Cell Carcinoma
  - Adenocarcinoma
  - Adenoid Cystic Carcinoma
  - Sinonasal Neuroendocrine Carcinoma and Undifferentiated Carcinoma
- Neuroectodermal Malignancies
  - Melanoma
  - Ewing's Sarcoma Family of Tumors
- Hematolymphoid Neoplasms
  - Lymphoma
  - B-Cell Type Lymphoma
  - Plasma Cell Neoplasm
  - Granulocytic Sarcoma or Chloroma
- Tumors of Soft Tissue, Bone and Cartilage
  - Rhabdomyosarcoma
  - Osteosarcoma
  - Chondrosarcoma
- Metastasis
- Miscellaneous

INTRODUCTION

- Sinonasal (SN) malignancies represent 3% of all the malignancies in head and neck regions.[1]
- Within the SN tract, the malignant tumors are more common as compared to benign tumors.
- The recent most World Health Organization classification for these malignant lesions has been discussed elsewhere in this book.
- Occupational exposure of dust, etc. significantly increases the risk of developing malignancies in SN area, while other predisposing conditions are previous radiation treatment, immunosuppression, etc.
- In addition to the primary neoplastic lesions of SN tract, there are many masses which have primary origin in the cranium or skull base or from the maxillary alveolus (Figs. 14.1A and B).

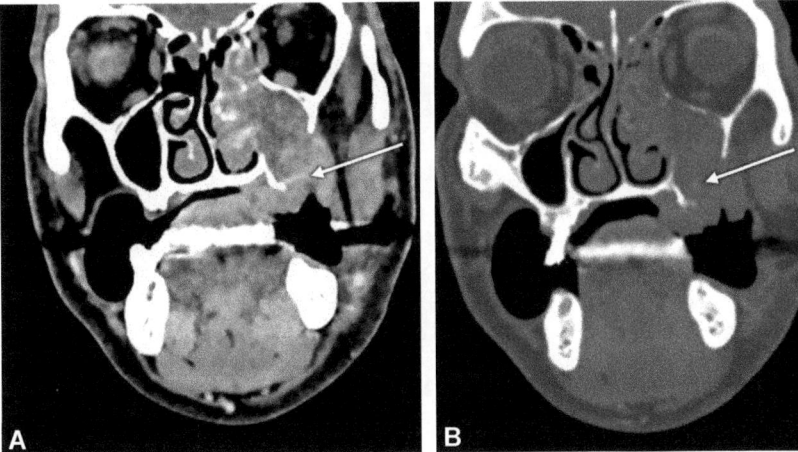

Figs. 14.1A and B: Carcinoma alveolus infiltrating maxillary sinus. Mass lesion centered over the left side maxillary alveolus causing destruction of floor (arrows in A and B) and medial wall of left maxillary sinus and soft tissue extension into maxillary antrum and left side nasal cavity. The epicenter of the mass lesion is in the left maxillary alveolus with secondary invasion of maxillary antrum. Also noted are the steak artifacts in the region of oral cavity.

- Sinonasal tumors need to be differentiated from other masses like inflammatory or infective lesions, hyperparathyroidism or osteonecrosis.
- Common malignancies in SN area are epithelial malignancies (squamous, adeno, neuroendocrine and undifferentiated carcinoma), melanoma, Ewing sarcoma (ES) family of tumors, hematolymphoid tumors (lymphoma, plasma cell neoplasm, granulocytic sarcoma), rhabdomyosarcoma (RMS), osteosarcoma, chondrosarcoma and metastases.

EPITHELIAL MALIGNANCIES

Squamous Cell Carcinoma

- Most common of these malignant lesions are seen in antrum followed by nasal cavity, ethmoid complex, sphenoid and frontal sinus in that order.
- Squamous cell carcinomas are the most common type of malignancy in SN area (50–80%) with highest incidence in 6th and 7th decades.
- Small tumors may be misdiagnosed as sinusitis and other inflammatory pathologies.

Imaging Features

- Large mass lesion with soft tissue attenuation, frequent necrosis and bone destruction showing heterogeneous enhancement (nonspecific appearance on imaging) (Figs. 14.2 and 14.3).

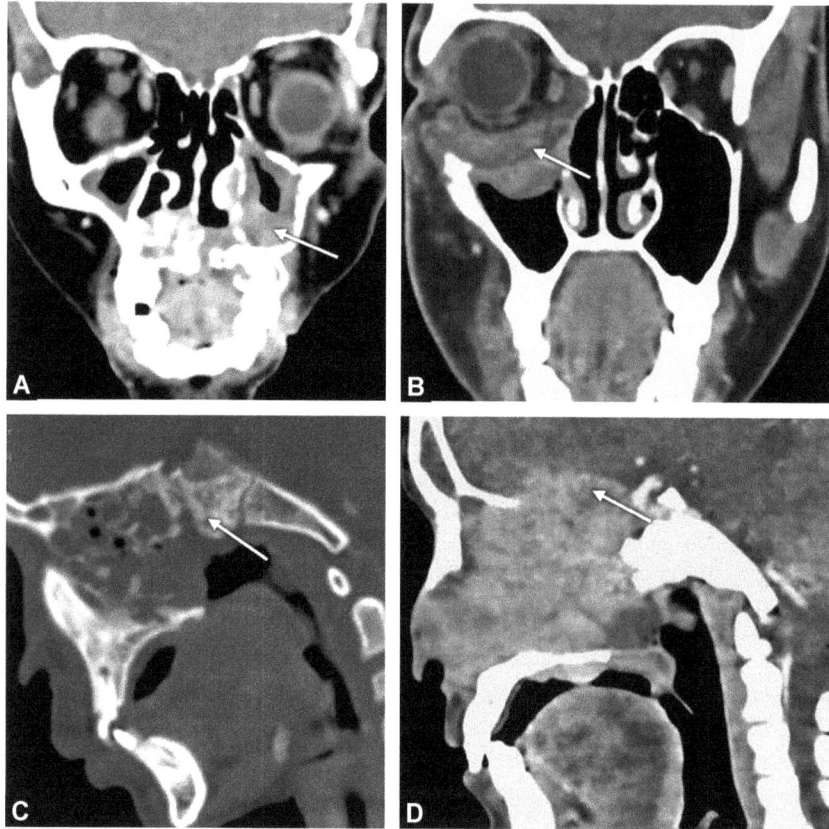

Figs. 14.2A to D: Maxillary sinus carcinoma—different stages. Irregular mucosal thickening and enhancement of the left side maxillary sinus (arrow in A). Also noted is the bone destruction seen in the walls of sinus—T2 tumor. Mass lesion infiltrating into right orbit (arrow in B) with associated bone destruction—T3 tumor. Mass lesion causing destruction of sphenoid sinus (arrow in C)—T4a tumor. Large mass lesion causing destruction of floor of anterior cranial fossa with intracranial extension (arrow in D)—T4b tumor.

- Because of anatomical separation, separate staging system exists for maxillary sinus carcinomas and ethmoidal carcinomas which are covered in Chapter 15.
- On T2-weighted images, it shows intermediate signal intensity, with more hyperintense areas represented by necrosis (Figs. 14.4A to C).
- Diffusion-weighted images (DWI) and contrast imaging help in differentiating the solid tumor part from the inspissated secretions in the blocked sinus cavity.
- Intracranial extension, intraorbital extension and perineural spread should be particularly searched for on imaging.
- Intracranial tumor extension is best evaluated with T1-weighted fat suppressed postcontrast imaging with thin sections and small field of view (FOV).

Chapter 14 Malignant Tumors of Sinonasal Cavities: Imaging

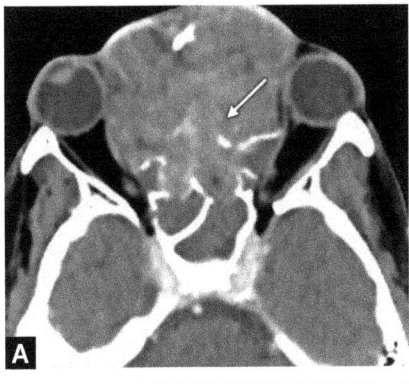
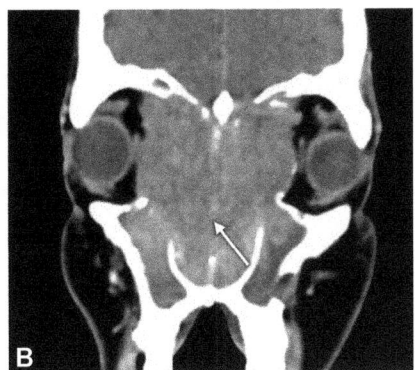
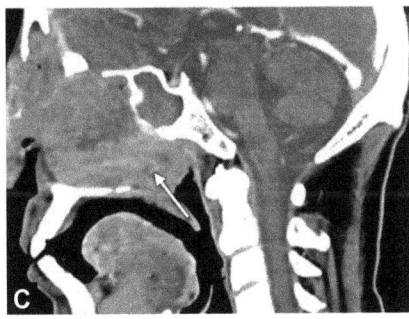

Figs. 14.3A to C: Nasopharyngeal carcinoma. Heterogeneous mass lesion (arrows in A to C) in nasopharynx and nasal cavity causing extensive bone destruction of the base of skull, all the paranasal sinuses and nasal turbinates. There is extension into bilateral orbits also.

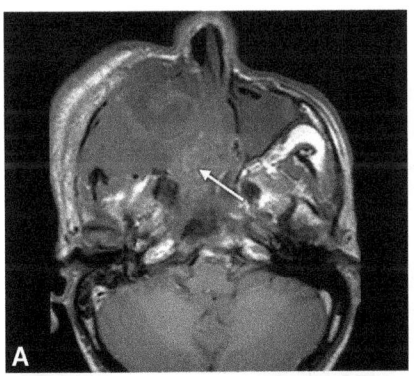
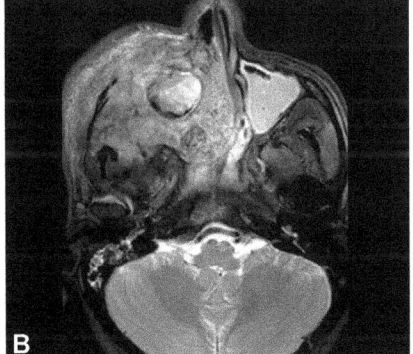
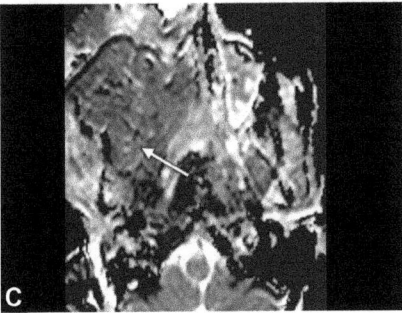

Figs. 14.4A to C: Squamous cell carcinoma of maxillary sinus. Heterogeneous mass lesion (arrows) involving the right maxillary sinus, infratemporal fossa and nasal cavity. (A) Lesion is isointense on T1w image; (B and C) hyperintense on T2w and showing significant diffusion restriction on ADC image—T4aN1M0—stage 4a.

- Positron emission tomography (PET) has limited role in SN tract tumor evaluation, e.g. for assessment of early regional or distant metastatic lesion identification.
- Low incidence of metastatic lymphadenopathy even if the tumor is quite bulky (~15%).
- Treatment may be surgery, irradiation or both with 5-year survival rate of approximately 62%.
- Curative surgery is not attempted, if there is involvement of central skull base, nasopharynx, pterygopalatine fossa, or regional or distant metastasis is present.

Adenocarcinoma

- Intestinal variety—more common in elderly, males and more associated with occupational exposure (ethmoid sinuses and nasal vault are more common areas).
- Nonintestinal variety—sporadic forms, more in females and commonly affects maxillary sinus.

Imaging Features

- Site—related to occupation—ethmoid sinus and nasal vault; in sporadic form, maxillary sinus.
- Nonspecific; large heterogeneous soft tissue with or without bone erosion.
- Has overlapping features with squamous cell carcinoma.
- On T2-weighted (T2w) images, it shows intermediate signal intensity, with necrotic areas showing hyperintensity.
- Diffusion-weighted imaging and contrast imaging help in differentiating solid tumor from inspissated secretions.

Adenoid Cystic Carcinoma

- Within the salivary glands, adenoid cystic carcinomas are the most common.
- Common in 5th decade with high recurrence rates (~60%) and prone to develop delayed recurrence (long latent period).
- Local recurrence is highest among SN malignancies.
- Common sites are maxillary sinus followed by nasal cavity.
- Polypoidal in appearance with *bone remodeling more common than bone destruction.*
- High signal on T2w images (Figs. 14.5A to C).
- Perineural spread, submucosal as well as subperiosteal spread is common.
- Perineural involvement is usually contiguous along the nerve and retrograde. Magnetic resonance imaging (MRI) is the modality of choice to detect perineural spread and it is characterized by thickening and irregularity of the involved nerve, abnormal enhancement compared to the normal nerve, obliteration of perineural fat and widening of neural foramina (Figs. 14.6A to D).[2]

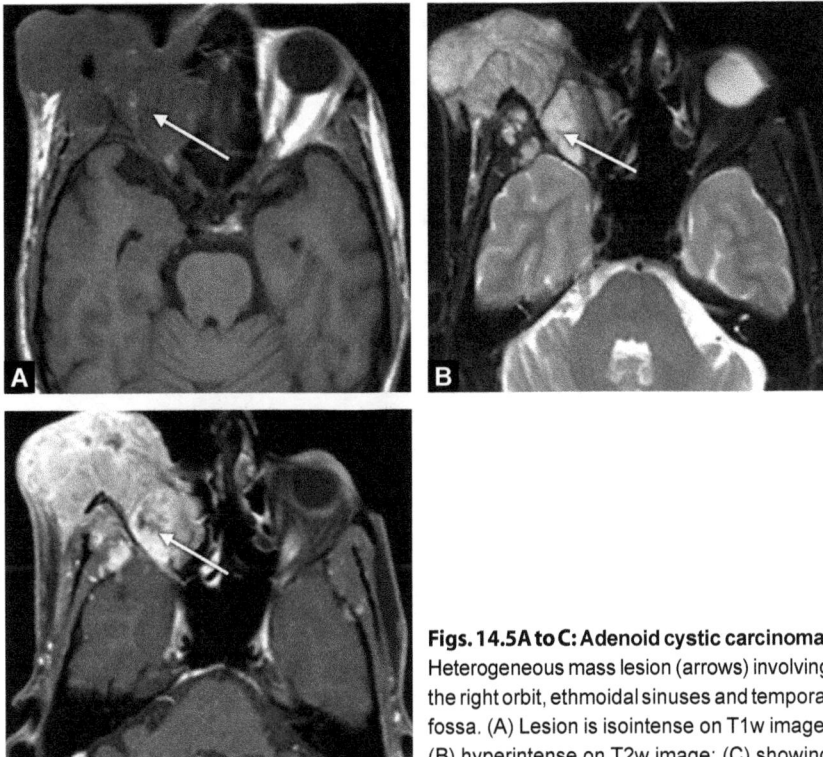

Figs. 14.5A to C: Adenoid cystic carcinoma. Heterogeneous mass lesion (arrows) involving the right orbit, ethmoidal sinuses and temporal fossa. (A) Lesion is isointense on T1w image; (B) hyperintense on T2w image; (C) showing intense enhancement on postcontrast image.

- Meckel's cave and cavernous sinus are the favored sites. It is important to recognize this complication because it is generally associated with local recurrence and poor survival.
- About half of these SN adenoid cystic tumors have distant metastasis to lungs, brain, bone and lymph nodes.
- Treatment of choice is wide local excision with or without local irradiation.

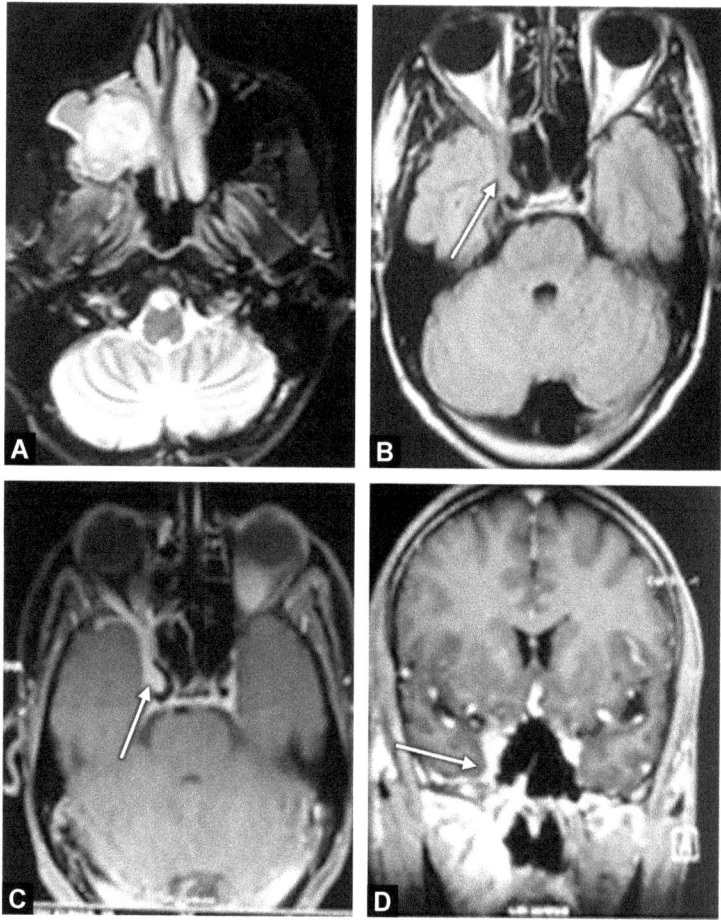

Figs. 14.6A to D: Adenoid cystic carcinoma with perineural invasion. (A) Mass lesion arising from right maxillary sinus which is hyperintense on T2w image. (B to D) Contiguous perineural extension of tumor (arrows) reaching up to the right cavernous sinus which is showing intense enhancement after contrast injection.

Sinonasal Neuroendocrine Carcinoma and Undifferentiated Carcinoma

- Both of these tumors are more undifferentiated as well as more aggressive.
- These lesions are more common in elderly age group (in 50–60 years).
- Imaging appearance largely comprises of more aggressive features like destruction of SN skeleton, invasion of orbit and skull base, nodal disease and metastasis at presentation (Fig. 14.7).

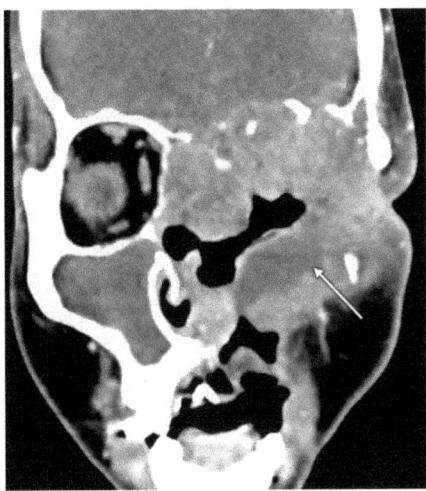

Fig. 14.7: Undifferentiated sinonasal carcinoma. Heterogeneous mass lesion with extensive destruction and invasion of ipsilateral orbit, sinuses, maxillary bone and floor of anterior cranial fossa with intracranial extension. The mass was sampled and histopathology showed undifferentiated sinonasal carcinoma—T4bN2bM0 Stage 4C.

NEUROECTODERMAL MALIGNANCIES

Melanoma

- In SN tract, usually the melanoma is of mucosal variety (unlike cutaneous elsewhere).
- Rare tumor of SN tract with poor prognosis.
- Low overall survival with frequent local as well as distant recurrence.

Imaging Features

- Site: The junction of mucosa and skin at anterior nasal septum, lateral nasal wall and inferior turbinate.
- Polypoid in appearance with well-defined margins.
- Bone remodeling is more common as compared to bone erosion.
- *The peculiar signal on MRI is homogenously hyperintense on T1WI and isointense to low signal intensity of T2w images (melanin or hemorrhage).*
- Treatment: Wide local excision with or without postoperative radiation therapy.
- The average survival time is only 2–3 years.

Ewing's Sarcoma Family of Tumors

- Ewing sarcoma is a highly aggressive small round cell tumor.
- Only small percentage (1–4 %) of all ES occur in the SN tract.
- Most common in mandible followed by maxilla and calvarium.
- Ewing sarcoma and primitive neuroectodermal tumor (PNET), both have common chromosomal translocation.

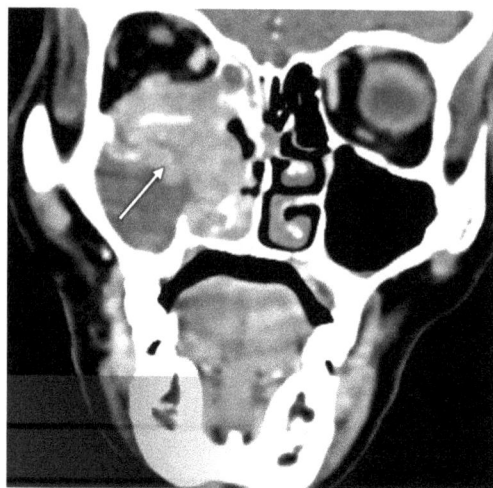

Fig. 14.8: Primitive neuroectodermal tumor of maxilla. Relatively homogeneous mass lesion (arrow) arising from right maxillary sinus with destruction of medial wall and roof and contiguous extension into right orbit, nasal cavity and ethmoidal sinuses. Homogeneous mass lesion with bone as epicenter is the typical appearance.

- On imaging, aggressive destructive soft tissue with typical onion peel type of periosteal reaction; less often sunburst type of periosteal reaction can also be seen (Fig. 14.8).
- Treatment: Local excision with radiotherapy, if local residual lesion is present, chemotherapy for micrometastases.
- Significant improvement in survival rate of these tumors (from 10% to 60–70%) in recent times.

HEMATOLYMPHOID NEOPLASMS

Lymphoma
- Sinonasal tract is uncommon site for lymphomas.
- B-cell, T-cell type and natural killer (NK) cell type varieties can affect SN tract.
- NK cell type occurs in nasal cavity whereas B-cell type occurs in maxillary sinus.
- NK cell type occurs as sheet of soft tissue which may mimic granulomatous infection or Wegener granulomatosis or carcinoma (Figs. 14.9A and B).
- NK cell type is usually not associated with cervical lymphadenopathy.
- Hypo- to isointense on T2w and hypointense on T1w images.
- Bone destruction and erosion without sclerosis.
- Association with *Epstein-Barr* virus.
- Poor prognosis.

B-cell Type Lymphoma
- Occurs more commonly in maxillary sinus (Figs. 14.10A and B).
- *Causes more of bone remodeling as compared to destruction.*

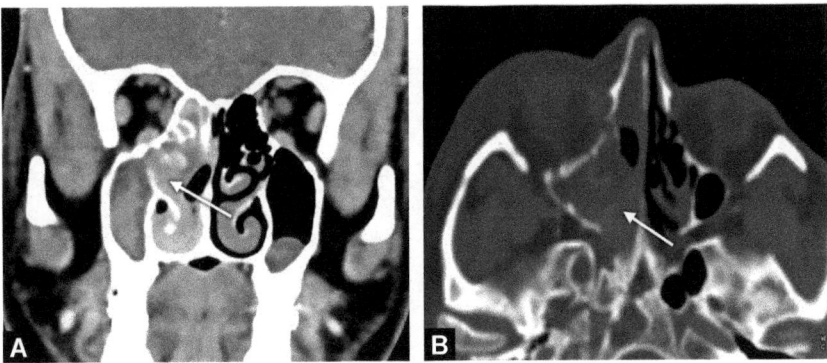

Figs. 14.9A and B: Natural killer T-cell lymphoma. Mass lesion seen in the right nasal cavity with destruction of nasal turbinates (arrows in A and B). Obstruction to the osteomeatal complex causing opacification of right maxillary antrum.

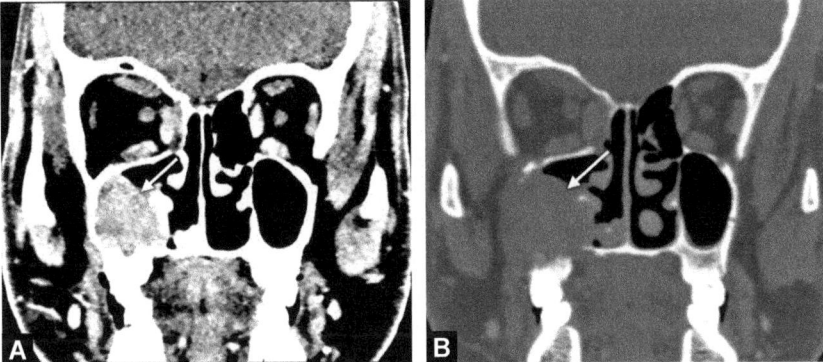

Figs. 14.10A and B: Diffuse large B-cell lymphoma. Homogeneous enhancing mass lesion (arrows in A and B) in the right side maxillary sinus with extensive bone destruction. No necrosis or calcification seen in the lesion which is typical for lymphoma.

- Intermediate signal on T2w images (rather than hypointensity as seen with NK cell type).
- Moderate enhancement.
- Burkitt's lymphoma is a type of B-cell lymphoma involving facial skeleton apart from other parts of lymphatic system.
- Role of imaging in SN lymphomas is to recognize the primary site of disease, to localize the site for biopsy and if radiotherapy is planned, then to map the lesion in its entirety.

Plasma Cell Neoplasm

- May manifest as part of multiple myeloma (MM) or truly solitary plasmacytoma.
- On imaging, multiple punched out lytic bone lesions will be seen in MM, lytic bone lesion with associated soft tissue in plasmacytoma or only soft tissue, if it is extramedullary plasmacytoma.

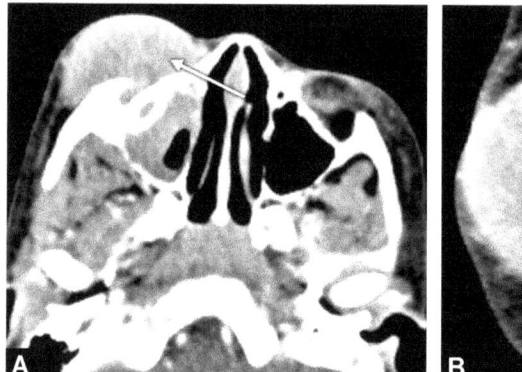
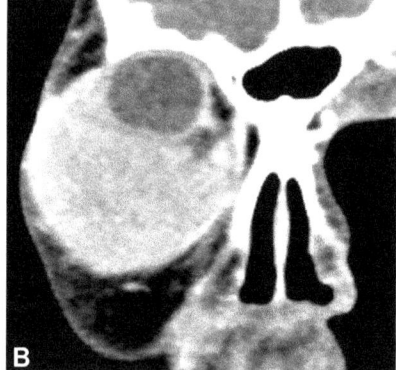

Figs. 14.11A and B: Granulocytic sarcoma of orbit. Homogeneous intensely enhancing mass lesion arising from the right orbit with contiguous extension into right maxillary sinus (arrow in A). Clinical background of leukemia and homogeneous mass lesion with enhancement are the clues to diagnosis.

- The soft tissue component usually enhances homogeneously.
- Moderate enhancement with intermediate signal on T2w images.

Granulocytic Sarcoma or Chloroma

- These are soft tissue lesions which develop as a spectrum of myeloproliferative disorders.
- Word "chloroma" indicate green color (on gross specimen).
- Seen in around 3% patients of acute leukemias.
- Can involve any part of head and neck, also in SN tract.
- On imaging, enhancing relatively homogeneous masses with infiltrative margins (Figs. 14.11A and B).[3]
- On MRI, intermediate signal on both T1 and T2w images.

TUMORS OF SOFT TISSUE, BONE AND CARTILAGE

Rhabdomyosarcoma

- In pediatric population, RMS is the most common SN malignancy.
- It has a quite aggressive behavior.
- Early metastases to nodes and lungs are common.
- These are usually of quite advanced stage at presentation with extensive involvement of multiple compartments in sinuses.
- Botryoid rhabdomyosarcoma is a subtype of RMS which has a polypoid appearance on clinical examination. It has the most favorable outcome amongst all subtypes of RMS.

Imaging Findings

- Large soft tissue mass with heterogeneous enhancement.
- Bone destruction is common with invasion into the adjacent compartments.

- On MRI, these lesions are isointense to hyperintense on T1w images and heterogeneously hyperintense on T2w images.

Osteosarcoma
- In SN tract, the onset of osteosarcoma is slightly late (one decade later than long bones).
- Osteosarcoma can be primary or secondary to other preexisting conditions like Paget's disease, previous radiation therapy, etc.

Imaging Findings
- Most common site is maxilla.
- Aggressive periosteal reaction is commonly seen along with large soft tissue mass. Presence of osteoid matrix on radiograph or computed tomography (CT) is typical.
- On MRI, the tumor is predominantly T2 hyperintense. Hypointense signal can also be seen due to new bone formation.

Chondrosarcoma
- Primary chondrosarcoma of SN tract are uncommon.
- Secondary chondrosarcoma occur after radiation therapy, or in association with Maffucci syndrome or Ollier disease.

Imaging Features
- Alveolar process of maxilla and nasal septum are most common sites.
- Large soft tissue mass lesion with stippled calcification seen on CT (Figs. 14.12A and B).
- Because of high content of water in chondroid matrix, chondrosarcomas are hyperintense signal on T2w images.
- Heterogeneous appearance on postcontrast images due to enhancement of the fibrovascular core and nonenhancement of chondroid matrix.

METASTASIS
- Metastasis to SN tract is quite rare.
- Most common site is maxillary sinus.
- Renal cell carcinoma, breast, lung, thyroid and prostate are the common primaries.
- Lesions may be either multiple or single.
- Imaging characteristics are nonspecific; however, if the primary is thyroid malignancy or renal cell carcinoma, it may present with large enhancing soft tissue.

MISCELLANEOUS
In addition to these above mentioned neoplasms of SN tract, there are other neoplasms which can extend into the SN area because of direct anatomical contiguity, e.g. malignant lesions of retromolar trigone area, skin carcinomas

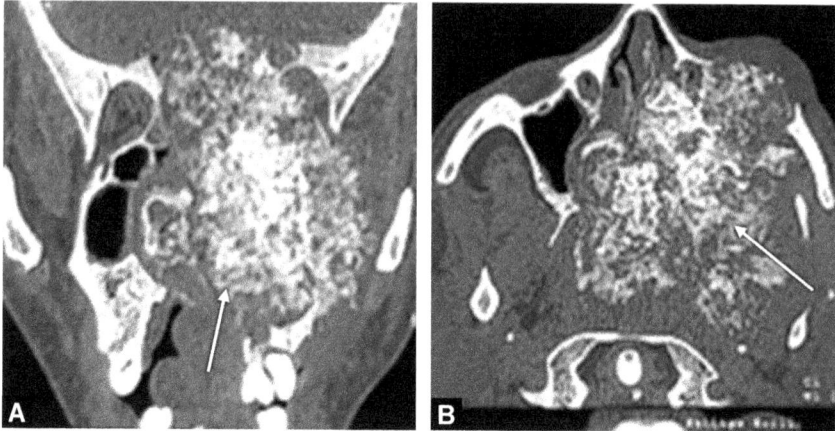

Figs. 14.12A and B: Chondrosarcoma. Large mass lesion (arrows in A and B) with extensive chondroid type of matrix seen involving the left side maxilla, orbit, masticator space and nasal cavity. There is also erosion of base of anterior cranial fossa with intracranial extension.

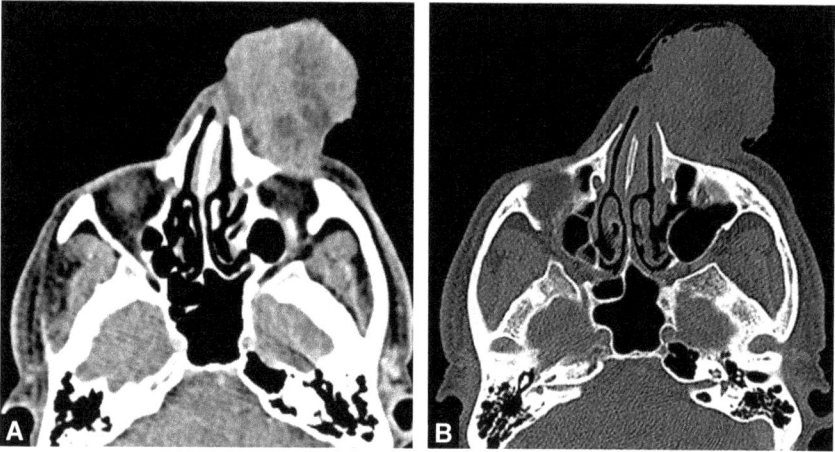

Figs. 14.13A and B: Basal cell carcinoma. Soft tissue mass arising from the area of medial canthus without underlying bone destruction.

of eye or cheek region (Figs. 14.13A and B) as well as aggressive lesions of orbit can also invade the SN tract. Once these tumors are large in size; it becomes difficult to differentiate the primary site of origin.

REFERENCES

1. Eggesbø HB. Imaging of sinonasal tumours. Cancer Imaging. 2012;12:136-52.
2. Sen S, Chandra A, Mukhopadhyay S, et al. Imaging approach to sinonasal neoplasms. Neuroimaging Clinics. 2015;25(4):577-93.
3. Guermazi A, Feger C, Rousselot P, et al. Granulocytic sarcoma (chloroma): imaging findings in adults and children. AJR Am J Roentgenol. 2002;178(2):319-25.

15 CHAPTER

Malignant Tumors of Nose and Paranasal Sinuses: Surgical Perspective

Rajeev Kumar, Hitesh Verma

- Introduction
- Clinical Presentation
- Local Examination
- Imaging
- Biopsy
- Classification
- Management
- Staging
  - Epithelial Tumors of Sinonasal Origin
    - Squamous Cell Carcinoma Staging System (AJCC 2017)
- Classification of Surgical Procedures
  - Medial Maxillectomy
  - Inferior or Infrastructural Maxillectomy
  - Posterior Maxillectomy
  - Total Maxillectomy
  - Craniofacial Resection
- Other Common Sinonasal Tumors
  - Adenocarcinoma
  - Adenoid Cystic Carcinoma
  - Olfactory Neuroblastoma

INTRODUCTION

- Malignant sinonasal tumors account 3% of all aerodigestive tract malignancies.[1]
- 5th and 6th decade of life is the most common age of presentation with male to female ratio as 2:1.[1]
- Maxillary sinus (55%) and nasal cavity (35%) is the most common site for origin of tumors.[1]
- The most common histological type of tumor is squamous cell carcinoma[1] followed by adenocarcinoma.
- Smoking, aflatoxin, heavy metal like chromium, nickel and polycyclic hydrocarbons are etiological factors.
- Occupational exposure to hard and soft wood increases chances of adenocarcinoma.[1]

CLINICAL PRESENTATION

- The presenting symptom will be depending on the area of involvement.
- Nasal obstruction and bleeding are the leading symptoms.

- Other symptoms are loosening of teeth, facial pain, facial swelling, proptosis, diplopia, neck swelling, etc.

LOCAL EXAMINATION

- Detailed endoscopic examination is mandatory for suspected malignancy patients.
- Proliferative irregular mass which bleeds on manipulation is the commonest finding in nasal cavity.
- Nonaxial proptosis, hard to soft swelling, ulceration of face skin, etc. can be found on examination.
- Enlarged level II lymph node is the commonest finding in neck, if tumor had metastasized.

IMAGING

- Both contrast-enhanced computed tomography (CECT) and contrast-enhanced magnetic resonance imaging (CEMRI) are required for accurate evaluation and staging purposes (*see* Chapter 14 for details).

BIOPSY

- For histological classification, tissue biopsy is mandatory.

CLASSIFICATION

Malignant sinonasal tumors are classified as per World Health Organization classification (*see* Chapter 10 for details).

MANAGEMENT

The treatment options for malignant sinonasal tumors are:
- Surgery
- Radiotherapy
- Chemotherapy.

The surgical options are discussed subsequently in this chapter. Nonsurgical options are discussed in Chapter 16.

STAGING

The decision for treatment depends upon stage of the tumor. American Joint Committee on Cancer (AJCC) staging system is used for malignant sinonasal tumors of epithelial tumors.

Epithelial Tumors of Sinonasal Origin

Squamous Cell Carcinoma Staging System (AJCC 2010)[1]

- For maxillary sinus malignancy [Tumor, node and metastasis (TNM) staging][2] (Table 15.1).

Table 15.1: Tumor, node and metastasis (TNM) staging for maxillary sinus malignancy.

TX: Primary tumor cannot be evaluated

T0: No primary tumor

Tis: Carcinoma in situ

T1: Tumor confined to maxillary sinus mucosa

T2: T1+ hard palate bone erosion or destruction and/or extension of tumor in the middle meatus

T3: T2+ involvement of posterior bony wall of maxillary sinus or subcutaneous tissues or medial and floor wall of orbit or pterygoid fossa or ethmoid sinuses

T4a: T3+ involvement of anterior orbital contents/cheek skin/pterygoid plates/infratemporal fossa/cribriform plate/sphenoid or frontal sinuses

T4b: T4a+ involvement of orbital apex/dura/brain/middle cranial fossa/cranial nerves other than V2, nasopharynx/clivus

Table 15.2: Tumor, node and metastasis (TNM) staging for nose and ethmoid sinuses.

TX: Primary tumor cannot be evaluated

T0: No primary tumor

Tis: Carcinoma in situ

T1: Tumor confined to any one subsite, with or without bony invasion

T2: T1+ one other subsite in a single region or involvement of an adjacent region within the nasoethmoidal complex

T3: T2+ involvement of the medial wall or floor of the orbit/maxillary sinus/hard palate/cribriform plate

T4a: T3+ involvement of anterior orbital contents/nose or cheek skin/ minimal extension to anterior cranial fossa/pterygoid plates/sphenoid or frontal sinuses

T4b: T4a+ involvement of orbital apex/dura/brain/middle cranial fossa/cranial nerves except V_2/nasopharynx/clivus

- For nose and ethmoid sinuses (TNM Staging) (Table 15.2).
- For regional neck nodes (Table 15.3):

Based upon the TNM stage, final stage of the tumor is assigned for treatment planning (Tables 15.4 to 15.6).

- Neck dissection can be combined with stage-wise treatment, if regional lymph node metastasis is present.
- The indications for combination of chemotherapy are involvement of resection limit, perineural invasion and distal metastasis.

Table 15.3: Tumor, node and metastasis (TNM) staging for regional neck nodes.

NX: Regional lymph nodes cannot be assessed
N0: No regional lymph node metastasis
N1: Single ipsilateral metastatic lymph node, ≤3 cm in size
N2a: Single ipsilateral metastatic lymph node, >3 cm but ≤6 cm in size
N2b: Multiple ipsilateral metastatic lymph node, ≤6 cm in size
N2c: Bilateral or contralateral metastatic lymph nodes, ≤6 cm in size
N3: Metastatic lymph node >6 cm in size

Table 15.4: Tumor, node and metastasis (TNM) staging for tumor.

Stage	
Stage 1	T1N0M0
Stage 2	T2N0M0
Stage 3	T3N0M0, T1-3N1M0
Stage 4a	T4aN0-2M0, T1-3N2M0
Stage 4b	T4b any N, M0, any T, N3, M0
Stage 4c	Any T, Any N, M1

Table 15.5: Staging system and treatment options for maxillary sinus malignancy.

Stage	Treatment plan
Stage 1	Wide local excision
Stage 2	Infrastructural maxillectomy
Stage 3	Total maxillectomy or extended total maxillectomy followed by radiotherapy
Stage 4a	Extended total maxillectomy with orbital exenteration followed by radiotherapy
Stage 4b	Palliative care or supportive care
Stage 4c	Palliative care or supportive care

Table 15.6: Staging system and treatment options for nose and ethmoid sinuses malignancy.

Stage	Treatment plan
Stage 1	Endoscopic excision/Lateral rhinotomy excision
Stage 2	Endoscopic excision/Lateral rhinotomy excision
Stage 3	Excision by open approach-extended ethmoidectomy follow by radiotherapy
Stage 4a	Extended ethmoidectomy with orbital exenteration follow by radiotherapy
Stage 4b	Palliative care or supportive care
Stage 4c	Palliative care or supportive care

CLASSIFICATION OF SURGICAL PROCEDURES

Medial Maxillectomy (Fig. 15.1)

- This surgical procedure entails removal of medial wall of maxilla from floor of orbit to floor of nose.
- This procedure is best suitable for tumors limited to medial wall of maxillary sinus and lateral wall of nasal cavity.
- This procedure can be done either through midfacial degloving approach or purely endoscopically.
- Medial maxillectomy can be combined with ethmoidectomy for tumors extending into ethmoids (Fig. 15.2).

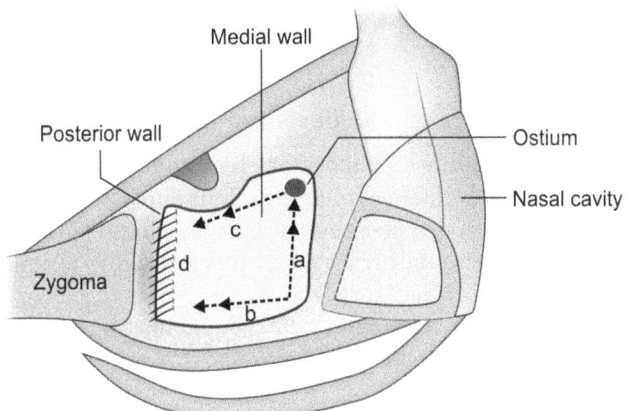

Fig. 15.1: Schematic diagram of medial maxillectomy, frontal view. (a: First bony cut; b: Second bony cut; c: Third bony cut; d: Fourth bony cut).

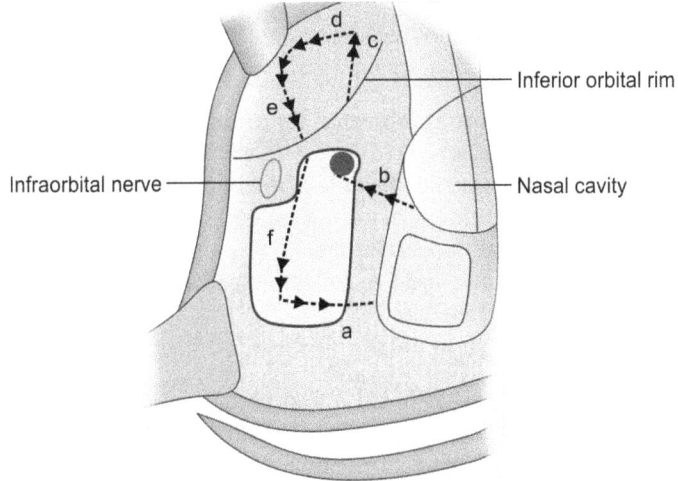

Fig. 15.2: Extended medial maxillectomy, frontal view. (a: First bony cut; b: Second bony cut; c: Third bony cut; d: Fourth bony cut; e: Fifth bony cut; f: Sixth bony cut).

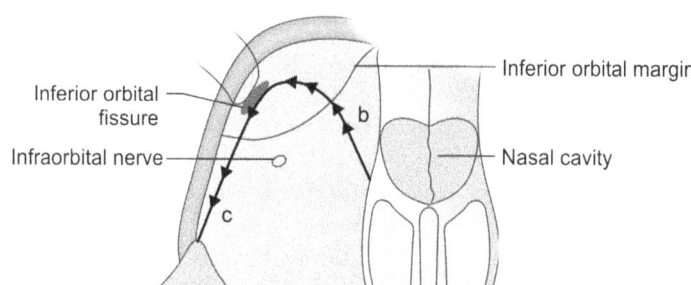

Fig. 15.3: Schematic diagram of total maxillectomy, frontal view. (a: First bony cut; b: Second bony cut; c: Third bony cut).

Inferior or Infrastructural Maxillectomy

- This surgical procedure is usually done for tumors limited to hard palate without gross involvement of maxillary sinus mucosa.
- It entails removal of part or complete removal of hard palate.
- The most common tumor resected by this procedure is squamous cell carcinoma.
- Others tumors like adenoid cystic carcinoma or mucoepidermoid carcinoma which are limited to palate only.

Posterior Maxillectomy

- This procedure is usually done for limited tumors of soft palate with minimal extension to hard palate.
- It entails removal of posterior aspect of hard palate, soft palate and part of posterior maxillary sinus.
- Usually done for squamous cell carcinoma of soft palate.

Total Maxillectomy (Fig. 15.3)

- This surgical procedure is indicated for tumors involving primarily the maxillary sinus mucosa.
- It entails complete removal of whole of the maxillary sinus in toto.
- The most common tumors requiring total maxillectomy are squamous cell carcinoma and adenocarcinoma.
- The palatal defect after total maxillectomy can be managed either by palatal prosthesis or free flap.

Craniofacial Resection

- The most advanced cases of nose and paranasal sinuses extending to cribriform plate with intracranial extension into anterior cranial fossa can be dealt with craniofacial resection.
- It entails complete removal of ethmoids, cribriform plate, and even dura.
- If required, a part of brain parenchyma can also be resected.

- Numerous extensions of this procedure can be done for complete disease removal.
- These include total maxillectomy, medial maxillectomy and orbital exenteration, etc.

OTHER COMMON SINONASAL TUMORS

Adenocarcinoma
- It is the second most common tumor of sinonasal region.
- Occupational exposure of wood dust is the risk factor.
- Upper part of nasal cavity and ethmoid sinuses are the most common site of origin.
- Surgery is the treatment of choice. Radiotherapy is required for adjuvant therapy for locally advanced unresectable/residual tumors.

Adenoid Cystic Carcinoma
- It accounts for less than 5% of sinonasal malignancies.[1]
- Maxillary sinus is most common site.
- It tends to grow slowly and usually present with prolonged history of facial pain.
- It spreads by perineural and vascular invasion.
- Surgery is the treatment of choice.

Olfactory Neuroblastoma
- Basal cell of the olfactory neuroepithelium is the cell of origin.
- It accounts for 5% of sinonasal malignancies.[1]
- It has slight female preponderance with bimodal age distribution with peaks at 20 years and 50 years.
- It can cause paraneoplastic syndromes, such as Cushing's syndrome, syndrome of inappropriate antidiuretic hormone secretion (SIADH) and hypertension by secreting vasoactive peptides.
- Surgery is the treatment of choice. Radiotherapy and chemotherapy has role in adjuvant setting.

CONCLUSION

Clinical features of malignant sinonasal tumors can be confused for common benign nasal conditions. High index of suspicion is required for early diagnosis. Usually patients present in advanced stage. Surgery is the primary treatment of choice. Radiotherapy and chemotherapy is useful in adjuvant setting.

ACKNOWLEDGMENT

Authors would like to acknowledge Dr. Smriti Panda for drawing schematic diagrams for various types of maxillectomies in this chapter.

REFERENCES

1. Mcmonagle BA, Gleeson M. Nasal cavity and paranasal sinus malignancy. In: Hibbert J, Gleeson M (Eds.). Scott Brown Otorhinolaryngology Head and Neck Surgery, 7th Edition. London: Hodder Arnold; 2008. pp. 2417-36.
2. Hermanek P, Hutter RVP, Sobin LH, Wagner G, Witteking C (Eds.). TNM Atlas: Illustrated Guide to the TNM/pTNM Classification of Malignant Tumors, 4th Edition. Berlin: Springer-Verlag, 1997.

16
CHAPTER

Radiation and Chemotherapy in Management of Malignant Sinonasal Tumors

Dodul Mondal

- Introduction
- Risk Factors
- Routes of Spread
  - Local Invasion
  - Lymphatic Spread Pathway
- Management
  - Indications for Radiotherapy in Sinonasal Malignancy
- Principles of Radiotherapy Planning
- Site-specific Radiotherapy Management and Technical Details
- Complications and Sequelae of Treatment

INTRODUCTION

- Tumors of nasal cavity and paranasal sinuses are complex and uncommon.
- Maxillary sinus cancers are most common followed by nasal cavity cancers.
- Cancers of frontal, ethmoid and sphenoid sinus are extremely uncommon.
- Most sinonasal cancers occur in south Asian countries and in Japan.

RISK FACTORS

These tumors show interesting association between histology, occupational exposure and different chemical agents (Table 16.1).

Table 16.1: Risk factors for sinonasal cancers.	
Histology/Location	Chemical exposure/Risk factor
Adenocarcinoma	Wood dust, glues
Squamous cell carcinoma	Nickel
Maxillary cancer	Thorotrast
Nasal cavity	Smoking, alcohol, human papillomavirus, Epstein-Barr virus

ROUTES OF SPREAD

- Tumors grow to a significantly large size before detection because of free space within sinonasal cavity.
- Most spread by local contiguous invasion. This is important during radiotherapy planning and deciding radiation treatment volume.
- Lymphatic spread is uncommon even in advanced stage.

Local Invasion

- Local spread by sinonasal malignancies is detailed in Table 16.2.
- Adenoid cystic carcinomas (ADCA) are known to spread thorough nerve roots and trigeminal nerve is often involved.

Table 16.2: Local invasion by sinonasal malignancies.		
Tumor location		Local spread
Nasal vestibule		Upper lip and nasal cavity are most frequently involved by local extension; gingivolabial sulcus, premaxillary space, floor of nose and nasal septum. Very large tumors can spread to opposite side of face.
Nasal cavity	Roof	Spreads thorough ethmoid, cribriform plate and orbit to involve anterior cranial fossa, subcutaneous tissue and skin.
	Floor	Hard and soft palate, maxillary antrum.
	Lateral wall	Maxillary antrum, ethmoid cells, orbit, pterygopalatine fossa, and nasopharynx.
Ethmoid sinus		Nasal cavity, orbit, maxillary antrum, nasopharynx, sphenoid sinus and anterior cranial fossa.
Suprastructure of maxillary antrum		Nasal cavity, ethmoid cells, orbit, pterygopalatine fossa, infratemporal fossa, and base of skull.
Infrastructure of maxillary antrum		Palate, alveolar process, gingivobuccal sulcus, soft tissue of the cheek, nasal cavity, masseter muscle, pterygopalatine space, and pterygoid fossa.
Sphenoid sinus		Most commonly involves cranial nerves (III, IV, V1, V2, VI) at cavernous sinus, nasal cavity and brain.

Lymphatic Spread Pathway (Table 16.3)

Lymphatic spread is uncommon and mostly determined by organ or contiguous structure involvement.[1,2]

Table 16.3: Lymphatic spread.	
Primary site of tumor	Possible nodal involvement
Nasal vestibule	Ipsilateral IB most common. Submandibular, facial, preauricular less commonly involved.
Nasal cavity	IB, retropharyngeal
Maxilla	IB, II

MANAGEMENT

- Clinical presentation, staging, diagnosis and surgical perspectives have already been discussed in Chapter 15.
- A general guideline involving all anatomical site and stage is unwise and not recommended.

Indications for Radiotherapy in Sinonasal Malignancy

Indications of different types of radiotherapy are described in Table 16.4.

Principles of Radiotherapy Planning

- Rigid thermoplastic head and neck mask is used for immobilization during planning and daily treatment.
- Planning CT scan is usually done in supine position with extended neck.
- Contrast MRI is highly recommended for better soft tissue and neuroanatomy details.
- All available helpful images should be fused with planning CT scan for better tumor delineation.
- Important normal organs requiring all precautions to reduce dose to them are: normal uninvolved brain, temporal lobes, hippocampus,

Table 16.4: Indications of radiotherapy in sinonasal malignancy.	
Definitive radiotherapy	• Early tumors usually T1, T2, N0. • Tumors of nasal vestibule and columella even when very small are usually treated with nonsurgical method because of significant facial deformity produced by surgery. • Sphenoid sinus malignancy • Unresectable tumor due to local infiltration or comorbidities.
Palliative radiotherapy[3]	• Patients having extremely poor general condition or incurable disease may benefit from palliative treatment.
Concurrent chemoradiotherapy	• Stages III and IV unresectable tumor, positive margin, high grade and neuroendocrine tumors.[4]
Adjuvant radiotherapy	• All resected tumors other than very early tumors • Close margin • Positive margin • High T stage • High grade tumor • Perineural invasion (PNI) • Lymphovascular invasion (LVSI) • Lymph node involvement • Incomplete resection or tumor spillage • Concurrent cisplatin can be considered after margin positive resection.
Elective neck node irradiation	• Advanced tumors, squamous or undifferentiated histology should be treated with elective irradiation.

Table 16.5: Modes of radiotherapy treatment.	
Mode	Definition
Brachytherapy	Sealed radiation sources are inserted within the tumor or placed at very close proximity of the tumor
External beam radiotherapy	Radiation source remains at a distance from the patient
Intensity-modulated radiotherapy[5]	Type of conformal radiation where multiple radiation beams are used from different angles to target the tumor. Each radiation beam is subdivided into multiple beamlets of different intensity.

brainstem, spinal cord, cochlea, optic chiasm, optic nerves, eyeballs, retina, lacrimal gland, parotid gland, lens and oral cavity.
- Modes of radiotherapy are detailed in Table 16.5.

Site-specific Radiotherapy Management and Technical Details (Table 16.6) (Figs. 16.1A to F)

The site specific management for nasal vestibule and maxillary sinus is detailed in Table 16.6.

For esthesioneuroblastoma, the treatment recommendations are discussed in chapter 15.

Table 16.6: Site-specific radiotherapy management.			
Nasal vestibule	Definitive radiation	Gross tumor with margin, elective nodes	50 Gy
		Boost to primary tumor with margin	16–20 Gy
		Boost to gross nodes with margin	16–20 Gy
	Adjuvant radiation	Postoperative[6] tumor bed depending on margin status	60–66 Gy
		Uninvolved nodal region	50 Gy
Maxillary sinus	Definitive	Gross tumor as determined by clinical examination, imaging or prechemotherapy tumor extension.	66–70 Gy
		Gross tumor volume (GTV) + 1 – 1.5 cm margin	66–70 Gy
		Clinical target volume (CTV)1 + 1 – 1.5 cm margin around the CTV1. If part of a sinus is involved, remaining of the sinus should be included in CTV2.	59–63 Gy
		Elective nodal regions, base of skull and nerve tract till the foramen at the base of skull	54–57 Gy
	Adjuvant	Gross residual tumor, sites of positive margin or extracapsular nodal extension	66–70 Gy
		Tumor bed + 1 – 1.5 cm margin	60 Gy
		Entire surgical bed	56–57 Gy
		Elective nodal regions, base of skull, nerve tract till foramen at base of skull, if pathology specimen shows presence of perineural involvement	54 Gy

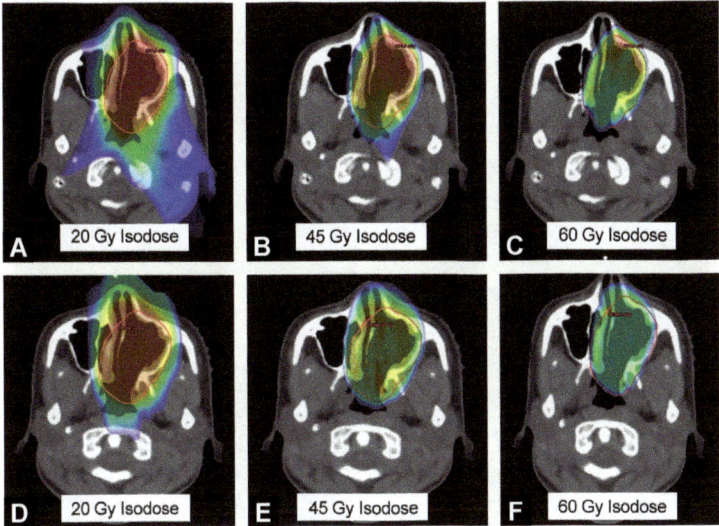

Figs. 16.1A to F: Comparative plan with photon beam intensity-modulated radiotherapy (IMRT) and double scatter proton beam therapy for adjuvant radiation of a nasal melanoma. The upper and lower panel shows photon IMRT and proton plan, respectively. The target coverage is comparable with both techniques, but proton beam is capable of excellent normal tissue sparing. The low dose isodose lines clearly separate from each other.
Courtesy: Rahul R Parikh, Rutgers Cancer Institute of New Jersey.

Complications and Sequelae of Treatment

- Chemotherapy and radiation are potentially toxic and should be used adequately and judiciously.
- Potential complications of radiation are mainly divided into acute and late radiation toxicity.
- Common acute toxicities are radiation dermatitis, nasal, oropharyngeal, laryngeal and esophageal mucositis; facial and nasal hair loss, loss of eyebrow and eyelash, congestion of eye, dryness of mouth, dysphagia, etc.
- Most acute radiation toxicities are symptomatically managed and usually start resolving weeks after radiation completion.
- Potential long-term side effects are mainly cataract, neuropathy, damage to optic structures, retinopathy, xerostomia, chronic dry eye syndrome, permanent loss of hair and soft tissue injury.
- Osteoradionecrosis (ORN), though not common with lower dose, can occur with higher dose. Mandible is the most common site but radionecrosis of other facial bones is also reported (Figs. 16.2A to D).
- Temporal lobe necrosis when dose to temporal lobe is very high.
- Both ORN and temporal lobe radionecrosis can pose challenge diagnostic dilemma with recurrence.
- Late sequelae are mostly dose and volume dependent and uncommon with modern radiation techniques in high volume academic centers.

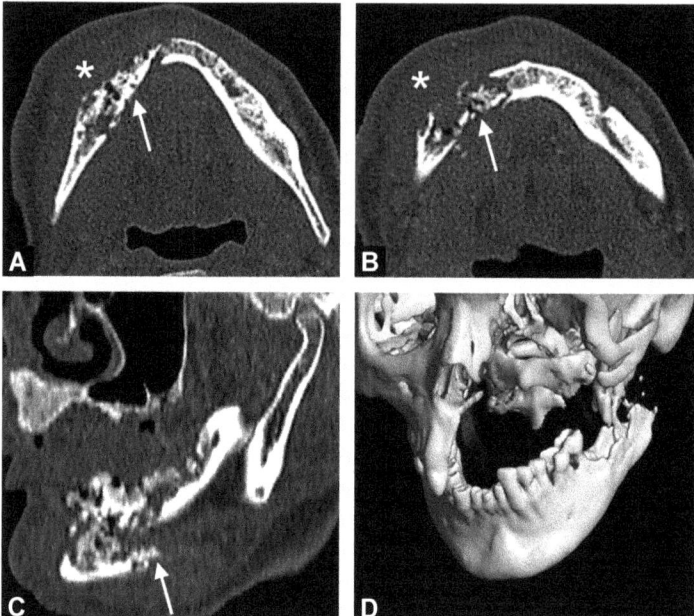

Figs. 16.2A to D: Osteoradionecrosis as a complication. (A and B) Axial bone window images. Irregular lytic-sclerotic destruction of mandible (arrows). Associated soft tissue (asterisks); (C) Sagittal bone window image (arrow); and (D) VRT image. Destruction of the angle and body of mandible extending till the alveolar margin.

CONCLUSION

- Sinonasal tumors are uncommon.
- Most present with advanced disease.
- Outcome is modest even with aggressive therapy.
- Surgical resection with adjuvant radiation and/or chemotherapy is standard for most tumors.
- Survival outcome has not changed significantly over the years; however, treatment related toxicity has been reduced providing better quality of life.
- Intensity-modulated radiotherapy should be the standard of care for radiation to sinonasal tumors.
- New modalities like proton beam therapy has provided hope to better tumor control and survival.

REFERENCES

1. Ang KK, Jiang GL, Frankenthaler RA, et al. Carcinomas of the nasal cavity. Radiother Oncol. 1992;24:163-8.
2. Le QT, Fu KK, Kaplan MJ, et al. Lymph node metastasis in maxillary sinus carcinoma. Int J Radiat Oncol Biol Phys. 2000;46:541-9.

3. Corry J, Peters LJ, Costa ID, et al. The 'QUAD SHOT'—a phase II study of palliative radiotherapy for incurable head and neck cancer. Radiother Oncol. 2005;77(2):137-42.
4. Robin TP, Jones BL, Gordon OM, et al. A comprehensive comparative analysis of treatment modalities for sinonasal malignancies. Cancer. 2017;123(16):3040-9.
5. Dirix P, Vanstraelen B, Jorissen M, et al. Intensity-modulated radiotherapy for sinonasal cancer: improved outcome compared to conventional radiotherapy. Int J Radiat Oncol Biol Phys. 2010;78(4):998-1004.
6. Hoppe BS, Stegman LD, Zelefsky MJ, et al. Treatment of nasal cavity and paranasal sinus cancer with modern radiotherapy techniques in the postoperative setting—the MSKCC experience. Int J Radiat Oncol Biol Phys. 2007;67(3): 691-702.

Section 4

Trauma

17. Imaging in Sinonasal Trauma
18. Imaging of Cerebrospinal Fluid Leaks
19. Sinonasal Trauma and Cerebrospinal Fluid Rhinorrhea: Surgical Aspects

CHAPTER 17

Imaging in Sinonasal Trauma

Manisha Jana, Ashu Seith Bhalla

- Introduction
- Classification, Anatomy
  - Key Concepts of Maxillofacial Trauma
- Specific Fractures
  - Complex Facial Injuries
    - Le Fort Fractures
  - Other Complex Fractures
    - Naso-orbitoethmoid Complex Fractures
    - Zygomaticomaxillary Complex Fractures
  - Fractures Involving Single Bone or Single Buttress
    - Frontal Sinus Fractures
    - Nasal Bone Fractures
    - Maxillary Sinus Fractures
    - Orbital Blowout Fractures
- Complications of Sinus Fractures
- Illustrative Case in a Reporting Format

INTRODUCTION

- Maxillofacial trauma encompasses a wide range of complex injuries. This chapter confines itself to those involving the sinonasal structures.
- Facial fractures may occur following blunt or penetrating trauma.
- Multidetector computed tomography is the modality of choice for delineating the complete extent of injury as well as the associated complications. It has currently replaced plain radiographs in this setting.

CLASSIFICATION, ANATOMY

Key Concepts of Maxillofacial Trauma

Classification is based on the concept of buttresses or pillars (Tables 17.1 and 17.2) which constitute the basic support of the facial form. This concept governs the surgical reconstruction. These buttresses are there both in horizontal and vertical planes.[1,2]

Table 17.1: Horizontal buttresses (Figs. 17.1A and B).

Upper transverse maxillary buttress	Nasofrontal suture > along inferior margin of orbit > zygomatic bone > zygomaticotemporal sutures > continues posteriorly as the floor of orbit
Lower transverse maxillary buttress	Runs along the maxillary alveolar process extending posteriorly to hard palate
Upper transverse mandibular buttress	Mandibular alveolar process > ramus > posterior margin
Lower transverse mandibular buttress	Inferior mandibular margin

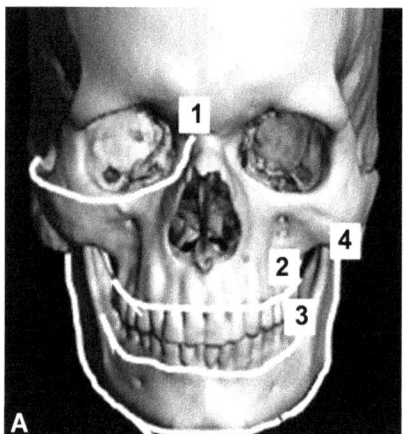 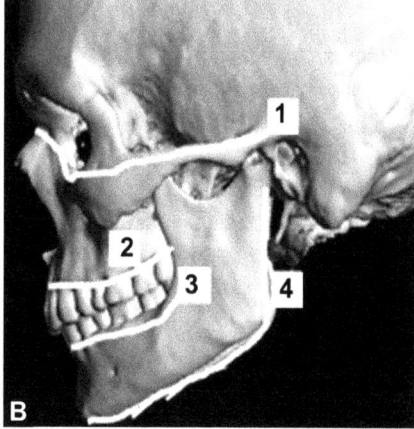

Figs. 17.1A and B: Horizontal buttresses. (1: Upper transverse maxillary buttress; 2: Lower transverse maxillary buttress; 3: Upper transverse mandibular buttress; 4: Lower transverse mandibular buttress).

Table 17.2: Vertical buttresses (Figs. 17.2A and B).

Medial maxillary buttress	Nasofrontal suture > lateral border of pyriform aperture > maxillary alveolar process > extends posteriorly including medial walls of orbit and maxillary sinus
Lateral maxillary buttress	Zygomaticofrontal suture > along lateral wall of orbit > body of zygomatic bone > maxillary alveolar process near the alveolus > extends posteriorly along lateral walls of orbit and maxillary sinus
Posterior maxillary buttress	Pterygoid plates > connects skull base (sphenoid) to maxilla

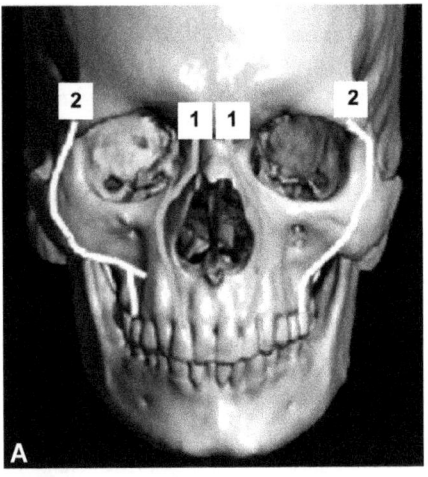

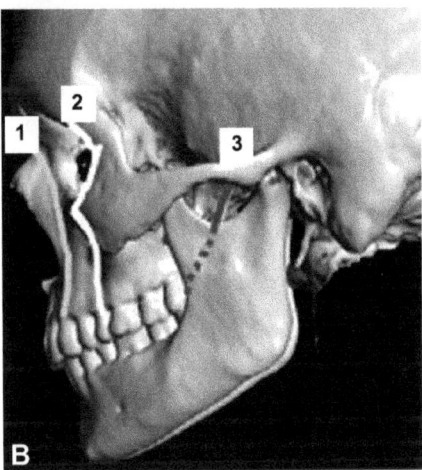

Figs. 17.2A and B: Vertical buttresses. (1: Medial maxillary buttress; 2: Lateral maxillary buttress; 3: Posterior maxillary buttress).

SPECIFIC FRACTURES

Sinonasal fractures may be part of more complex facial fractures involving multiple buttresses (Le Fort fractures); or occur as less severe isolated injuries.

Complex Facial Injuries

Complex facial injuries include Le Fort fractures, nasoorbitoethmoid (NOE) fractures, and zygomaticomaxillary complex fractures.

Le Fort Fractures (Table 17.3 and Figs. 17.3 to 17.8)

- These are complex maxillofacial fractures involving multiple facial bones, and often occur as a consequence of high impact force on the midface.
- A combination of different types may be seen on two sides of the face (Figs 17.7 and 17.8).

Type/synonym	Extent/area involved	Structures involved	Best plane
Type 1/Guerin fracture Floating plate (Fig. 17.4)	Horizontal fracture Inferior maxillary buttress (hard palate) separated from rest of the face and skull base	Maxillary sinus wall (anterior, medial and lateral) Pyriform aperture Nasal septum Pterygoid plates	• Coronal • 3D images
Type 2/Pyramidal (Fig. 17.5)	Maxillary fragment pyramidal in shape with apex at nasofrontal suture May move independent of rest of face	Medial orbital wall Floor of orbit Zygomaticomaxillary suture Zygomatic bone spared	• Axial • Coronal oblique
Type 3/ Craniofacial dissociation (Fig. 17.6)	Complete separation of face from skull base	Nasofrontal suture > medial orbital wall > lateral orbital wall > zygomatic bone Only type to involve lateral orbital wall and zygomatic bone	• Axial • Coronal

Table 17.3: Types of Le Fort fractures (Figs. 17.3 to 17.8).

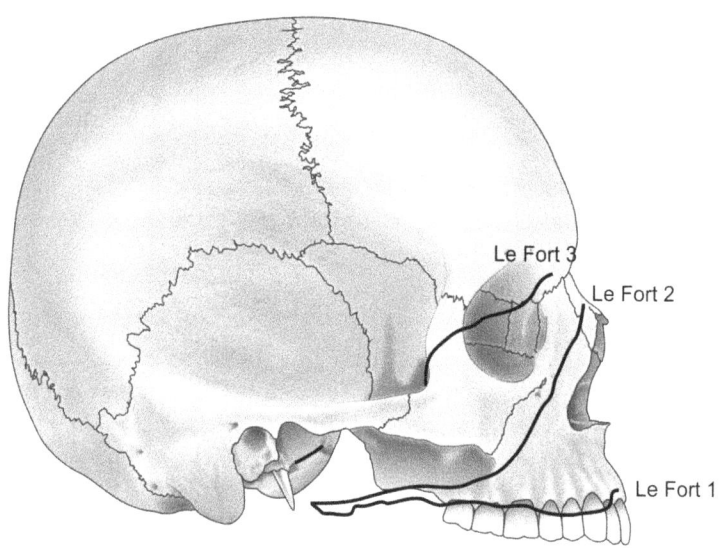

Fig. 17.3: Types of Le Fort fractures.

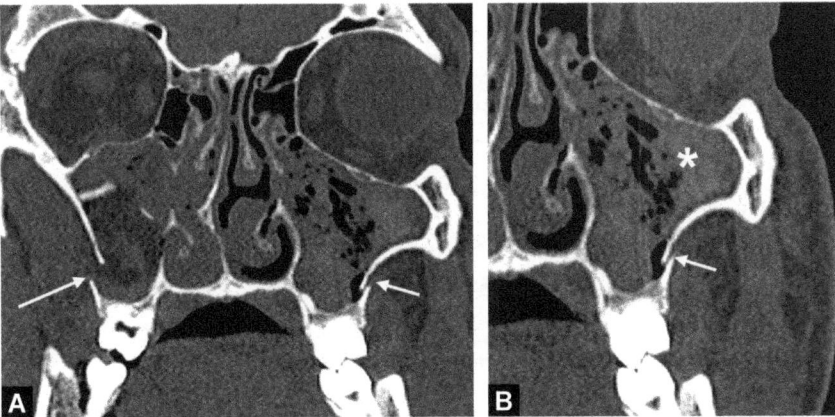

Figs. 17.4A and B: Le Fort type 1 fracture. Fracture line through inferior maxillary buttresses (arrows) and hemosinus (asterisk).

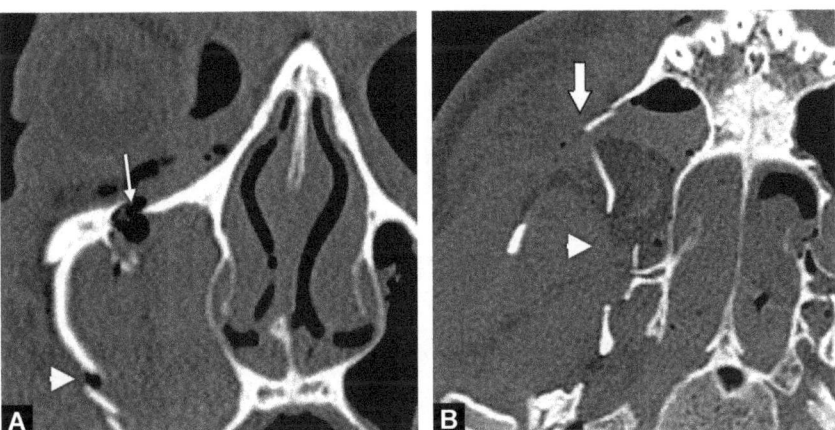

Figs. 17.5A and B: Le Fort type 2 fracture. (A) Fracture line through inferior orbital rim (arrow), (B) lateral maxillary wall (arrowhead) and anterior maxillary wall (block arrow).

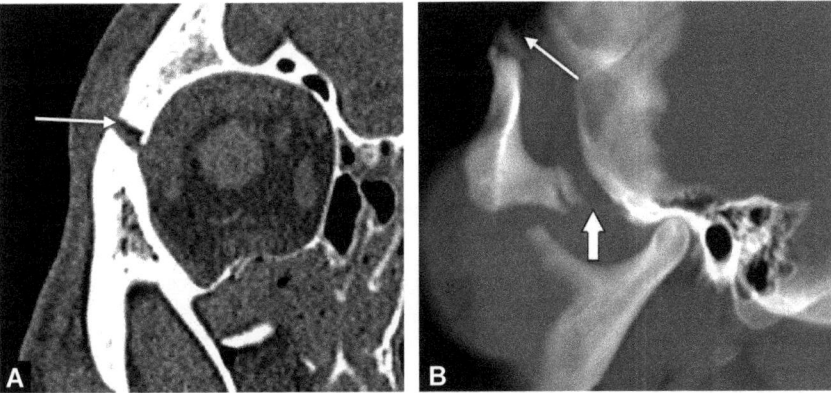

Figs. 17.6A and B: Le Fort type 3 fracture. Fracture line through lateral orbital wall (arrows), and the zygomatic bone (block arrow).

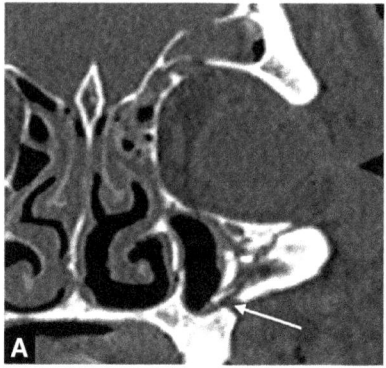
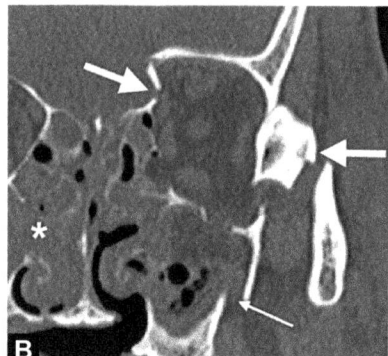
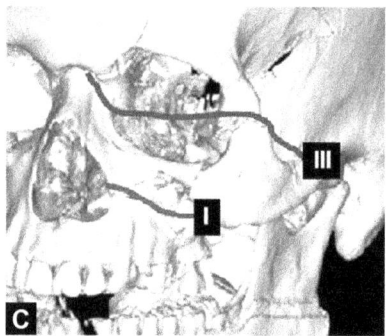

Figs. 17.7A to C: Combined Le Fort type 1 and 3 fracture. (A) Horizontal Le Fort I fracture line (arrow); (B) Le Fort III fracture involving medial and lateral orbital wall and zygoma (thick arrows). Hemosinus (asterisk); (C) Le Fort III fracture line (III) and Le Fort I fracture line (I).

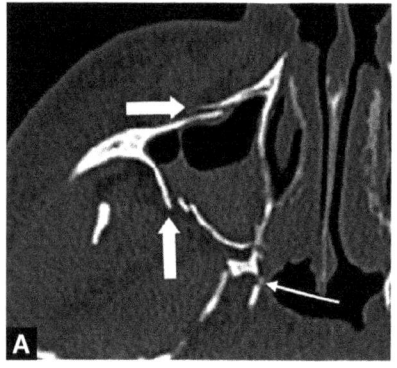
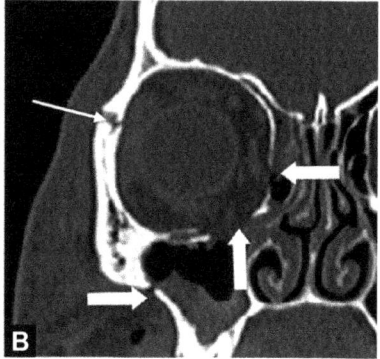
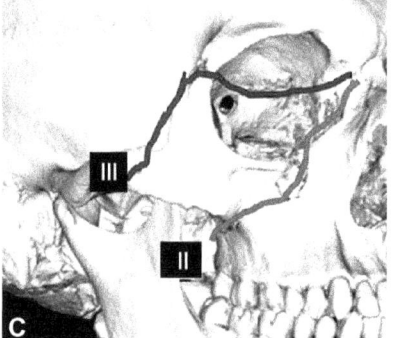

Figs. 17.8A to C: Combined Le Fort type 2 and 3 fracture. (A) Fracture in posterior maxillary wall (block arrows) and pterygoid plate (thin arrow); (B) Le Fort II fracture involving medial and inferior orbital wall, and lateral maxillary wall (block arrows); (C) Lateral orbital wall fracture as a part of Le Fort III fracture. Le Fort III fracture line (III). Le Fort II fracture line (II).

Other Complex Fractures

Naso-orbitoethmoid Complex Fractures

- These are comminuted fractures, involving unilateral or bilateral maxillary buttresses which occur as a consequence of high impact force to the nose.
- They involve nasal bones, nasal septum, medial orbital walls and ethmoid sinuses. The nasoorbitoethmoid area is involved in this type of injury (Fig. 17.9).
- These fractures are subclassified into three types (Markowitz and Manson classification) based on whether medial canthal tendon is involved or not.[3] Medial canthal tendon cannot be directly visualized on CT; however, when the fracture is comminuted, it is more likely to cause avulsion of the tendon which inserts on the medial orbital wall.
- *Type 1*: Single large NOE fragment bearing the medial canthal tendon (Fig. 17.10).
- *Type 2*: Comminuted NOE fragment, but medial canthal tendon remains attached to one fragment.
- *Type 3*: Comminuted fracture, medial canthal tendon is detached (Figs. 17.11A and B).

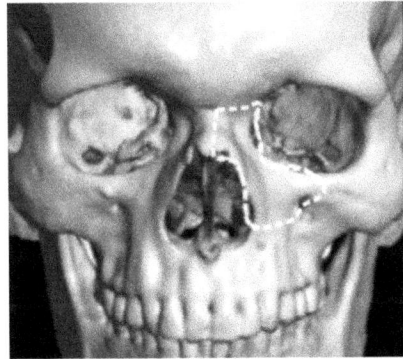

Fig. 17.9: Nasoorbitoethmoid complex (dashed line).

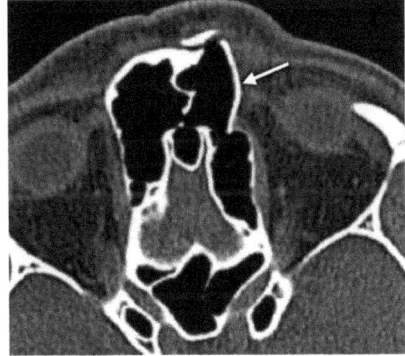

Fig. 17.10: Type 1 nasoorbitoethmoid fracture (arrow).

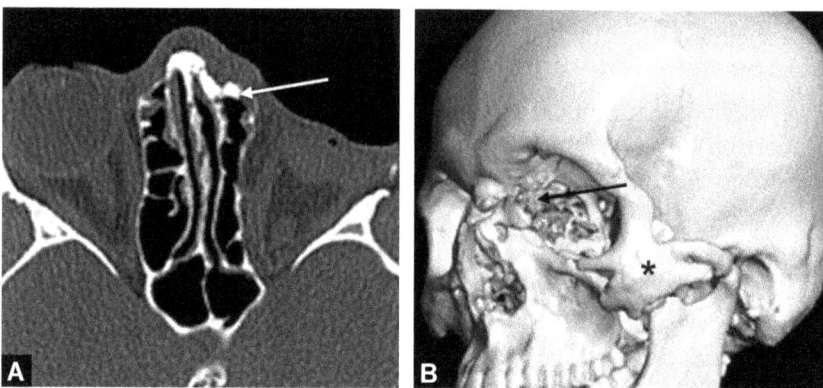

Figs. 17.11A and B: Type 3 nasoorbitoethmoid fracture (arrows) with **tetrapod fracture** (asterisk).

Zygomaticomaxillary Complex Fractures

- *Synonym*: Tetrapod or quadripod fracture.
- Mechanism of injury for these injuries is direct blow to malar eminence.
- Zygomatic bone becomes dissociated from the rest of face or calvarium (Figs. 17.12A and B).
- Result in orbital complications and mastication difficulties.

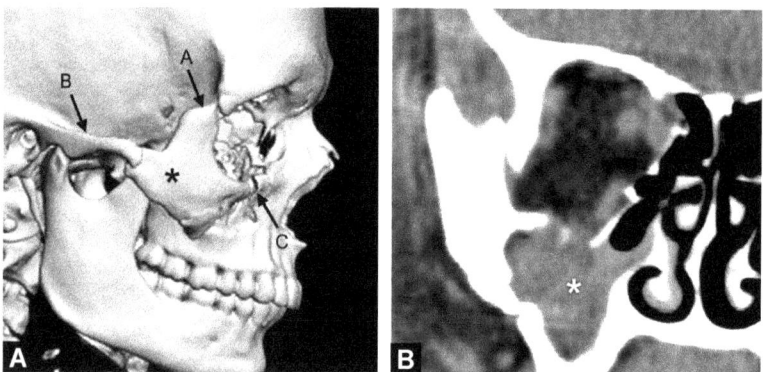

Figs. 17.12A and B: (A) **Tetrapod fracture** (asterisk); (B) Hemosinus (white asterisk). (A: Zygomaticofrontal suture; B: Zygomaticotemporal suture; C: Zygomaticomaxillary suture).

Fractures Involving Single Bone or Single Buttress

Frontal Sinus Fractures

- Frontal sinus walls are thin and hence are often involved in injuries involving the upper jaw region, and the anterior wall is frequently involved.
- Posterior wall fractures are more ominous as these are associated with cranial complications.
- Inferomedially placed fractures result in obstruction of nasolacrimal duct and impaired drainage (Figs. 17.13A and B).

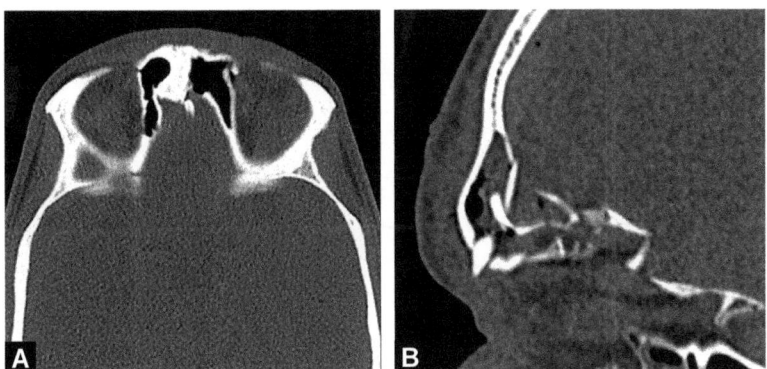

Figs. 17.13A and B: (A) **Frontal sinus fracture** (bilateral); (B) Left frontal sinus posterior wall fracture.

Nasal Bone Fractures

- These are the commonest facial fractures, as nasal bone is thin and superficially located.
- Mechanism of injury may be an anterior or lateral blunt force.
- Classification (based on the anatomical plane): These are divided into three types:
  - *Type 1*: Below the anterior nasal spine, septum not involved.
  - *Type 2*: Septum and anterior nasal spine also involved.
  - *Type 3*: Septum, orbital bone involved. Intracranial structures may be involved.
- Nasal septum injury may be associated with disruption of perichondrium and hematoma formation. As a long-term sequelae, this can result in ischemia, cartilage necrosis and septal perforation.

Imaging:
- Plain radiographs are most frequently used.
  - Low kVp settings and coned view are required (Fig. 17.14).
  - Ancillary views such as axial view, lateral and Water's view are complementary to confirm diagnosis.

- Radiological signs include a horizontal lucency with displaced or overlapping fragments.
- *Imaging pitfall*: Nasomaxillary suture or nasociliary groove may be mistaken for fracture (Figs. 17.15 and 17.16).
- Vertical lucent lines which are grooves for anterior ethmoidal nerves can also be confused as fractures.
- Computed tomography is more accurate than radiographs.
- High resolution ultrasonography has also been advocated especially in children.

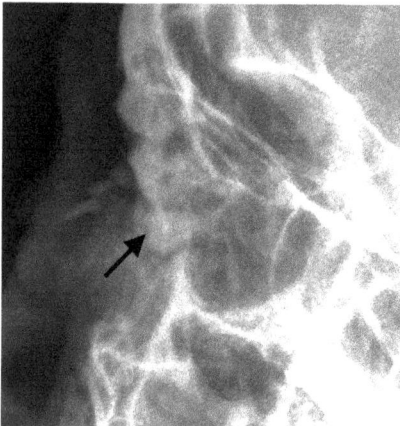

Fig. 17.14: Right nasal bone **comminuted fracture.**

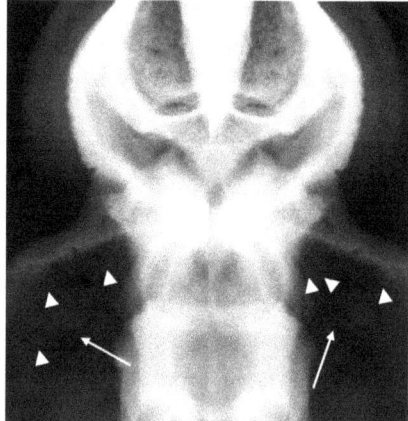

Fig. 17.15: Lateral radiograph of **normal** right (a) and left (b) **nasal bones** showing nasomaxillary suture (arrows) and nasociliary groove (arrowheads).

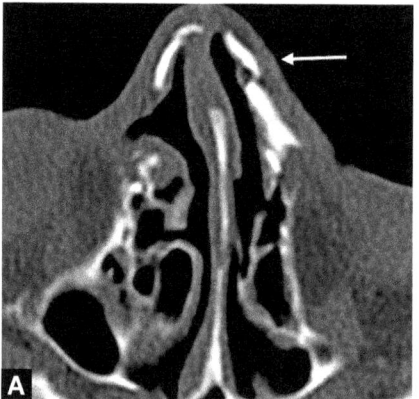
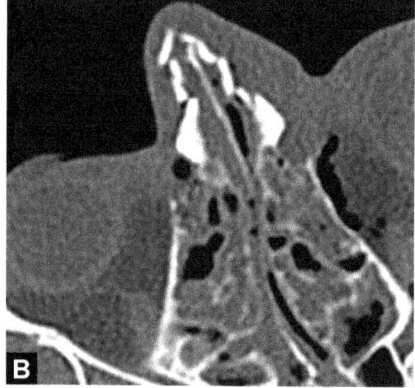

Figs. 17.16A and B: (A) Left nasal bone fracture associated with **nasoorbitoethmoid fracture** (arrow); (B) Bilateral **nasal bone comminuted fracture**.

Maxillary Sinus Fractures (Figs. 17.17A and B)

- Isolated displaced or undisplaced fractures of the anterior and lateral walls of the maxillary sinus may be seen in lesser degrees of trauma.
- As the maxillary alveolar process constitutes the floor of the sinus, its fractures involve the maxillary sinus too.
- Similarly orbital trauma involving its floor affects the sinus.
- Posterior maxillary fractures occur as part of the Le Fort fractures involving pterygoid plates and even sphenoid sinus.

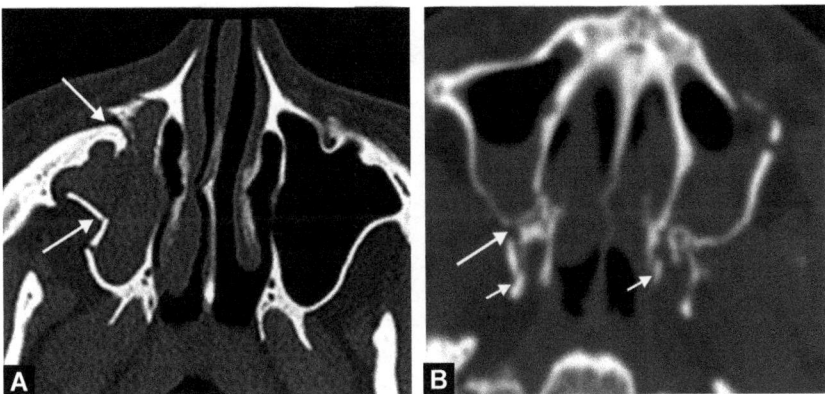

Figs. 17.17A and B: (A) Anterior and lateral wall of right **maxillary sinus fractures** (arrows). (B) Posterior maxillary fracture involving pterygoid tubercle (arrow) and pterygoid plates (small arrows).

Orbital Blowout Fractures

- Isolated fractures of the orbit result from direct blunt force received on the globe. This causes outward displacement of its walls with resultant increase in orbital volume and enophthalmos.
- Most commonly affected wall is the inferior, followed by the medial wall.
- The fractured inferior wall protrudes into the maxillary sinus along with the orbital fat, with or without the inferior rectus muscle (Figs. 17.18A and B).
- Medial wall injury involves the adjoining ethmoid sinuses (Figs. 17.19A and B).

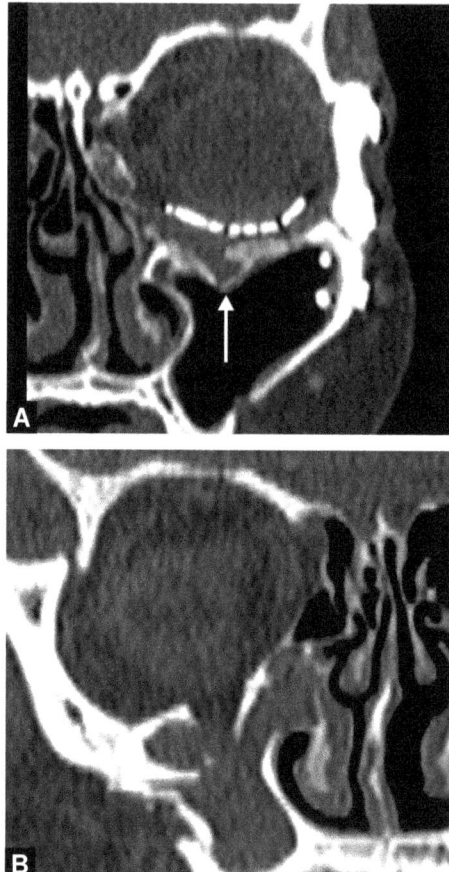

Figs. 17.18A and B: (A) Left **inferior orbital wall blowout fracture**, post repair. Note the infraorbital nerve entrapment (arrow). (B) Right inferior orbital blowout fracture.

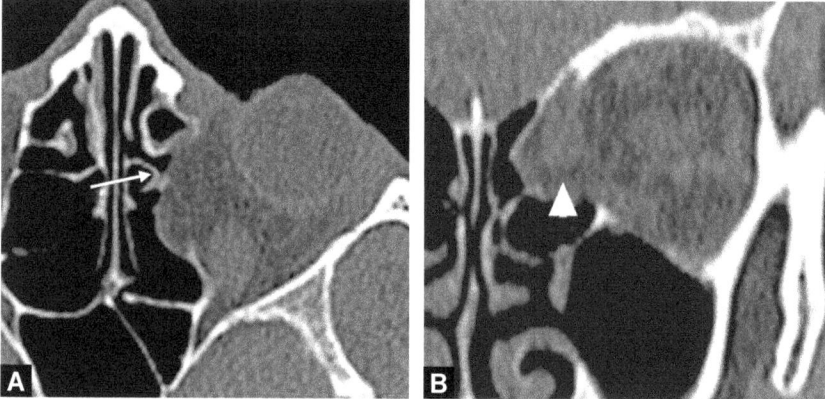

Figs. 17.19A and B: (A) Left-sided **medial wall orbital blowout fracture** (arrow). (B) Medial rectus muscle entrapment (arrowhead).

COMPLICATIONS OF SINUS FRACTURES

- In the acute phase, sinuses are opacified due to hemorrhage (*hemosinus*). As the hemosinus resolves, residual soft tissue or mucosal thickening remains.
- *Pneumocephalus* (intracranial air) may result from sinus fractures of ethmoid and frontal sinuses that violate the skull base.

Region-wise complications of these fractures are enlisted in Tables 17.4 and 17.5 and illustrative care.

Table 17.4: Complications of the complex facial fractures.	
Fracture type	Complications
Nasoorbitoethmoid (NOE) complex fractures	• Enophthalmos (as the orbital volume increases) • Cerebrospinal fluid rhinorrhea (due to cribriform plate disruption) (Figs. 17.20A and B) • Telecanthus (due to avulsion of medial canthal tendon) • Epistaxis (following injury to anterior/posterior ethmoidal arteries) • Lacrimal sac/duct injury leading to epiphora, dacryocystitis (Figs. 17.21A and B) • Intracranial infection (meningitis, epidural abscess, cerebral abscess) • Orbital apex syndrome • Optic nerve injury • Globe injury (vision loss)
Zygomaticomaxillary complex fracture (tetrapod fracture)	• Increased orbital volume and enophthalmos • Other orbital complications like globe injury/extraocular muscle injury, hematoma • Orbital apex syndrome • Superior orbital fissure syndrome • Difficulty in mastication

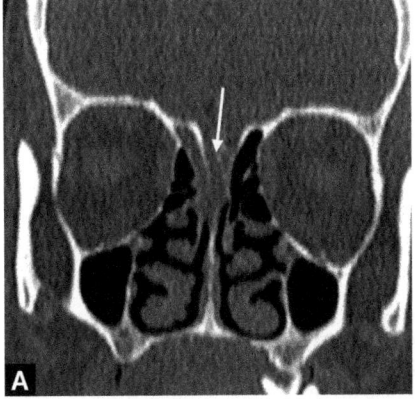 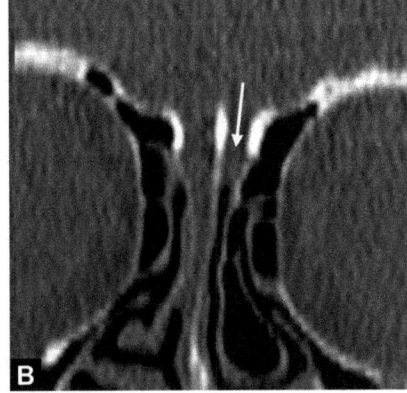

Figs. 17.20A and B: (A) Cerebrospinal fluid rhinorrhea secondary to traumatic defect in right cribriform plate (arrow); (B) Magnified image showing the defect (arrow).

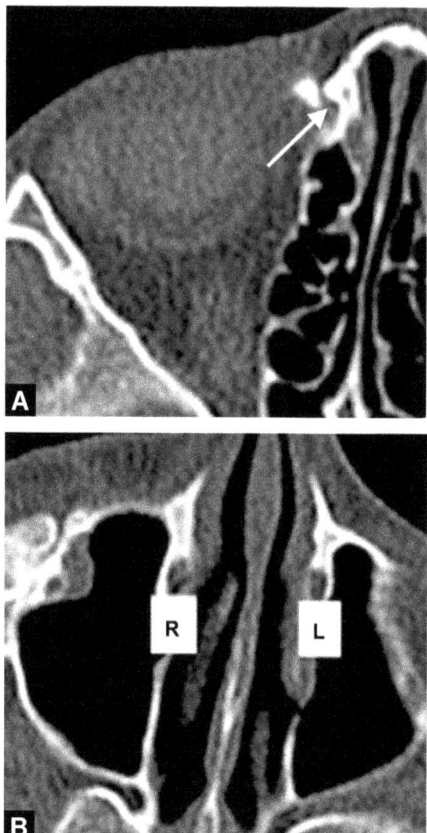

Figs. 17.21A and B: (A) Right-sided canalicular block by a fracture fragment (arrow); (B) Note normal right (R) and left (L) bony NLDs.

Table 17.5: Complications of the facial fractures involving single bone or single buttress.	
Frontal sinus fractures	• Cerebrospinal fluid rhinorrhea • Brain herniation, intracranial infection (posterior wall fractures) • Nasofrontal duct obstruction and mucocele (medially located fractures)
Nasal bone fracture involving septal cartilage	• Septal hematoma and impaired breathing • Secondary infection, abscess leading to septal perforation
Maxillary sinus roof fractures (orbital blowout fractures)	• Extraocular muscle entrapment following herniation • Infraorbital nerve injury • Globe injury
Posterior maxillary fractures	• Pterygoid plate disruption, sphenoid bone extension leading to carotid artery injury/carotid cavernous fistula • Skull base foramina disruption (e.g. foramen ovale)
Maxillary alveolar process fractures	• Dental complications (tooth avulsion, tooth fractures, etc.) • Secondary infection of sinus (due to oral flora)

Illustrative Case

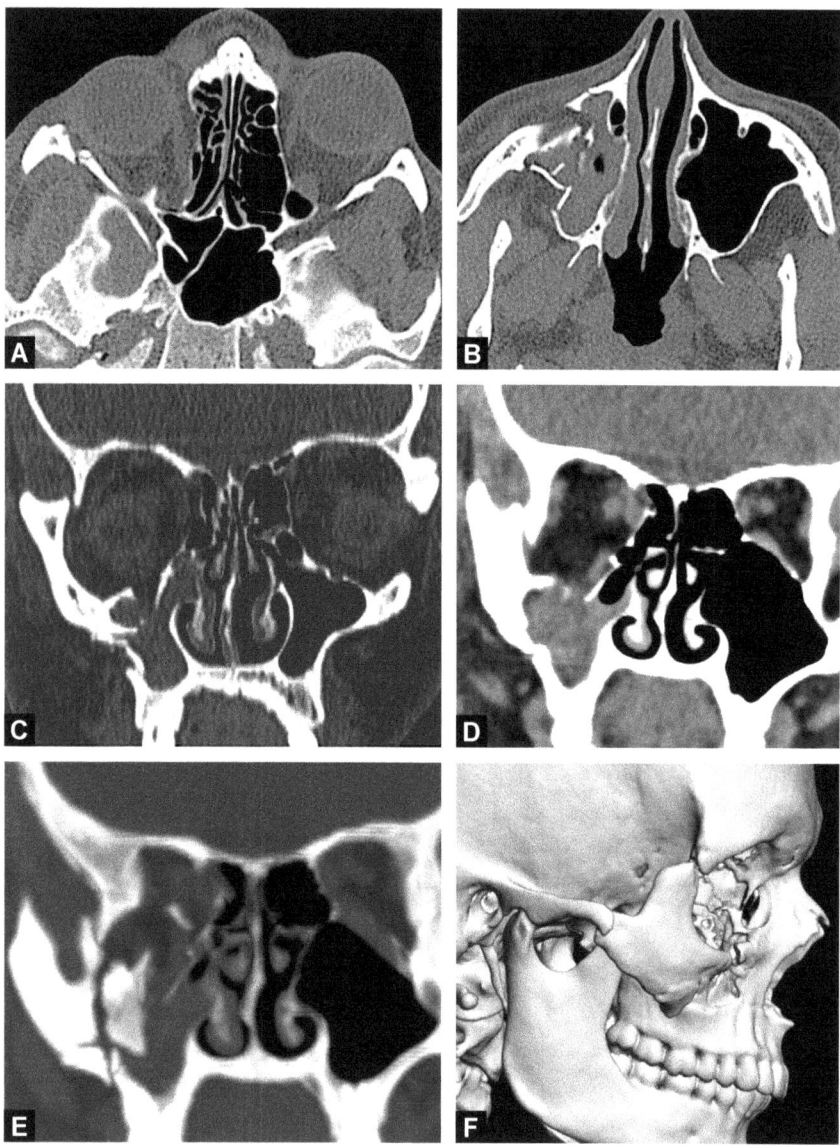

Figs. 17.22A to F

ILLUSTRATIVE CASE IN A REPORTING FORMAT

Structures Involved

Table 17.6

	RT	LT		RT	LT
Frontal sinus					
- Anterior table	N	N			
- Posterior table			Sphenoid sinus		
- Sinus floor	N	N	- Anterior wall	N	N
- Frontonasal duct	N	N	- Roof	N	N
- Sinus opacification	N	N	Posterior wall	N	N
Sinus expansion					
	N	N			
	N	N			
Ethmoid sinus and bone			Zygomatic bone		
- Sinus septae	N	N	- Arch	N	N
- Cribriform plate	N	N	- Zygomaticomaxillary suture	F	N
Fovea ethmoidalis	N	N			
Orbit			Mandible		
- Medial wall (lamina papyracea)	F	N	- Condyle	N	N
			- Ramus	N	N
- Lateral wall	F	N	Symphysis menti		
- Roof	N	N			
- Floor	F	N			
- Optic canal	N	N			
- Superior orbital fissure	N	N			
Inferior orbital fissure	N	N			
Maxillary sinus	O		Nasal cavity		
- Anterior wall	F	N	- Turbinates (superior, middle, inferior)	N	N
- Roof	F	N			
- Posteromedial wall	N	N	- Nasal septum		
Posterolateral wall	F	N	Nasal bone	N	N
Pterygoid plates	N	N	Intracranial complications	None	
Pterygopalatine fossa	N	N			

(N: Normal; F: Fracture; if displaced add D; O: Obstructed).
Impression: Right sided zygomaticomaxillary complex fracture, medial orbital wall fracture; with right maxillary hemosinus, right enophthalmos and inferior orbital nerve entrapment.

REFERENCES

1. Winegar BA, Murillo H, Tantiwongkosi B. Spectrum of critical imaging findings in complex facial skeletal trauma. Radiographics. 2013;33(1):3-19.
2. Avery LL, Susarla SM, Novelline RA. Multidetector and three-dimensional CT evaluation of the patient with maxillofacial injury. Radiol Clin North Am. 2011;49(1):183-203.
3. Markowitz BL, Manson PN. Panfacial fractures: organization of treatment. Clin Plast Surg. 1989;16(1):105-14.

CHAPTER 18

Imaging of Cerebrospinal Fluid Leaks

Atin Kumar, Ajay Garg

- Introduction
- Clinical and Laboratory Workup
- Clinical Course
- Role of Imaging
- Imaging Modalities
  - Plain High-resolution Computed Tomography Skull Base
    - *Role*
    - *Technique*
    - *Findings*
    - *Pitfall*
  - Computed Tomography Cisternography
    - *Role*
    - *Technique*
    - *Findings*
    - *Pitfalls*
    - *Disadvantages*
  - Magnetic Resonance Cisternography (Plain)
    - *Role*
    - *Technique*
    - *Findings*
    - *Pitfalls*
  - Contrast Magnetic Resonance Cisternography
    - *Role*
    - *Technique*
    - *Findings*
    - *Advantages*
    - *Pitfall*
  - Radionuclide Cisternography
- Etiology
  - Accidental Trauma
  - Iatrogenic Trauma
  - Secondary Leaks
  - Spontaneous Leaks
- Protocol for Evaluation

INTRODUCTION

- Cerebrospinal fluid (CSF) leak or fistula is an abnormal communication of the sterile subarachnoid space with the sinonasal, sphenoid or tympanomastoid cavities caused by the presence of both an osseous and a dural defect.
- It presents clinically with rhinorrhea or otorrhea.
- It may allow the flora of the sinonasal cavity or the middle ear to spread to the intracranial compartment and lead to meningitis.
- Hence, it requires an early diagnosis and timely repair.

CLINICAL AND LABORATORY WORKUP

- Rule out other causes of nasal discharge such as allergic rhinitis, polyps, sinusitis or tumors.
- Biochemical examination of fluid for beta-2 transferrin levels which is a highly specific protein for CSF. If facility for testing is not available, then indirect method of confirmation of CSF is by evaluation of glucose and protein levels.

CLINICAL COURSE

- Most of the acute leaks resolve spontaneously with conservative management, sometimes aided by decreasing CSF pressure by a lumbar or external ventricular drain.
- Surgery required for nonhealing, long duration leaks (usually more than 7-10 days) or for associated conditions
- Imaging required as a preclude for surgery.

ROLE OF IMAGING

- To localize the exact site of the leak.
- To diagnose any associated condition such as a tumor or encephalocele.
- To provide a roadmap for surgery.

IMAGING MODALITIES

Plain High-resolution Computed Tomography Skull Base (Figs. 18.1A and B)

Role

- This is the first line of imaging and has an excellent accuracy with a sensitivity of 84-95%.
- Best investigation to exactly delineate the defect as well as the surgical anatomy for planning and guidance.
- Can be done even when the patient is not actively leaking.

Technique

- High-resolution thin sections through the face and skull base including the mastoids in supine position.
- Multiplanar reformats done in coronal and sagittal plane.

Findings

- Detects site of bony defect or fractures.

Indirect signs include pneumocephalus, meningoencephaloceles and fluid in paranasal sinuses just beneath the site of defects.

Pitfall

- The bony defect detected may not be associated with a dural defect.

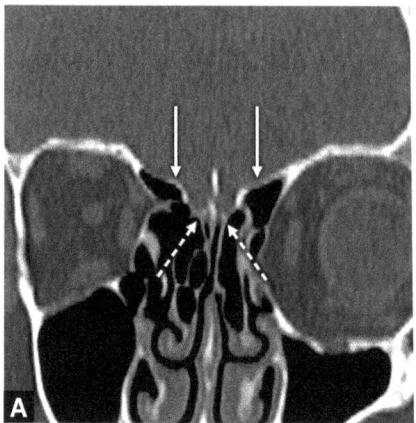 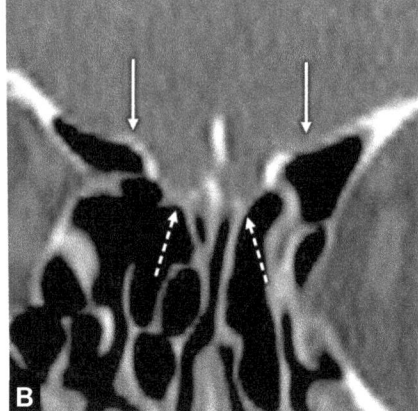

Figs. 18.1A and B: Normal high-resolution computed tomography (HRCT) skull base. Coronal reformatted CT image (A) (magnified in B) shows cribriform plates (dotted arrows) are joined to the roof of ethmoids (fovea ethmoidalis) (white arrows) by a thin bone of lateral lamella.

Computed Tomography Cisternography (CT Cisternography)

Role

- It is the most accurate method for investigation of active CSF leak with a sensitivity of 72–81% for detection of leaks.
- It is done when the patient is having an active leak.
- Considered as a gold standard.
- Done in cases where there are multiple fractures.

Technique

- Cotton pledgets are placed in both nostrils of the patient.
- Take initial precontrast thin section multidetector computed tomography. (MDCT) in prone position.
- Perform lumbar puncture with adequate sterile precautions.
- Instill 10 mL of iodinated nonionic contrast (Iohexol) under fluoroscopic guidance.
- Keep the patient in reverse Trendelenburg position for 15 minutes to allow the contrast to reach cranium and distribute freely.
- Obtain thin sections computed tomography (CT) of skull base in coronal plane with patient lying prone (Figs. 18.2A and B).

Findings

- Cerebrospinal fluid leaks are seen as areas of contrast pooling in the paranasal sinuses or nasal cavity adjacent to the site of defect.
- Often the direct contrast column is seen extending through the bony defect.
- Can measure Hounsfield unit values in suspected regions and compare with precontrast images–a 2-fold increase in attenuation confirms the leak.

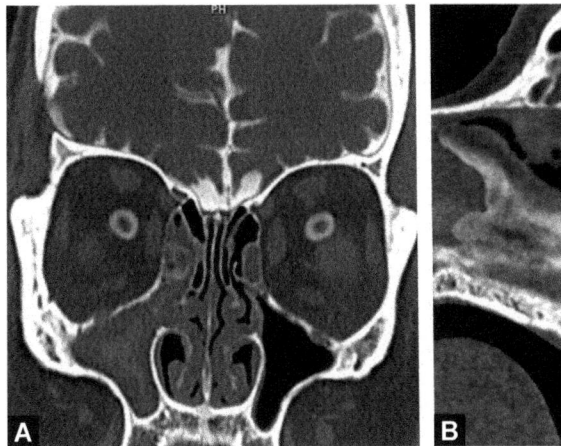
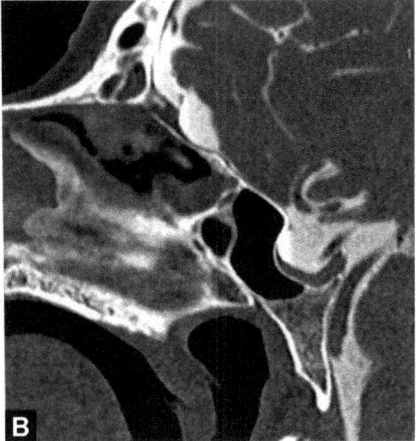

Figs. 18.2A and B: Normal CT cisternography. (A) Coronal and (B) Sagittal reformatted images. The contrast is seen to opacify the sulcal spaces within the intracranial compartment with intact base of skull. No contrast is seen to leak into the nasal cavity or paranasal sinuses.

- If doubtful, repeat localized section with change in patient position. The contrast will change in position.
- If high flow leak is present, the intracranial contrast may show a washout in the ipsilateral compartment.
- Change in position of contrast with change in patient position
- Souffle effect.

Pitfalls

- Low flow fistulas or thin hairline fractures may not be demonstrated due to higher viscosity of contrast.
- Inadequate contrast distribution in region of interest either due to improper technique or adhesions in subarachnoid space secondary to bleed.
- Difficult to appreciate small amount of dilute contrast medium adjacent to a surrounding bony structure or sometimes highly dense contrast which mimics bone.

Disadvantages

- High radiation.
- Risks associated with lumbar puncture.
- Adverse reactions to contrast.

Magnetic Resonance Cisternography (Plain) (MR Cisternography) (Fig. 18.3A)

Role

- A nonradiating and noninvasive method with a sensitivity of 94% for detecting leaks.

- It is good for characterization of the contents of the leak–can diagnose meningoencephaloceles by detecting meninges and brain tissue within. Intravenous contrast can be helpful for seeing dural enhancement in case of suspected meningoencephalocele.

Technique

- Predominantly utilizes heavily T2-weighted 3D sequences [constructive interference in steady-state (CISS) or driven equilibrium (DRIVE) or fast imaging employing steady-state acquisition (FIESTA)]
- Done in prone position.

Findings

- Detects leak as a hyperintense signal intensity within the paranasal sinuses in continuation with CSF with an overlying defect at the bone-dura interface.
- The signal of the leak is matching that of the CSF. The signal of fluid due to rhinosinusitis, if present, is usually slightly less hyperintense and does not parallel that of CSF.
- Herniation of brain content can also be detected.

Pitfalls

- Indirect method of detecting leaks as fluid intensity in the sinuses is presumed to be of CSF.
- Sometimes difficult to differentiate from secretions in sinuses.

Contrast Magnetic Resonance Cisternography (Fig.18.3B)

Role

- This is performed with intrathecal administration of MR contrast agent and has a sensitivity close to 100% for high-flow leaks.
- Used as a problem solving tool as off-label use of gadolinium contrast.

Technique

- About 0.5–1 mL of intrathecal gadolinium contrast (Gd-DTPA) injected after lumbar puncture followed by same positional maneuvers as in CT cisternography.
- Magnetic resonance (MR) is typically done after an hour of intrathecal contrast administration. However, the window for imaging is reported to be up to 24 hours.
- T1-weighted 3D sequence is obtained in coronal plane with patient lying prone.

Findings

- Shows CSF leaks as continuous column of hyperintense signal CSF on T1 image from intracranial compartment to within the paranasal sinuses through the defect in bone-dura interface.

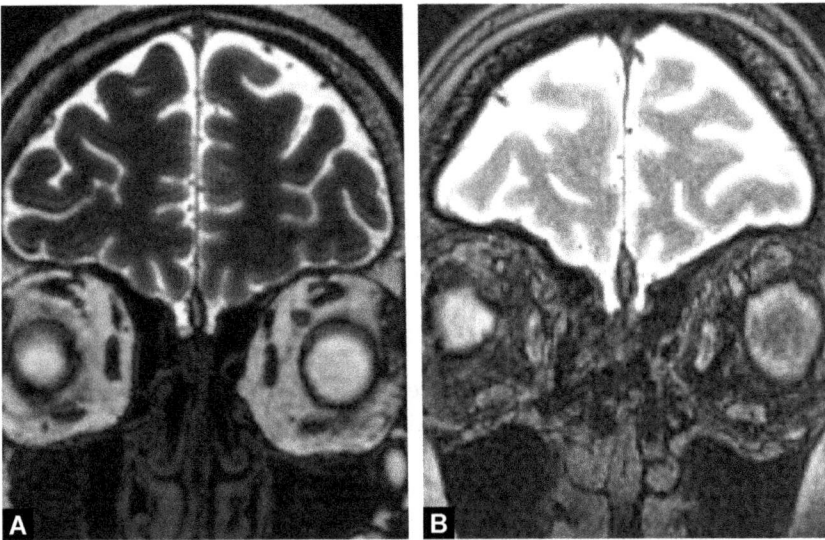

Figs. 18.3A and B: (A) Normal plain magnetic resonance cisternography; and (B) Contrast magnetic resonance cisternography. Coronal reformatted images. The constructive interference in steady-state (CISS) sequence shows: (A) the hyperintense cerebrospinal fluid in sulcal spaces limited to the intracranial compartment. In the contrast study (B) gadolinium is seen to opacify the sulcal spaces within the intracranial compartment with intact base of skull on this T1 weighted coronal MR image. No contrast is seen to leak into the nasal cavity or paranasal sinuses.

Advantages

- Nonradiating
- Better than plain MR cisternography for detection.
- Lower dosage and better CSF distribution of contrast compared to CT cisternography.
- Contrast stays longer in CSF. Hence, imaging can be done up to 24 hours–helps to detect intermittent leaks.

Pitfall

- Safety of the intrathecal contrast not well established–not approved by the United States Food and Drug Administration for potential risk of neurotoxicity. However, many European studies have shown no significant adverse effects with off-label use.

Radionuclide Cisternography

- Performed after intrathecal administration of technitium-99 labeled diethylenetriaminepentaacetic acid (DTPA).
- The radioactivity is measured after 24–48 hours in the pledgets placed in the nasal cavity for confirming presence of CSF leak.
- More helpful for confirming presence of CSF leak and not so good for detection of site of leak.
- Rarely used now in clinical practice.

ETIOLOGY

The numerous causes of CSF rhinorrhea are:
- *Trauma*: accidental or iatrogenic
- Secondary leaks
  - Tumor related
  - Congenital defects
  - Postradiation or chemotherapy
- Spontaneous leaks.

Accidental Trauma (Figs. 18.4 to 18.6)

- It is the most common etiology seen in 10–30% of all skull base fractures.
- The patients present early within the first few days.
- Most common sites—cribriform plates, ethmoid roof, frontal sinus, sphenoid sinus, tegmen tympani.
- Cerebrospinal fluid may leak into the sinonasal cavity (in frontobasal fractures) or into the middle ear cavity and mastoid air cells (in temporal bone trauma).
- Acute CSF rhinorrhea (80%) or otorrhea is the usual clinical presentation.
- Most posttraumatic CSF leaks heal spontaneously with conservative management.
- Meningitis may be seen in up to 50% of cases, if the leak does not resolve spontaneously or is not repaired.
- Persistent leaks for longer than 7–10 days, in spite of CSF diversion, require intracranial or endoscopic repair.
- Larger skull base defects (>1.5 cm) or severely comminuted fractures, with meningoencephalocele, also require surgical repair.

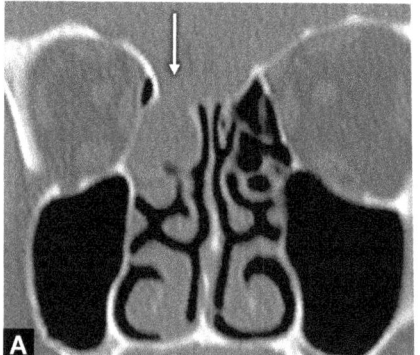 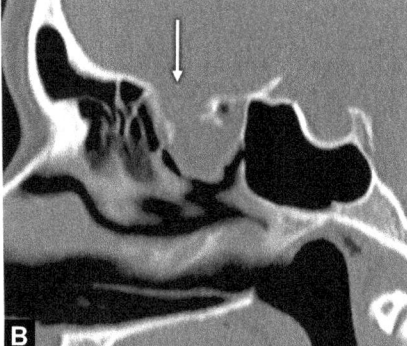

Figs. 18.4A and B: Fracture anterior skull base. (A) Coronal and (B) Sagittal reformatted high-resolution computed tomography skull base images in an 18-year-old male with road traffic injury shows a bony defect at the right ethmoid roof (arrows) with fluid density seen in ethmoid sinus just beneath the defect.

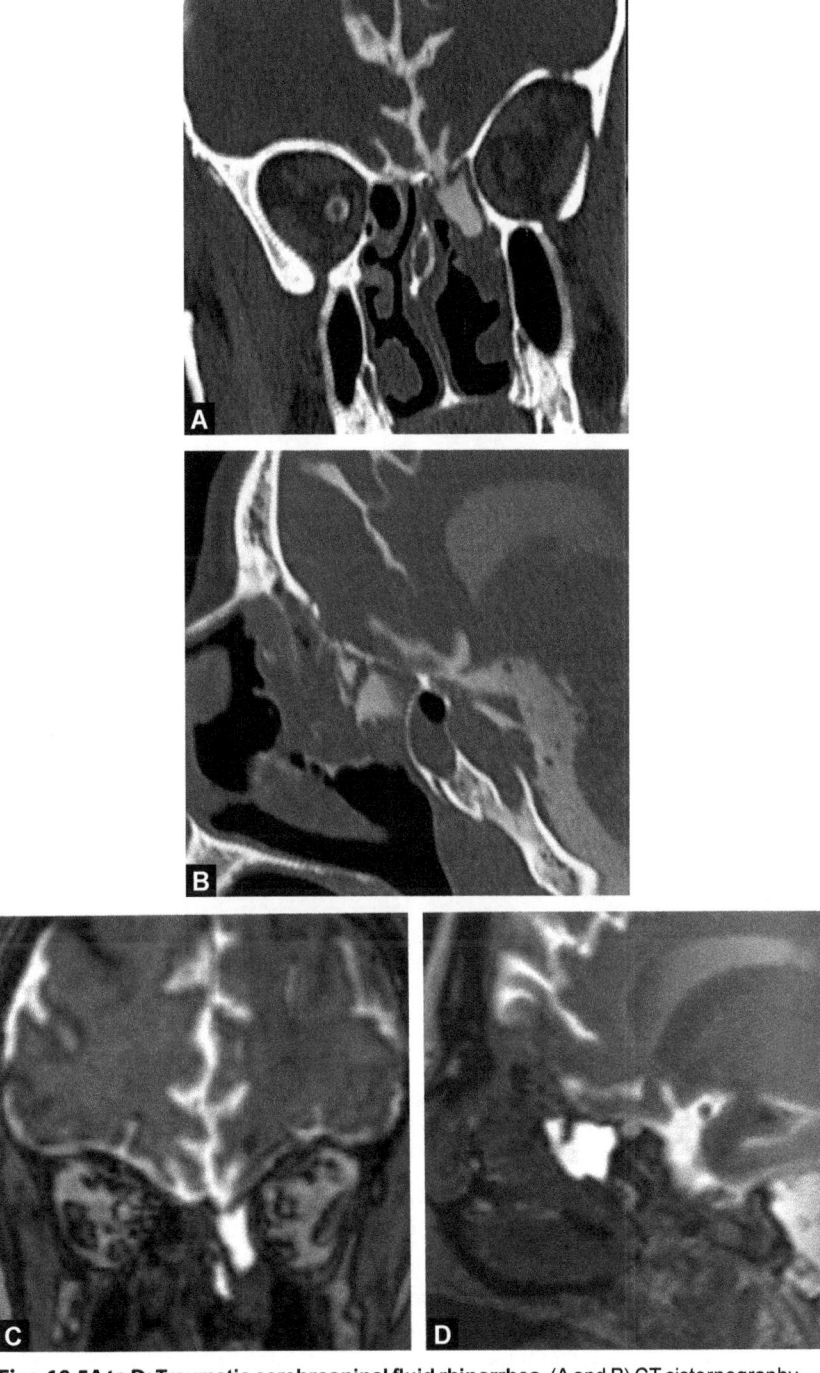

Figs. 18.5A to D: Traumatic cerebrospinal fluid rhinorrhea. (A and B) CT cisternography—bony defect at the left ethmoid roof with contrast column extending from intracranial compartment to the ethmoid sinus; (C and D) Contrast MR cisternography—confirms the findings of CT.

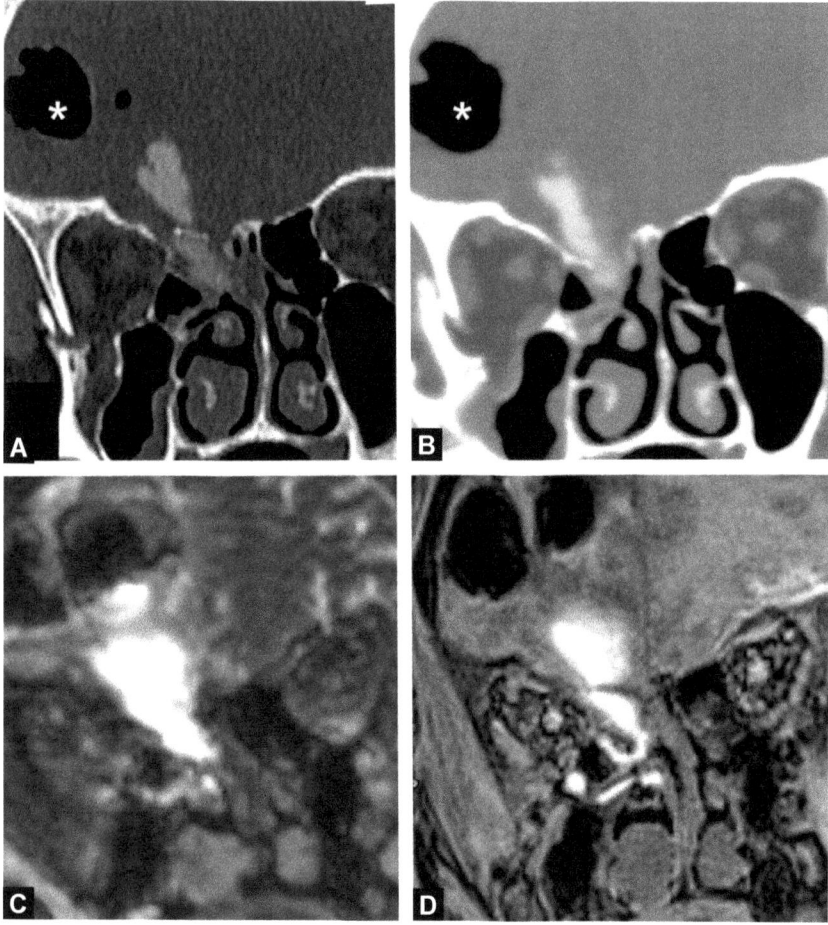

Figs. 18.6A to D: Traumatic cerebrospinal fluid rhinorrhea. (A and B) CT cisternography. Bony defect at the right ethmoid roof with contrast column extending from intracranial compartment to the ethmoid sinus. Pneumocephalus (star) seen in brain. Fracture of lateral orbital wall on right side; (C and D) Contrast MR cisternography shows contrast extending from intracranial compartment to the ethmoid sinus and nasal cavity.

Iatrogenic Trauma (Figs. 18.7A and B)

- Secondary to neurosurgical or otolaryngological procedures along skull base, mostly endoscopic and endonasal procedures. It can also occur following craniotomy.
- Common sites—cribriform plates along vertical insertion of middle turbinate, frontal sinuses and regions of variant anatomy including pneumatization of skull base.
- Accounts for 16% of all traumatic CSF rhinorrhea cases.
- Present within first 2 weeks following the operative procedure.

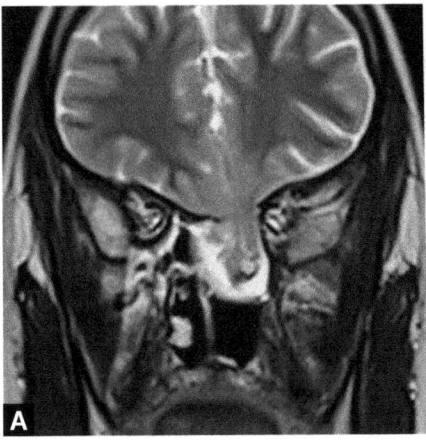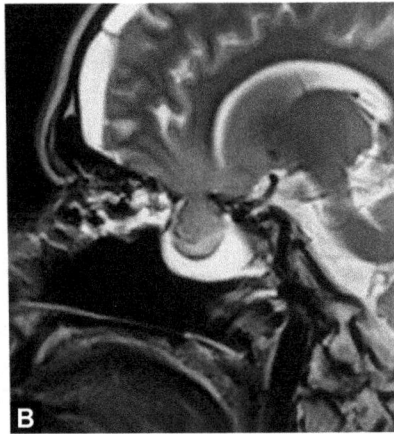

Figs. 18.7A and B: Iatrogenic leak. (A) Coronal; and (B) Sagittal MR images in a 27-year-old male who underwent transsphenoidal skull base surgery 2 months back shows a defect in the roof of the sphenoid sinus with cerebrospinal fluid and brain herniation consistent with encephalocele.

- Usually resolve spontaneously with conservative measures.
- Presence of packs or hemorrhage secondary to the procedure may hamper the interpretation of CT cisternography.

Secondary Leaks

- It refers to the leaks of nontraumatic etiology but with a definite pathologic cause.
- Etiologies include erosion by tumors, mucoceles, postradiation changes, osteonecrosis, congenital (encephaloceles, persistent canals through skull base) (Figs. 18.8A and B).
- Its identification is important for surgical management.

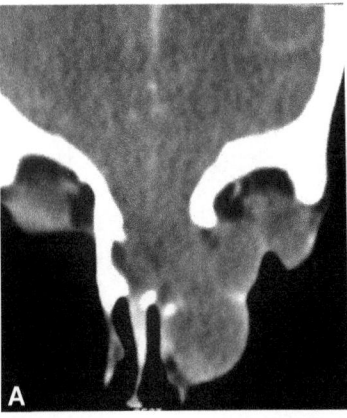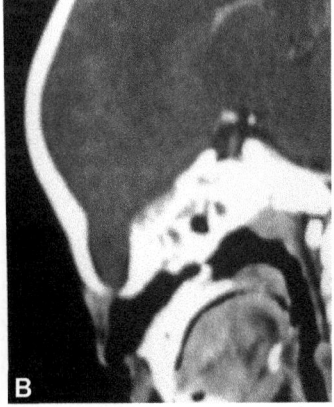

Figs. 18.8A and B: Congenital frontoethmoidal encephalocele. (A) Coronal; and (B) Sagittal reformatted CT images. A large defect is seen in anterior skull base through which brain parenchyma is herniating into the ethmoid sinuses.

Spontaneous Leaks

- Cerebrospinal fluid leaks occurring without any identifiable cause such as trauma, surgery, underlying lesion or congenital abnormality.
- It may represent 4–40% of all CSF leaks.
- Most often these patients present with clinical features of raised intracranial pressure and are found to have idiopathic intracranial hypertension (IIH) (Figs. 18.9A and B).Imaging required to rule out any cause of raised intracranial pressure and to evaluate for features of IIH (given in Table 18.1).
- Empty sella, widening of optic sheath with tortuosity, scleral flattening at posterior aspect, scalloping of inner calvarial table, widening of skull base foramina, meningoceles, low-lying cerebellar tonsils with inferiorly displaced brainstem and cerebellum. MR venography may reveal stenosis of transverse sinuses.
- Most common sites of leak are cribriform plate or ethmoid roof.

Table 18.1: Radiological signs of idiopathic intracranial hypertension.
• Empty sella
• Widening of optic sheath with tortuosity
• Scleral flattening at posterior aspect
• Scalloping of inner calvarial table
• Widening of skull base foramina
• Meningoceles
• Low-lying cerebellar tonsils with inferiorly displaced brainstem and cerebellum
• Stenosis of transverse sinuses on magnetic resonance venography

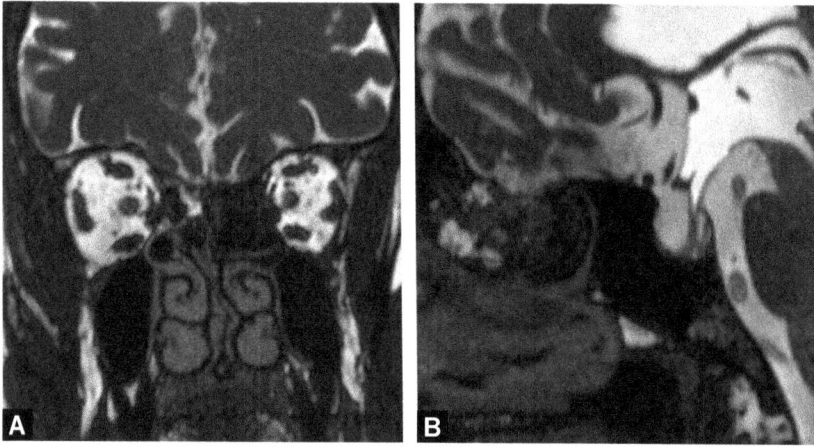

Figs. 18.9A and B: Intracranial idiopathic hypertension in a 45-year-old female patient with spontaneous cerebrospinal fluid (CSF) rhinorrhea. Coronal MR cisternography CISS image (A) shows a fluid signal intensity column in the right ethmoid sinus suggestive of CSF leak. (B) Empty sella seen on the sagittal image.

- Management requires surgery for the defect as well as medication to decrease intracranial pressure so as to prevent future recurrences.

PROTOCOL FOR EVALUATION (FLOWCHART 18.1)

- Most leaks usually resolve either spontaneously or conservative measures including lumbar drain placement by 7-10 days. Imaging is required if persistent leak present.
- Plain high-resolution computed tomography (HRCT) skull base is the first imaging modality. If shows a clear defect in skull base at a single site which is correlating clinically with side of leak, then no more investigation is required. The surgery can be planned based on CT.
- If the HRCT shows multiple defects or if the site of defect is equivocal, then further evaluation is done based on how strong is the suspicion for

Flowchart 18.1: Algorithm for workup of cerebrospinal fluid (CSF) rhinorrhea.

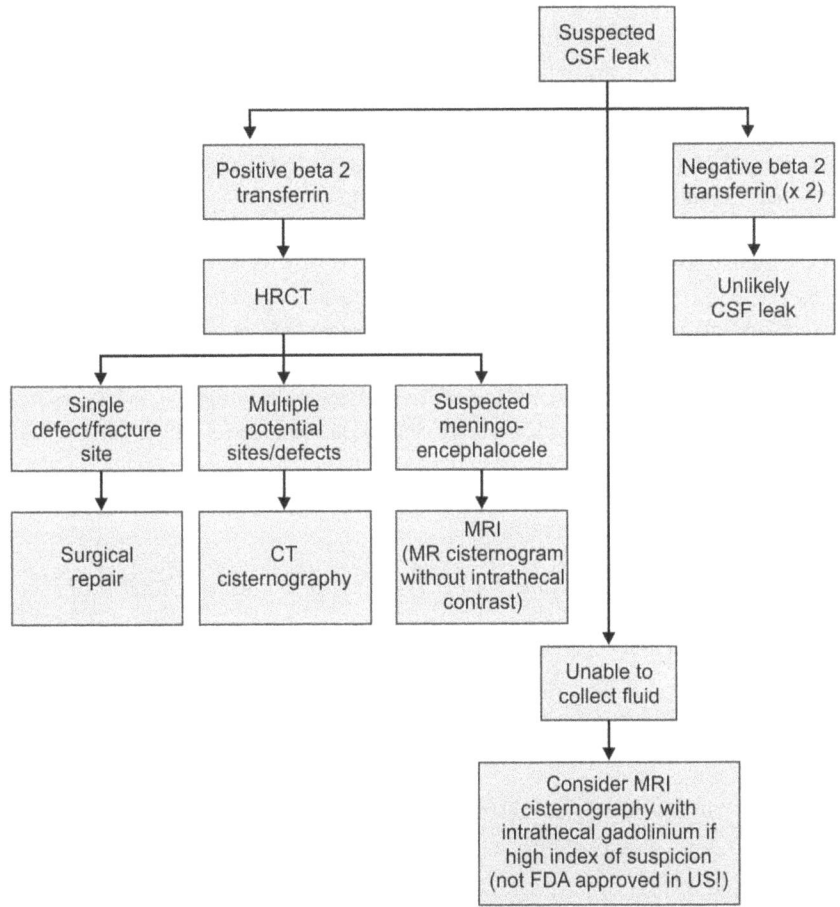

(HRCT: high-resolution computed tomography; FDA: Food and Drug Administration)

CSF rhinorrhea. If it is a confirmed CSF leak clinically and biochemically, then CT cisternography can be done as the next investigation. If there is a doubt whether it is CSF rhinorrhea or not, then plain MR cisternography can be done as the next investigation being noninvasive and nonradiating.
- If plain HRCT findings reveal a possibility of an encephalocele or a tumor or congenital defect, then MR cisternography should be done after it with or without intravenous contrast.
- MR cisternography with intrathecal contrast is reserved as a problem-solving tool (off-label use).
- Contrast CT and MR cisternography are particularly useful in the setting of multiple defects and in recurrence following surgery.

BIBLIOGRAPHY

1. Algin O, Hakyemez, B, Gokalp G, et al. The contribution of 3D-CISS and contrast-enhanced MR cisternography in detecting cerebrospinal fluid leak in patients with rhinorrhea. Br J Radiol. 2010;83:225-32.
2. Baugnon KL, Hudgins PA. Skull base fractures and their complications. Neuroimaging Clin N Am. 2014;24(3):439-65.
3. Connor SE. Imaging of skull-base cephalocoeles and cerebrospinal fluid leaks. Clin Radiol. 2010;65(10):832-41.
4. Lloyd KM, DelGaudio JM, Hudgins PA. Imaging of skull base cerebrospinal fluid leaks in adults. Radiology. 2008;248(3):725-36.
5. Reddy M, Baugnon K. Imaging of cerebrospinal fluid rhinorrhea and otorrhea. Radiol Clin North Am. 2017;55(1):167-87.
6. Selcuk H, Albayram S, Ozer H, et al. Intrathecal gadolinium-enhanced MR cisternography in the evaluation of CSF leakage. AJNR Am J Neuroradiol. 2010;31(1):71-5.
7. Sherif C1, Di Ieva A, Gibson D, et al. A management algorithm for cerebrospinal fluid leak associated with anterior skull base fractures: detailed clinical and radiological follow-up. Neurosurg Rev. 2012;35:227-38.
8. Wang EW1, Vandergrift WA, Schlosser RJ. Spontaneous CSF leaks. Otolaryngol Clin North Am. 2011;44(4):845-56.

19
CHAPTER

Sinonasal Trauma and Cerebrospinal Fluid Rhinorrhea: Surgical Aspects

Kapil Sikka, Alok Thakkar

- Causes
- Evaluation and Approach to Patient with Facial Trauma
  - Soft Tissue Injuries of Face
  - Bony Sinonasal Injuries
    - Upper-third Face Fractures
    - Middle-third Face Fractures
- General Principles in Managing Facial Fractures
- Cerebrospinal Fluid Rhinorrhea
  - Symptoms
  - Signs
  - Investigations
  - Management

CAUSES

- Face is a commonly injured part of body. The common causes being road traffic accidents, interpersonal violence, injuries at workplace and home (falls and machine related injuries). Some places also witness serious injuries related to animal bites.
- Seat belts, and airbags, though have played significant protective role, facial injuries are common after road traffic accidents involving 50% of survivors.
- Management is challenging because of close proximity and possible direct impact on vital structures like upper airway, larynx, trachea, carotid artery, etc. This chapter will primarily focus on the diagnosis and management of sinonasal injuries with fractures and cerebrospinal fluid (CSF) rhinorrhea.

EVALUATION AND APPROACH TO PATIENT WITH FACIAL TRAUMA

- All major injury patients require general systemic evaluation as per advanced trauma life support (ATLS) protocols.
- Airway, spine, thoracic, cardiac and major abdominal injuries can be life threatening and take precedence.

- Careful history regarding mode of injury and exact recapitulation of events can provide a useful clue to severity and also aid in management.
- General examination for evaluation of systemic injuries and corresponding referrals is important.
- Local examination should focus on evaluation of skin and soft tissue lacerations over face. Antibiotic and tetanus prophylaxis needs to be individualized on case-to-case basis. Adequate wound assessment at times requires local or general anesthesia. Thorough wound irrigation with saline or an antiseptic aids in assessment and also to identify and remove debris and foreign bodies.
- Bony eminences and contours should be palpated for deformity, step-offs and mobility. These include the skull, orbit, zygoma, maxilla, mandible and palate.
- Some critical injuries to the eyelid, nasolacrimal duct, facial nerve, parotid duct are often missed and fare badly, if not dealt immediately.
- Eye and ear examination should be performed, and any abnormality should be assessed by an expert. Blood in ear canal, abnormal conjunctival congestion, hematoma behind the ear, etc. can be evidences of more serious skull base fracture.
- Disruption of canalicular apparatus should be suspected in eyelid injuries. Vision and ocular mobility should be grossly assessed and documented.
- Imaging may be ordered in case there is suspicion of deep injury or undetected fractures. Foreign bodies like glass or metallic pieces may be identified with imaging while some like wood may be missed. Very careful evidence of head injury should be obtained. Overt CSF rhinorrhea, nasal and ear bleed, vomiting, visual blurring, diplopia or inequality of pupil size should warrant prompt radiology to identify skull fractures and underlying brain injury.

Soft Tissue Injuries of Face

- Soft tissue injuries can be abrasions, lacerations or avulsions.
- Basic concepts of cosmetic and functional repair need to be applied while evaluating and repairing these wounds. Concepts of tattooing, wound contraction and scarring should be kept in mind.
- Appropriate suture material and/or adhesive is paramount for appropriate results.
- Special consideration and expert consultation should be sought in injuries involving critical areas like eyelids, lips, salivary glands and facial nerve.
- Ears and nose soft tissue injuries should be handled with respect and care because of high risk of deformities due to cartilage loss and risk of perichondritis and deformity.

Bony Sinonasal Injuries

Face is arbitrarily divided into upper third formed by frontal bones, middle third by maxilla, ethmoids and zygoma, and lower third by mandible.

Upper-third Face Fractures
- They may be only anterior wall fractures where they are mostly of cosmetic concern or involves posterior wall also where intracranial injuries must be investigated and treated.

Middle-third Face Fractures
- Middle-third fractures involve the maxilla, zygoma and the ethmoids. Due consideration to orbit, dental occlusion and skull base needs to be given for adequate management. Conventionally, middle third fractures are classified by Le Fort fracture classification (Chapter 17).
- *Lower-third (mandible fractures):* Mostly due consideration needs to be given to anatomic region of fracture and whether the bone is dentulous or edentulous. Dental occlusion is important consideration for management.

GENERAL PRINCIPLES IN MANAGING FACIAL FRACTURES
- Computed tomography scan is the single most important diagnostic modality for evaluating the extent of fractures and their management. Plain radiographs, though frequently employed for simple nasal fractures, are unnecessary.
- As already highlighted, the life-threatening injuries of brain, abdomen and thorax take precedence over fracture fixations. General principles of management are same as mentioned in soft tissue injuries.
- Incisions may be customized to allow the access to the area and facilitate elevation and fixation of fracture fragments. These include:
  - Bicoronal incision for frontal and upper third fractures
  - Temporal hairline (Gillies incision) for zygomatic fractures
  - Upper lid blepharoplasty incision is used for frontozygomatic area
  - Orbital floor through transconjunctival incision
  - Maxilla and fragments through the sublabial and gingivobuccal incisions.
- Areas called as pillars or buttresses require due consideration for adequate results after fracture fixation (also see Chapter 17). These include horizontal and vertical buttresses. These are important to provide support to facial architecture during jaw movements. Most repairs are performed using titanium plates and screws.
- Dental occlusion is paramount in severe midface fractures and is established by use of arch bars.
- Upper third fractures involve frontal sinus and often get complicated by sinusitis. If the repair hampers the outflow, cranialization or obliteration may be considered.

CEREBROSPINAL FLUID RHINORRHEA (CSF RHINORRHEA)
- Causes of CSF rhinorrhea can be traumatic or nontraumatic. Most common cause of CSF rhinorrhea is trauma, either accidents or injury

to skull base during operative procedures (nasal and neurosurgical procedures).
- Nontraumatic causes include neoplastic or nonneoplastic intracranial hypertension, skull base osteomyelitis, etc.
- Idiopathic CSF rhinorrhea is rare and most have etiology like benign intracranial hypertension associated.

Symptoms
- Clear watery discharge typically unilateral but can be bilateral. The discharge is more when patient bends forward (teapot sign).
- The more common conditions like allergic rhinitis may produce similar watery discharge and differentiating the two can be challenging.

Signs
- "Halo sign" is an important clinical sign. A halo around a blood spot is indicative of CSF.
- An associated meningocele or meningoencephalocele may be visualized on endoscopy.

Investigations
Investigations should be aimed at confirming the fluid to be CSF and evaluation of exact site of leak. Frequently false negative, estimation of sugar in collected nasal fluid can help differentiate it from nasal fluid.
- B_2 transferrin, though a more accurate test for confirmation, is not readily available and is costly.
- Intrathecal agents like fluorescein (0.1 mL of 10% in 10 mL of patient's own CSF). Radioactive iodine labeled serum albumen or other radioisotopes can be used for *radionuclide cisternography*.
- Imaging is detailed in Chapter 18, and is critical to localize the site of leak.

Management
- *Conservative management:* Traumatic CSF leaks often heal without surgical management. Head end elevation, avoidance of straining, tapping of CSF with lumbar catheters are often successful, if strictly employed for 1-2 weeks.
- *Surgical management:* Leaks which fail conservative management and spontaneous leaks frequently require surgical repair. Conventional transcranial repair is rarely required nowadays as most cases can be handled endoscopically. Accurate identification of site of leak is paramount before embarking on surgical correction. The area is adequately exposed and surrounding mucosa elevated. Any meningoencephalocele is reduced by bipolar cauterization.
- The area is suitably grafted. Choice of graft material varies. We have been using fascia lata placed in onlay or underlay fashion with excellent results. Larger defects require cartilage or bone for bony defect reconstruction. Fascia layer is supplemented with diced abdominal fat or glue.

- Nasal packs are kept for 3-4 days. Patients are nursed with antibiotics, mannitol (to lower CSF pressure), and stool softeners.
- Revisions and recurrences may require transcranial repair.

BIBLIOGRAPHY

1. Chegar BE, Tatum SA. Nasal fractures. In: Flint PW, Haughey BH (Eds). Cummings Otolaryngology-Head and Neck Surgery, 6th edition. Canada: Elsevier; 2014. pp. 583-97.
2. Citardi MJ, Fakhri S. Cerebrospinal fluid rhinorrhea. In: Flint PW, Haughey BH (Eds). Cummings Otolaryngology-Head and Neck Surgery, 6th edition. Canada: Elsevier; 2014. pp. 944-58.
3. Hill JD, Stoddard DJ, Hamilton GS. Facial trauma: soft tissue lacerations and burns. In: Flint PW, Haughey BH (Eds). Cummings Otolaryngology-Head and Neck Surgery, 6th edition. Canada: Elsevier; 2014. pp: 383-402.
4. Kellman RM. Maxillofacial trauma. In: Flint PW, Haughey BH (Eds). Cummings Otolaryngology-Head and Neck Surgery, 6th edition. Canada: Elsevier; 2014. pp. 403-31.

Section 5

Congenital/Pediatric Diseases

20. Pediatric Sinonasal Disorders: Imaging
21. Pediatric Sinonasal Disorders: Surgical Perspective

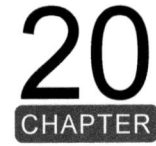

20
CHAPTER

Pediatric Sinonasal Disorders: Imaging

Priyanka Naranje

- Introduction
- Relevant Terminology, Anatomy, and Pitfalls
  - Terminology
  - Anatomy and Pitfalls
- Imaging Modalities
- Development of Paranasal Sinuses
  - Ethmoid Sinuses
  - Maxillary Sinuses
  - Sphenoid Sinuses
  - Frontal Sinuses
- Classification of Pediatric Sinonasal Disorders
- Congenital Pediatric Sinonasal Disorders
  - Anterior Neuropore
  - Midface Anomalies
    - Proboscis Lateralis
    - Nasal Cavity Anomalies
    - Choanal Atresia
    - Nasolacrimal Apparatus Anomalies
- Infective or Inflammatory Pediatric Sinonasal Disorders
  - Rhinosinusiti
    - Acute Sinusitis
    - Chronic Sinusitis
- Tumors and Tumor-like Conditions
  - Infantile Frontonasal Capillary Hemangioma
  - Teratoma
  - Hamartoma
  - Lipoblastoma
  - Sinonasal Nerve Sheath Tumors
  - Hemophilic Pseudotumor
  - Sinonasal Chloroma
- Miscellaneous
  - Chronic Adenoid Hypertrophy
- Illustrative Cases
  - Nasal Cavity Masses
  - Masses Presenting in Frontonasal Region
  - Medial Canthus Masses
  - Sinus Masses

INTRODUCTION

- A wide variety of conditions affect the nose, nasal cavity, and paranasal sinuses in children. Many conditions, such as nasal congenital deformities, anterior nasal cavity, or superficial frontonasal masses can be seen on clinical examination. However, these require imaging

evaluation for extent, determining possible intracranial extension, differential diagnosis, and need for biopsy.
- Biopsy is hazardous in several conditions, such as encephalocele and proliferating hemangioma. Contrast-enhanced computed tomography (CECT) and magnetic resonance (MR) imaging are complementary examinations, and although MR imaging is now the preferred examination for evaluating many of these lesions, CT may be necessary to further assess bone changes.

RELEVANT TERMINOLOGY, ANATOMY, AND PITFALLS

Terminology

It is important to make note of various relevant surface anatomical definitions as below:
- *Midface*: It is the region located between the forehead superiorly and upper lip inferiorly.
- *Glabella*: Part of forehead between the eyebrows (above the nose).
- *Nasion*: It is a point just below the glabella, bony depression in the midline where the two nasal bones and frontal bone meet.
- *Root of nose*: Depressed part of nose just below the nasion.
- *Nasofrontal region*: It is a generic term used to refer to anterior neuropore anomalies projecting in the region of glabella or root of nose and lower forehead.

Anatomy and Pitfalls

- Cribriform plate is nonossified in neonates—must not be misinterpreted as being deficient (Figs. 20.1A and B).
- Cribriform plate begins to ossify between 2 months and 8 months.
- Perpendicular plate of ethmoid begins to ossify between 4 months and 11 months.
- There is normally a midline gap between the two nasal bones—may be misinterpreted as a dermal sinus tract.
- Heterogeneous fatty marrow replacement of the sphenoid between 7 months and 2 years may mimic a sphenoid lesion.
- *Foramen cecum*:
  - It is a gap situated between crista galli and frontal bone.
  - Normal width—up to 10 mm (mean being 4 mm).
  - It appears as soft tissue density on CT and shows low to intermediate signal intensity on magnetic resonance imaging (MRI).
- *Crista galli*: Normal measurement is 1-8 mm (mean 3 mm)
  - CT density and MR signal intensity are same as bone marrow.
  - Age of ossification—1 year.
  - Fatty replacement may be seen in majority of children and is seen by 14 years in all.
  - Fatty signal can be mistaken for dermoid cyst.

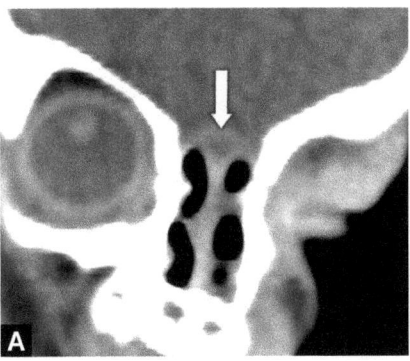 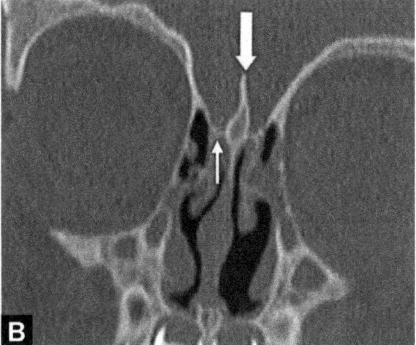

Figs. 20.1A and B: Unossified crista galli infant (A) and normal appearance (B) of ossified crista galli (thick arrows) and cribriform plate (thin arrow) of a 6-year-old child.

- *Measurements*:
  - *Posterior choana*: Normal size is up to 0.34 cm in children less than 2 years.
  - *Vomer*: Normally width of posteroinferior vomer is less than 0.23 cm, maximum is 0.55 cm in children less than 8 years.

IMAGING MODALITIES

- Plain radiograph has a very limited utility with poor sensitivity and specificity.
- *Computed tomography*—suffices for choanal atresia, pyriform aperture (PA) stenosis, nasolacrimal duct (NLD) anomalies, complications of acute sinusitis, recurrent/chronic infection not responding to treatment, evaluation of osteomeatal complex, surgical planning, bony tumors or destruction, and facial trauma.
- *Magnetic resonance imaging*—is preferred in midline mass lesions, intracranial complications of sinusitis, and sinonasal tumors. However, CT is often required in addition to delineate the bony defect of the anterior skull base (ASB). MR imaging sequences that are ideal for assessing nasal lesions include multiplanar thin-section T1-weighted imaging, T2-weighted imaging with fat saturation, contrast material-enhanced T1-weighted imaging with fat saturation, and diffusion-weighted imaging.

DEVELOPMENT OF PARANASAL SINUSES

- Paranasal sinuses form as diverticula from the walls of the nasal cavities.
- The original openings of the diverticula persist as the ostia of the sinuses.
- Sinuses expand and get pneumatized as the child grows (Table 20.1; Figs. 20.2 and 20.3).

260 Section 5 Congenital/Pediatric Diseases

Table 20.1: Time of appearance and maturation of paranasal sinuses.		
Paranasal sinuses	Appear at	Attain full size
Ethmoid	Present at birth	At puberty (16–18 years)
Maxillary	Present but rudimentary at birth	
Sphenoid	7 months to 2 years	
Frontal	6–8 years	

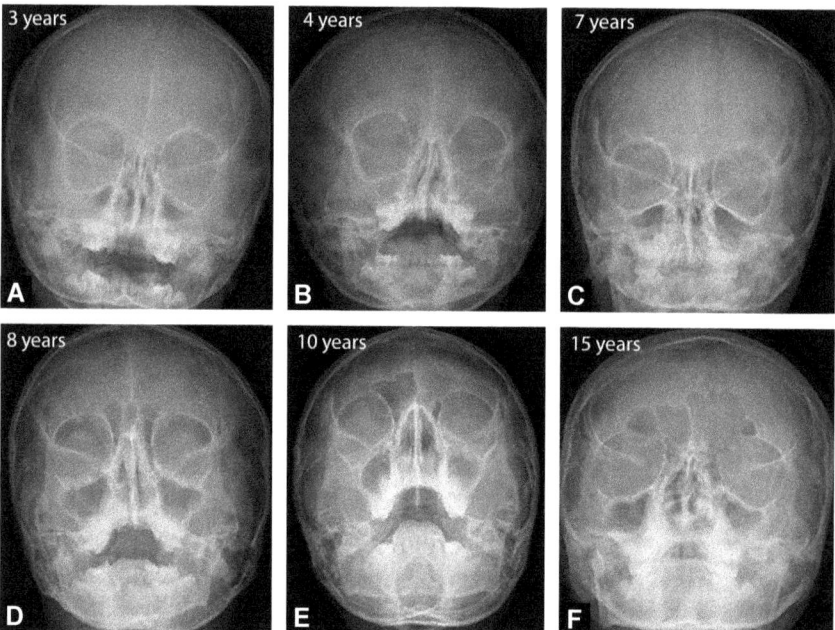

Figs. 20.2A to F: Radiographic development of paranasal sinuses according to age (A). At 3 years, bilateral maxillary sinuses are partially pneumatized and their progressive enlargement with age is seen in subsequent radiographs (B to F). Beginning of pneumatization of the frontal sinuses is noted attaining the full size by 15 years (F).

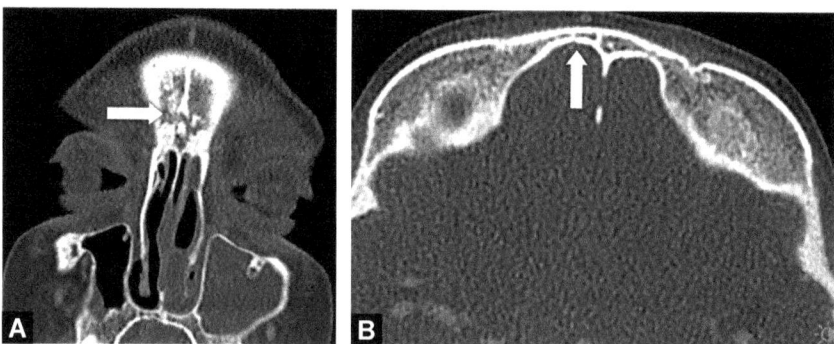

Figs. 20.3A and B: Hypoplastic frontal sinus at 11 years. Computed tomography (CT) images coronal (A) and axial (B) shows nonpneumatized frontal sinuses at 11 years of age (arrows).

- Familiarity with the normal chronology of these events is important to prevent misinterpretation of partially developed/nonpneumatized sinuses as sinusitis.

Ethmoid Sinuses
- Present at birth and pneumatization progresses in all the directions until the age of 12 years.

Maxillary Sinuses
- The early phase of pneumatization is directed laterally and posteriorly in 0–3 years, whereas the later phase proceeds inferiorly toward the maxillary teeth at 6–12 years of age.

Sphenoid Sinuses
- Undeveloped at birth, aeration begins 7 months to 2 years in anterior portion of sinus and progresses posteriorly, laterally, and inferiorly. It reaches the nerve of pterygoid canal in 6–7 years; finally reaching the anterior wall of clivus/anterior clinoids and is completed by 9–12 years.

Frontal Sinuses
- Not present at birth and begin to pneumatized at 6 years of age and expanding superiorly, laterally, and medially, continue to grow in adolescence (*see* Figs. 20.2 and 20.3).

CLASSIFICATION OF PEDIATRIC SINONASAL DISORDERS

Congenital anomalies are divided based on embryology into anterior neuropore/midface/nasobuccal region abnormalities (also *see* Chapters 21 and 23). For the purpose of imaging approach we have clubbed these according to various etiologies (Table 20.2). Similarly, the "tumors" have been clubbed according to the age of presentation (Flowchart 20.1).

SPECIFIC DISORDERS

CONGENITAL PEDIATRIC SINONASAL DISORDERS

Anterior Neuropore

Anterior neuropore abnormalities projecting in nasofrontal region include:[1]
- Nasal glioma
- Nasal encephalocele
- Dermoid cyst
- Epidermoid cyst
- Nasal dermal sinus.

These entities have been discussed in detail in Chapters 21 and 23 and illustrative cases are shown at the end of this chapter.

Midface Anomalies

Developmental errors of the central midface region include:

Table 20.2: Classification of pediatric sinonasal disorders.

Congenital	Inflammatory/infective	Tumors and tumor-like conditions	Craniofacial syndromes	Miscellaneous

Anterior neuropore abnormalities projecting in nasofrontal region:
• Nasal glioma
• Nasal encephalocele
• Dermoid cyst
• Epidermoid cyst
• Nasal dermal sinus
 	
Midface anomalies:
• Aplasias
• Hypoplasias
• Hyperplasias
 	
Nasal cavity anomalies:
• Choanal atresia
• CNPAS
 	
Midfacial clefts: Beyond the scope of this book
 	
Nasolacrimal (NLD) apparatus anomalies
	Rhinosinusitis:
	• Acute/chronic (bacterial/fungal)
	• Allergic/infective
	
	Inflammatory diseases:
	• Granulomatous polyangitis
	• Sarcoidosis
		Neonates/infants:
		• Hemangioma
		• Teratoma
		• Hamartoma
		• Lipoblastoma
		• Lipoma
		• Chondroid hamartoma
		• Fibroma
		
		Older child:
		• Benign
		  – Fibro-osseous lesions
		  – Juvenile nasopharyngeal angiofibroma
		  – Nerve sheath tumor
		  – Hemophilic pseudotumor
		• Malignant:
		  – Rhabdomyosarcoma
		  – Lymphoma
		  – Granulocytic sarcoma
		  – Primitive neuroectodermal tumor (PNET)
		  – Carcinoma
		  – Esthesioneuroblastoma
			• Apert syndrome
			• Crouzon syndrome
			
			• Treacher Collins syndrome
			• Carpenter syndrome
				Adenoid hypertrophy
				
				Nasolabial cysts

(CNPAS: Congenital nasal pyriform aperture stenosis).

Flowchart 20.1: Differential diagnosis of pediatric sinonasal masses.

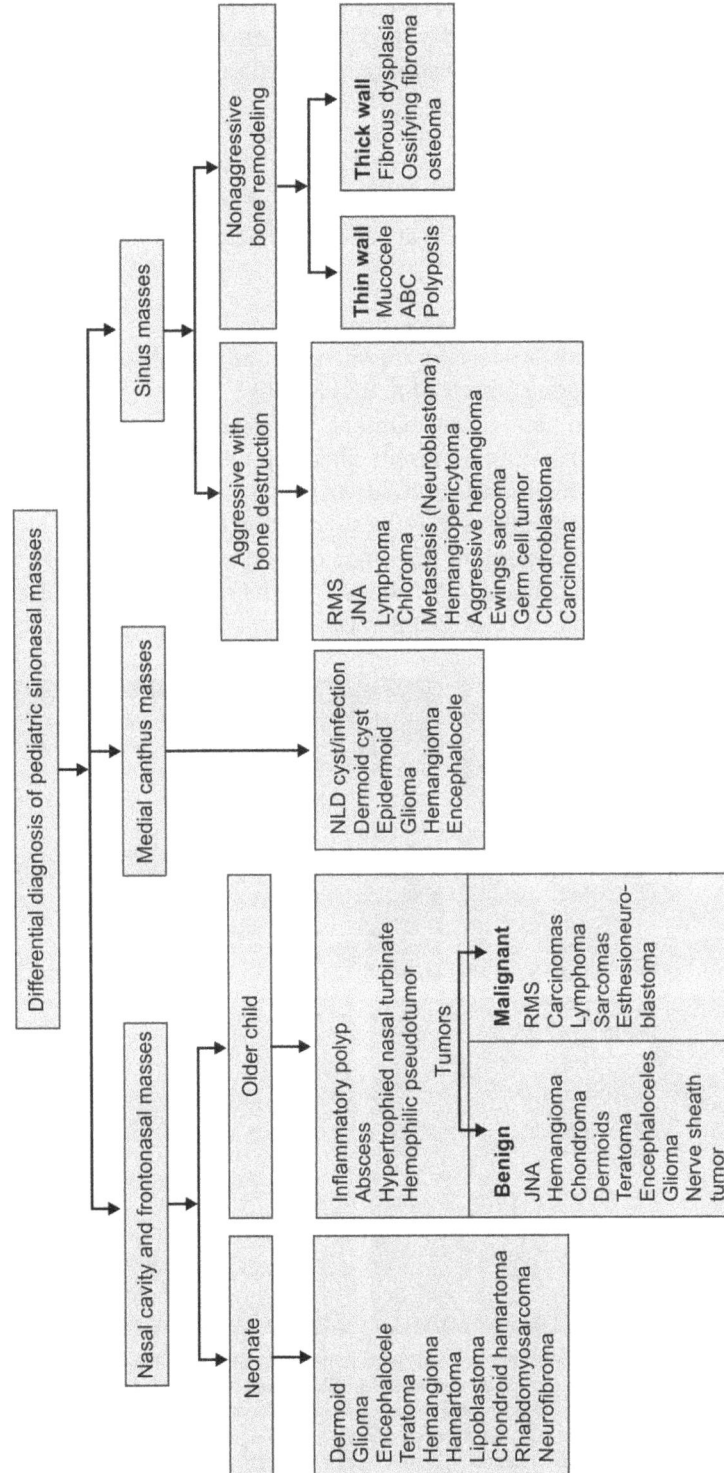

(RMS: Rhabdomyosarcoma; JNA: Juvenile nasopharyngeal angiofibroma; NLD: Nasolacrimal duct).

- *Aplasias*—arhinia and heminasal aplasia.
- *Hypoplasias*—nasal bone hypoplasia (Fig. 20.4A)/agenesis, hypoplastic anterior nasal spine, hypoplastic nares, nasal cavity, and maxillary sinus hypoplasia.
- *Hyperplasias*—polyrhinia, supernumerary nostril, and proboscis lateralis.

The pathogenesis of these entities is discussed in Chapter 21 and imaging features of some of the conditions are discussed below.

Proboscis Lateralis

- Rare hyperplastic midface malformation.
- External nose fails to develop on one side and is replaced by a tubular structure emanating from the medial canthus.
- Associated with faulty development of ipsilateral paranasal sinuses and nasolacrimal system, absent olfactory nerve, olfactory lobe, and cribriform plate on the affected side.
- Computed tomography reveals the single nasal cavity in normal location and an ectopic opening of the other nose at medial canthus location. Associated malformations of sinuses and cribriform plate are well demonstrated on CT (Figs. 20.4B to D).

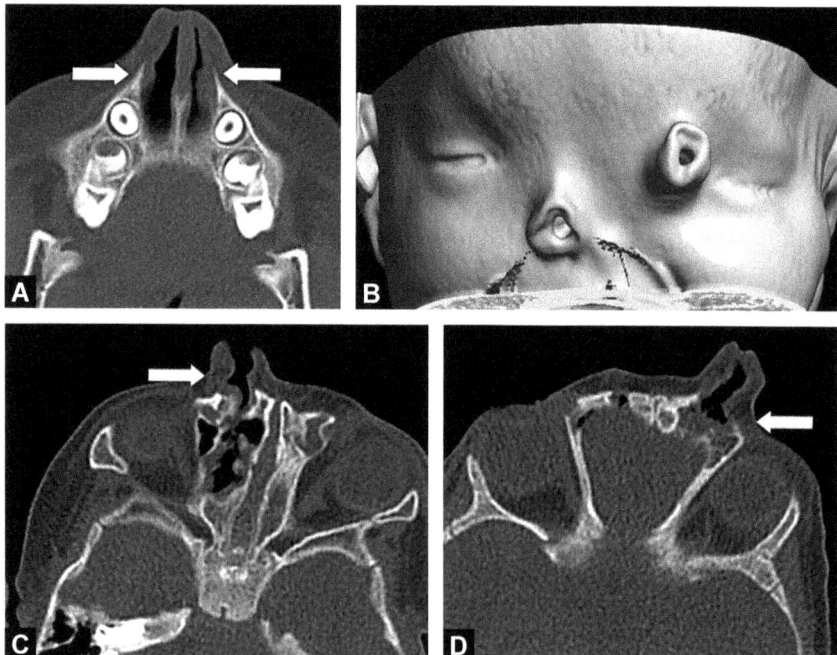

Figs. 20.4A to D: (A) Case of hypoplastic nasal bones. Arrows depict the shortened bilateral nasal bones. (B to D) Case of proboscis lateralis. (B) Surface rendered image shows the two widely separated nasal openings and left nasal opening is seen at the level of left medial canthus. (C) Computed tomography (CT) axial image shows normal right nasal cavity (arrow). (D) Left nasal opening is seen to be blind ending (arrow) with a defect in left frontal bone.

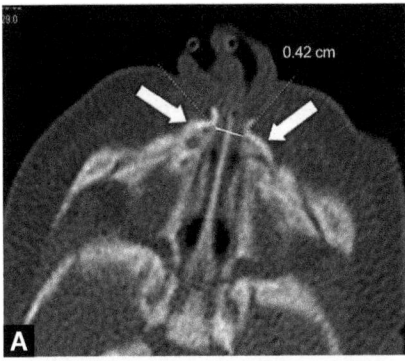
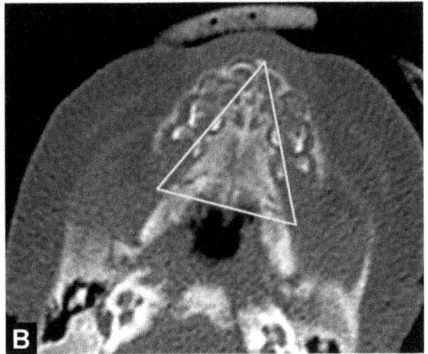
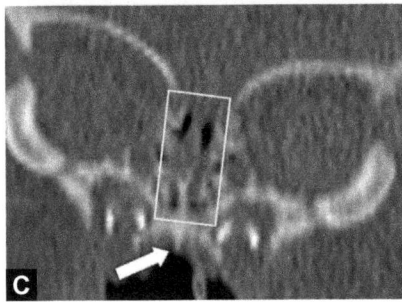

Figs. 20.5A to C: Congenital nasal pyriform aperture stenosis (CNPAS). (A) Medial bowing and overgrowth of medial nasal process of the maxilla (arrow), narrowing of anterior pyriform aperture of less 11 mm (arrows). (B) Triangular-shaped hard palate. (C) Bony ridge in the undersurface of hard palate (arrow) and "box"-shaped anterior aperture (box).

Nasal Cavity Anomalies

Congenital nasal pyriform aperture stenosis:[2]

- Congenital nasal pyriform aperture stenosis (CNPAS) is a congenital anomaly characterized by narrowing of the *anterior* bony nasal passage, most often bilateral.
- *Pathogenesis*: It results from the deficiency of primary palate derived from midline mesodermal tissue, with dysplasia/overgrowth of nasal processes of maxilla.
- *Clinical features*:
  - Presents in newborns or infants in first few months of life.
  - Constitutes one-fifth to one-third of cases of congenital airway obstruction.
  - Presents with respiratory distress, which may be triggered after respiratory infection. Cyanosis may be present.
  - It is difficult to pass nasogastric tube in these neonates.
  - *Imaging*—best modality is multidetector computed tomography (MDCT) mainly *axial and coronal* planes (Figs. 20.5A to C).
    Imaging findings include:
    ▶ Medial deviation of anterior maxillae with inward bowing of the maxillary spines.
    ▶ Thickening of nasal processes.

- For narrowing of the PA, less than 11 mm in term infant is considered diagnostic.
- No standard measurements exist for the normal PA; few studies quote PA width 13.4–15.6 mm as normal and PA area of 0.7–1.1 cm² as normal. In CNPAS, the PA width is reduced to 4.8–7.0 mm and PA area is reduced to 0.2–0.4 cm².
- *Abnormal maxillary dentition*: Solitary median maxillary central incisor syndrome (SMMCI) is seen in 75% of cases.
- Triangle-shaped palate seen as a bony ridge along the oral surface of hard palate on coronal images.
- Posterior choanae are normal.
- The anterior aperture is "box"-shaped as opposed to normal triangular shape.
- Associated with holoprosencephaly, hypopituitarism, absent olfactory bulbs [brain MRI/cranial ultrasonography (USG) recommended routinely].
- *Management*:
  - It generally has a good prognosis, as the nasal cavity grows eventually and obstruction is relieved.
  - Severe cases having persistent respiratory difficulty and poor weight gain may require surgical reconstruction with stent placement, sublabial resection of the anteromedial maxilla, or reconstruction of the anterior nasal passage.

Choanal Atresia[3]

- Choanal atresia is the most common nasal congenital anomaly.
- It is more often unilateral then bilateral.
- Choanal openings refer to a pair of posterior apertures of the nasal cavity that open into the nasopharynx.
- *Terminology*:
  - *Atresia*: Complete obstruction of the posterior choanal openings.
  - *Stenosis*: Narrowing of the posterior choanal opening/nasal passage.

There are three types:
1. *Bony (85–90%)*: This is the most common variant.
2. Membranous (10–15%).
3. Mixed/osseomembranous is a combined type of abnormality.

Pathogenesis:
- Failure of perforation of embryonic oronasal membrane at 7th week.
- Retinoic acid receptor developmental error also implicated.

Associated syndromes: CHARGE syndrome (most important), Apert syndrome, Crouzon syndrome, and DiGeorge syndrome.

Clinical features:
- *Bilateral*: Neonate/infant with respiratory distress, aggravated by feeding, failure to pass nasogastric tube beyond 3–4 cm, usually associated with syndromes.

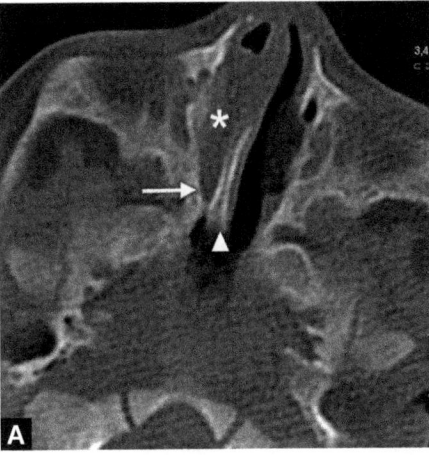 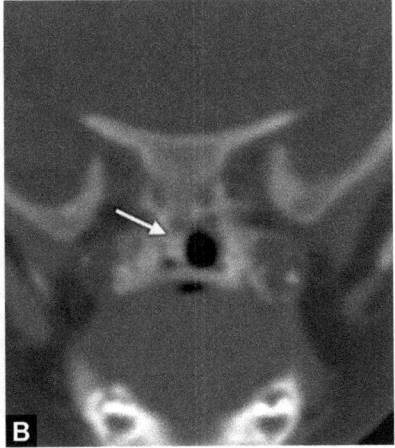

Figs. 20.6A and B: Unilateral bony choanal atresia. (A) Computed tomography (CT) axial image showing medial bowing of posterior lateral nasal walls (arrow), thick vomer (arrowhead), nasal cavity filled with fluid (asterisk). (B) Coronal CT shows bony plate occluding the posterior choana (arrow).

- *Unilateral*: Child/young adult with chronic purulent unilateral rhinorrhea with mild respiratory difficulty, usually isolated anomaly.

Imaging modality:
- Best modality is thin section MDCT interpreted in *axial and sagittal* planes with 3D reconstruction for surgical planning.
- CT should be performed after suctioning and after instillation of nasal decongestants.

Imaging findings (Figs. 20.6A and B):
- Medial bowing of the posterior lateral nasal walls (posterior maxilla).
- Thickening of vomer—may fuse with maxilla.
- *Bony type*—bony plate occludes the choana.
- *Membranous type*—soft tissue membrane (which may be thin and strand like or thick and plug like) occludes the choana.
- Nasal cavity may be filled with soft tissue/fluid/inferior turbinates.
- *Size criteria*: Thickening of vomer more than 2.4 mm; narrowing of choanae less than 3.4 mm.

Management:
- In a newborn with bilateral atresia there is a need to establish immediate oral airway.
- In choanal stenosis, conservative management can be done, allowing natural growth of nasal cavity.
- For unilateral obstruction, definitive treatment delayed up to 6-9 years (midface develops).
- For bilateral obstruction, surgical management is necessary. Common surgeries performed include:
  - Endoscopic perforation of thin membranes

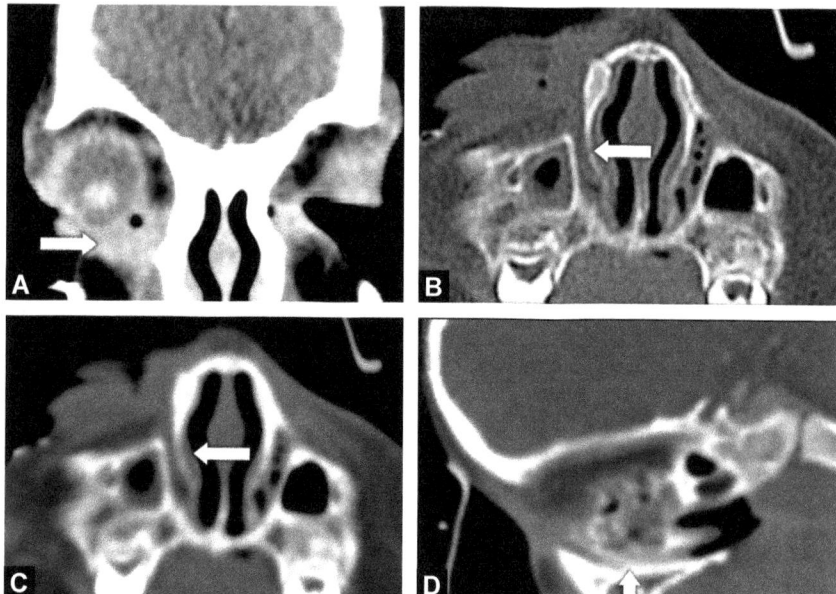

Figs. 20.7A to D: Nasolacrimal duct (NLD) stenosis. (A) Right medial canthus is swollen secondary to dacryocystitis (arrow). (B and C) Coronal oblique images show mild narrowing of the proximal right NLD compared to left side (arrows). (D) Sagittal oblique image showing the narrowed NLD with secretions (arrow).

- Transpalatal resection of vomer with choanal reconstruction
- Stent placement.

Nasolacrimal Apparatus Anomalies

- These include NLD stenosis, congenital dacryocystocele, and dacryocystitis.

Embryology: The valve of Hasner, located at the opening of the NLD within the nasal cavity, is imperforate in up to 70% of newborns resulting in NLD obstruction. Spontaneous opening of an imperforate valve of Hasner usually occurs within 6–12 months.

Nasolacrimal duct stenosis:
- It results from partial persistence of the Hasner membrane.
- *Imaging*—may be normal or show accumulation of secretions within an enlarged nasolacrimal duct proximal to stenosis (Figs. 20.7A to D).
- *Treatment*: Duct massage followed by duct probing or ductal intubation is done (depending on the response); 90% resolve within a year.

Congenital dacryocystocele:
- *Synonym*: Nasolacrimal duct mucoceles.
- These result due to obstruction of both the proximal and distal ends of the nasolacrimal duct.

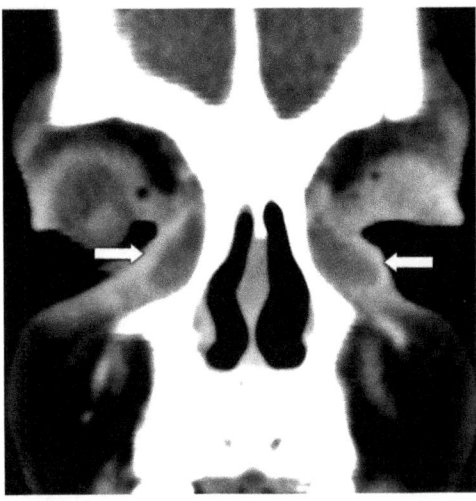

Fig. 20.8: Infected bilateral dacryocystoceles. Coronal contrast-enhanced computed tomography (CECT) image shows bilateral cystic dilatation of the nasolacrimal ducts (NLDs) with peripheral enhancement suggestive of secondary infection (arrows).

- *Pathogenesis*:
    - Distal block occurs due to an imperforate Hasner membrane.
    - Proximal block occurs due to nasolacrimal sac distension or an anatomic variation compresses proximal valve.
- *Clinical features*:
    - Patient presents with epiphora or cellulitis (preseptal).
    - Proximal lesion is seen as small, tense, and bluish medial canthus mass at birth or shortly after birth.
    - Distal lesion is seen as submucosal nasal cavity mass at inferior meatus, may even cause respiratory distress, if bilateral.
    - It is more frequent in females (female > male = 3:1).
- *Complications*: Nasal obstruction, infection (dacryocystitis), and rupture.

Imaging findings include (Fig. 20.8):

Computed tomography/MRI—both CT and MRI can be used, multiplanar reconstruction is important:

- Nasolacrimal duct dilatation.
- Well-defined, thin-walled mass with fluid attenuation/signal intensity involving the medial canthus or nasal cavity.
- Contiguity of the mass with the enlarged NLD can be demonstrated.
- Superior displacement of the inferior turbinate.
- Contralateral shift of the nasal septum.
- Postcontrast slight enhancement of the cyst wall (unless dacryocystitis when thick enhancement can be seen).

Treatment:

- Dacryocystoceles require prompt treatment due to a tendency to become infected and cause subsequent permanent damage to nasolacrimal system.

Table 20.3: Difference between congenital dacryocystocele and dermoid/epidermoid.		
	Congenital dacryocystocele	Dermoid/epidermoid
Location	Medial canthus	Lateral canthus (more common)
Fat density	Absent	Present in 50%
Rim enhancement	Usually absent	Thin rim enhancement common
Calcification	Absent	May be seen
Contiguity with NLD	Present	Absent

(NLD: Nasolacrimal duct).

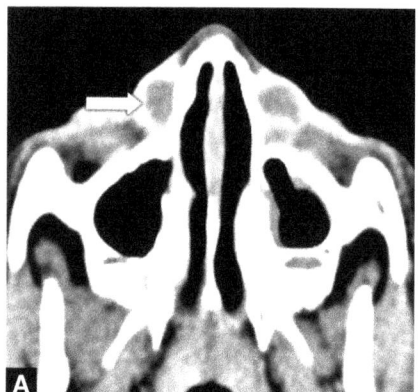 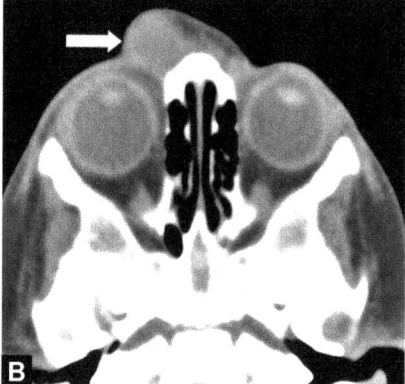

Figs. 20.9A and B: (A) Dacryocystocele versus (B) dermoid.

- *Graded treatment is done*: Manual pressure, probing—irrigation—endoscopic resection—marsupialization in severe cases, depending on the response.
- Dacryocystoceles closely resemble medial canthus dermoids, differentiating points are highlighted in Table 20.3 and corresponding Figures 20.9A and B.

INFECTIVE OR INFLAMMATORY PEDIATRIC SINONASAL DISORDERS

Rhinosinusitis

Role of imaging in acute sinusitis is limited to evaluation of suspected complications. Amongst complications, orbital complications such as cellulitis and subperiosteal abscess are more frequent in children.

Acute Sinusitis

- It is difficult to differentiate viral rhinosinusitis versus bacterial sinusitis on radiology.
- Imaging may show only opacification of sinuses. Although air-fluid levels are more commonly seen in acute sinusitis (Fig. 20.10A).

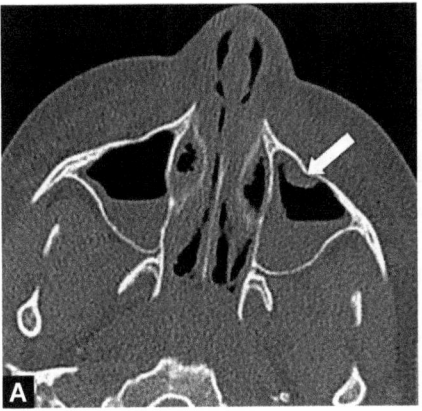
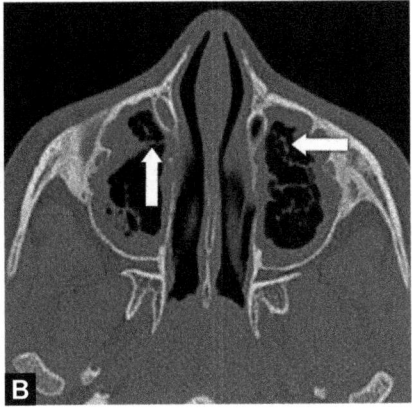

Figs. 20.10A and B: (A) Acute on chronic sinusitis 11 years/female. Air fluid levels seen in bilateral maxillary sinuses. Mucoperiosteal thickening (arrow) also noted in both maxillary sinuses. (B) Intrasinus synechiae. Chronic sinusitis can lead to formation of bands of scar tissue (arrows) stretching between lateral and medial surfaces of maxillary sinuses.

- Uncomplicated acute sinusitis is a clinical diagnosis (no imaging is required).

Complications of acute sinusitis:
1. *Subperiosteal abscess:*
   - Most common intraorbital complication in children.
   - If suspecting sinusitis complications, a CECT scan should be performed.
   - Orbital complications are frequently from ethmoid sinusitis.
2. *Osteomyelitis and Pott's puffy tumor:*
   - To find subtle osteomyelitis, pay attention to the bone adjacent to the area of most prominent soft tissue swelling.
   - MRI can show early phase of osteomyelitis as bone edema and enhancement.
3. Intracranial abscess
4. Intrasinus synechiae (Fig. 20.10B)
5. Subdural empyema
6. *Cavernous sinus thrombosis:* Cranial nerve palsy in the setting of orbital or sinus infection should raise the suspicion of this complication.
7. Pyomyositis
8. Infectious optic neuritis.

Chronic Sinusitis

- Pediatric chronic sinusitis may be associated with certain predisposing factors, which include:
  - Recurrent upper respiratory tract infection (URI)
  - Mucociliary deficiency, cystic fibrosis (CF) (seen in nearly 100% of children with CF)

- Allergy
- Gastroesophageal reflux disease
- Chronic systemic disorders, such as vasculitis and immunodeficiency.

TUMORS AND TUMOR-LIKE CONDITIONS

Tumors and tumor-like conditions encountered in neonates, infants, and older children according to the age of occurrence are enlisted in Table 20.2. The spectrum of tumors occurring in pediatric age group resemble those in adults and several individual entities, such as rhabdomyosarcoma, Juvenile nasopharyngeal angiofibroma, and lymphoma have been covered elsewhere in the book (*see* Chapters 12 and 14). Also see illustrative cases at the end of this chapter.

Some of the tumors and tumor-like conditions seen in pediatric age are discussed below.

Infantile Frontonasal Capillary Hemangioma[4]

- Hemangioma is the most common benign tumor in an infant.
- These show a proliferative growth phase (during the 1st year) and an involutional phase (after the 1st year). However, some of them may not involute (noninvoluting hemangioma).
- Clinical differential diagnosis is nasal glioma, as both might present with a bluish or reddish mass.
- *Association*: PHACE syndrome refers to—posterior fossa brain malformations, hemangioma, arterial anomalies, coarctation of the aorta, cardiac defects, and eye abnormalities.
- *Ultrasonography*—soft tissue mass with intense vascularity showing arterial flow channels representing feeding vessels.
- *Computed tomography*—intensely enhancing mass in subcutaneous plane in frontonasal region, nasal ala, nasolabial region, or anywhere within the nasal cavity. CT important to rule out bony involvement/bony origin, which is seen in intraosseous cavernous hemangiomas (Figs. 20.11A and B).
- The MRI shows a lobular mass, on T1WI mass is mildly hyperintense and is hyperintense on T2WI with hypointense internal flow voids.
- On contrast-enhanced magnetic resonance imaging (CEMRI), the mass show intense postcontrast enhancement. In the involuting stage, heterogeneous enhancement is noted.

Teratoma

- Teratomas are tumors containing elements from the three embryonic layers (ectoderm, mesoderm, and endoderm).
- These are frequently benign, though malignant forms may also occur.
- These may occur in the sinuses, within the nasal cavity or nasopharynx.
- Teratomas represent spontaneous and autonomous new growth of tissue foreign to a region.

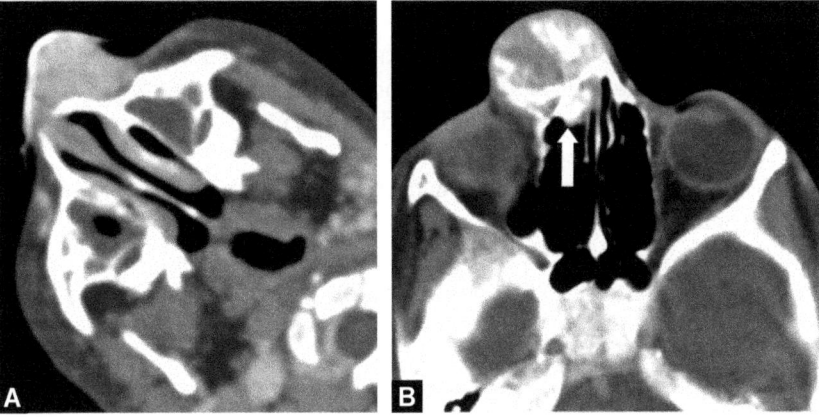

Figs. 20.11A and B: (A) Capillary hemangioma in a 3 years/female. Contrast-enhanced computed tomography (CECT) shows lobular, intensely enhancing mass in skin and subcutaneous tissue anterior to nasal bone on left side. (B) Nasal "bone" hemangioma in a 4 years/female. CECT images showing an avidly enhancing soft tissue density lesion with bone density within it giving "sun burst appearance" arising from right nasal bone.

- Clinically sessile or pedunculated masses, which may protrude through the mouth, are seen.
- Anencephaly, hemicrania, and palatal fissures may be associated.
- Can be detected in utero and are associated with polyhydramnios.
- Imaging findings include soft tissue mass with presence of calcification, fat, tooth, and may show cystic areas within. Majority of them do not show intracranial extension.
- Treatment is complete excision.

Hamartoma

- Hamartomas are rare lesions involving the abnormal growth of any of the three germinal layers, which are normally indigenous to a region.
- *Location*: Oral cavity, nasal cavity, tongue, nasopharynx, Eustachian tube, hypopharynx, or larynx.
- In nasal cavity, sites reported—septum, ethmoid, vestibule, and maxillary sinuses.
- In head and neck region, these are mostly composed of vascular tissue.
- Imaging findings are nonspecific. CT shows a well-marginated and homogenous soft tissue mass. It may or may not show enhancement and do not show calcification.
- These tumors have limited growth potential and surgical resection is the treatment of choice.

Lipoblastoma

- Rare benign and circumscribed mesenchymal tumors of embryonal fat.
- The CT and MRI—entire fat-containing tumor, cannot be distinguished from lipoma on imaging.

Sinonasal Nerve Sheath Tumors[5]

- These are uncommon lesions, which represent less than 4% of head and neck nerve sheath tumors (schwannomas).
- Affected age group varies from childhood to elderly (0–78 years with no sex or racial predilection).
- Symptoms are nonspecific, such as nasal obstruction, epistaxis, and anosmia.
- The CT shows an expansile and mildly enhancing mass with no bone remodeling may be appreciated.
- The MR imaging shows an intermediate T1 and variable T2 signal intensity (Figs. 20.12A to D).
- Sometimes intracranial extension through cribriform plate may be seen.
- Histopathology remains gold standard for diagnosis.

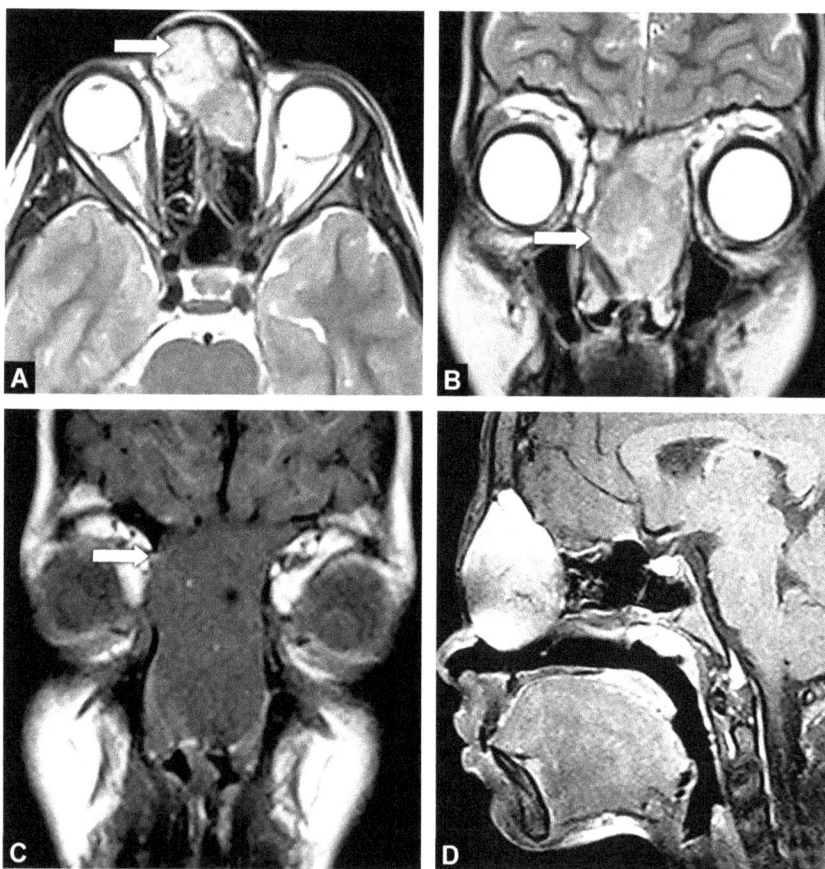

Figs. 20.12A to D: Nasal benign nerve sheath tumor. (A and B) Axial and coronal T2-weighted images show intermediate hyperintense mass in the nasal cavity with intracranial and extradural extension. (C) T1 coronal image shows hypointense signal. (D) T1 postcontrast shows homogenous enhancement.

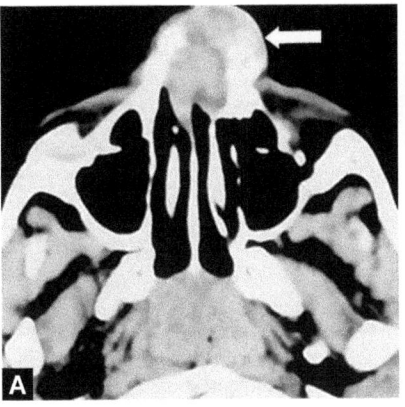
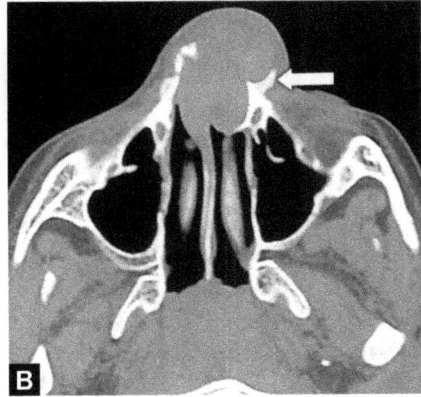

Figs. 20.13A and B: Hemophilic pseudotumor. (A) Noncontrast computed tomography (NCCT) showing an externally protruding large soft tissue mass with high density (arrow). (B) Bone window images shows erosion of anterior nasal septum and smooth scalloping of the adjoining bones (arrow).

Hemophilic Pseudotumor

- This is a complication of hemophilia and represents a chronic hematoma that expands slowly because of recurrent bleeding.
- Gets encapsulated by a thick fibrous tissue.
- Leads to slow pressure destruction of adjacent structures/bones.
- Pediatric sinonasal involvement rare (exact incidence not known).
- Clinically, these may sometimes present with rapidly expanding mass in undiagnosed patient.
- *Computed tomography scan*—demonstrates a high-density mass and mass effects on surrounding structures, especially bony changes of chronic pressure erosion/scalloping (Figs. 20.13A and B) are seen.
- *Magnetic resonance imaging*—delineates soft tissue extent and intramedullary extension within the bone.
- *Treatment*:
  - Factor VIII replacement + complete surgical excision of entire mass to prevent recurrence.
  - *Radiotherapy*: 600–2,350 cGy with or without factor replacement, where surgery is not feasible is shown to have good response.

Sinonasal Chloroma

- It is a rare malignant extramedullary neoplasm of myeloid precursor cells.
- *Synonym*: Granulocytic sarcoma or myeloid sarcoma.
- It is seen in acute myeloid leukemia (AML) or other myeloproliferative disorder.
- Seen in 3–9.1% of AML, preferentially in young patients or in children with no gender preference.
- Its presence is a sign of poor prognosis.
- It frequently involves bones and periosteum with associated soft tissue.

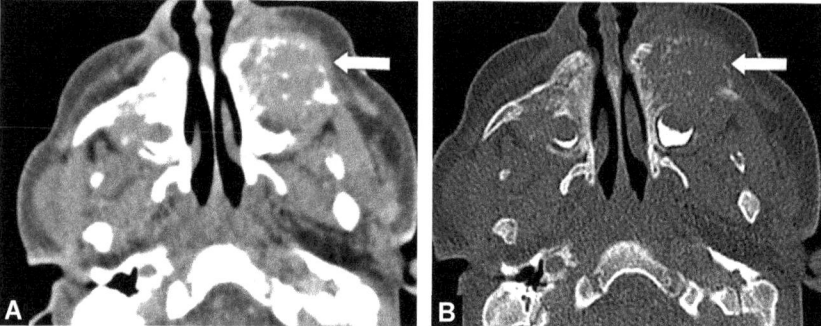

Figs. 20.14A and B: Left maxillary sinus granulocytic sarcoma in a child with acute myelocytic leukemia (AML). (A and B) Axial computed tomography (CT) images show hyperdense soft tissue mass in the left maxillary sinus causing lytic destruction of all the walls of the maxillary sinus (arrows).

- In the head and neck region, sites affected include soft palate, nasopharynx, orbit, salivary glands, scalp, face, jaw, lips, nasal cavity, maxilla, and temporal bone.
- The CT shows nonspecific soft tissue mass with homogenous contrast enhancement. When affecting the sinuses, it shows lytic destruction of the bony walls of the sinuses with infiltration into adjacent tissues (Figs. 20.14A and B).
- The MR shows T1 hypointense and T2 iso to hypointense signal within the soft tissue mass.
- Chloromas are radiosensitive and local radiotherapy in conjunction with chemotherapy is treatment of choice.

MISCELLANEOUS

Chronic Adenoid Hypertrophy

- Adenoids are situated in the nasopharynx and are small at birth, grow till 5 years of age and gradually get atrophied by adolescence.
- When enlarged, these may lead to obstructive sleep apnea.
- Lateral neck radiograph depicts the enlarged adenoid with obstruction of nasopharynx to variable extent (Figs. 20.15A and B).
- The size of the adenoids is less of a consideration than the degree to which they encroach on the nasopharyngeal airway.
- Adenoid grades based on airway to soft palate ratio are:
  1. Normal (airway-to-soft-palate ratio ≥1)
  2. Mild-to-moderate hypertrophy (airway-to-soft-palate ratio between 0.5 and 1)
  3. Severe hypertrophy (airway-to-soft-palate ratio <0.5).

Differential diagnosis of pediatric sinonasal masses according to the region of involvement is summarized in Flowchart 20.1.

Various congenital masses presenting in the region of root of nose are discussed in chapters 21, 23 and the current chapter. A brief imaging based approach for these masses is summarized in the Flowchart 20.2.

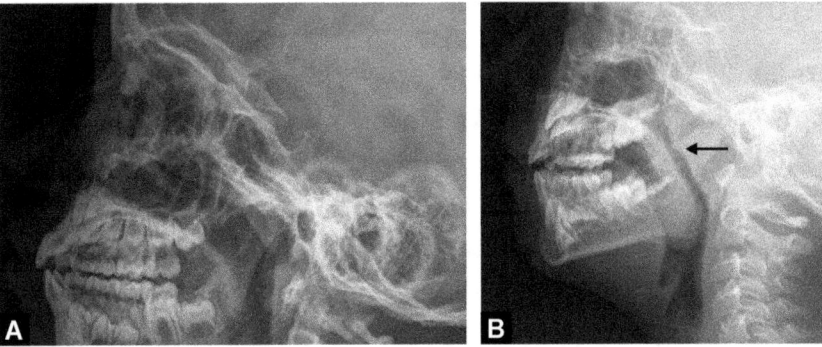

Figs. 20.15A and B: (A) Normal adenoid. No nasopharyngeal airway comprise seen. (B) Hypertrophied adenoids—showing thickening of posterior nasopharyngeal soft tissue, which is indenting and narrowing nasopharyngeal air column on posterior aspect (arrow).

Flowchart 20.2: Imaging approach to congenital masses presenting in the region of root of nose.

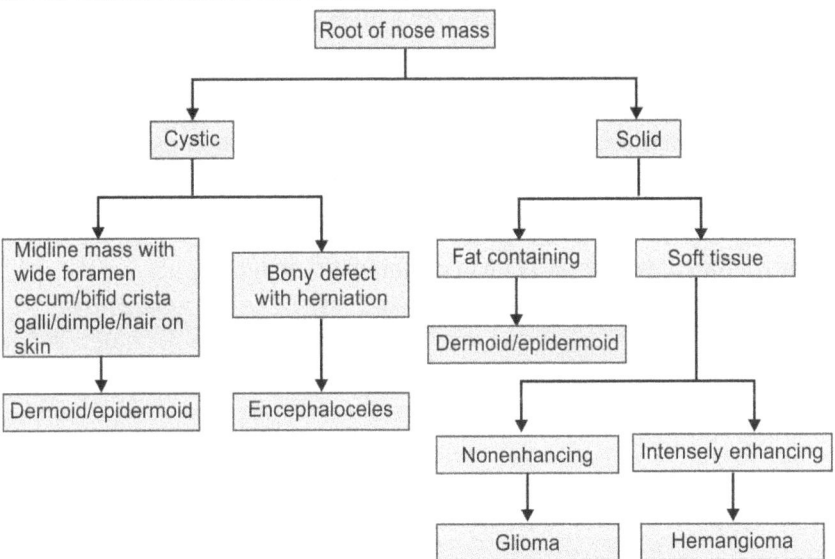

REFERENCES

1. Hedlund G. Congenital frontonasal masses: developmental anatomy, malformations, and MR imaging. Pediatr Radiol. 2006;36(7):647-62.
2. Visvanathan V, Wynne DM. Congenital nasal pyriform aperture stenosis: a report of 10 cases and literature review. Int J Pediatr Otorhinolaryngol. 2012;76(1):28-30.
3. Lowe LH, Booth TN, Joglar JM, et al. Midface anomalies in children. Radiographics. 2000;20(4):907-22.
4. Rodriguez DP, Orscheln ES, Koch BL. Masses of the nose, nasal cavity, and nasopharynx in children. Radiographics. 2017;37(6):1704-30.
5. Kim YS, Kim HJ, Kim CH, et al. CT and MR imaging findings of sinonasal schwannoma: a review of 12 cases. Am J Neuroradiol. 2013;34(3):628-33.

ILLUSTRATIVE CASES

Nasal Cavity Masses

Case 1: Intranasal Dermoid Cyst

A and *B*. Computed tomography (CT) images depict a cystic well-defined mass in the anterior nasal cavity in the midline septum (arrows).

C. The intracranial extension is suggested by the presence of bifid crista galli (arrow).

> **Imaging pearl**
>
> Apart from these, CT may show a large (>3 mm in diameter) foramen cecum in the case of intracranial extension.

Case 2: Nasal Dermal Sinus Tract

A. Plain radiograph lateral view shows marker at the site of dimple at the tip of the nose (arrow).

B. Contrast injection from this site opacified a linear tract coursing up to the level of foramen cecum (arrow). The intracranial portion usually remains extra-axial involving the dura and falx cerebri.

C. Sagittal T1 postcontrast MR image shows similar enhancing linear tract (arrow) from the nasal cavity up to the foramen cecum.

> **Imaging pearl**
>
> The transcranial tract mostly courses through the foramen cecum, and less commonly through crista galli or cribriform plate.

Chapter 20 Pediatric Sinonasal Disorders: Imaging

Case 1 (Figs. 20.16A to C)   *Case 2 (Figs. 20.17A to C)*

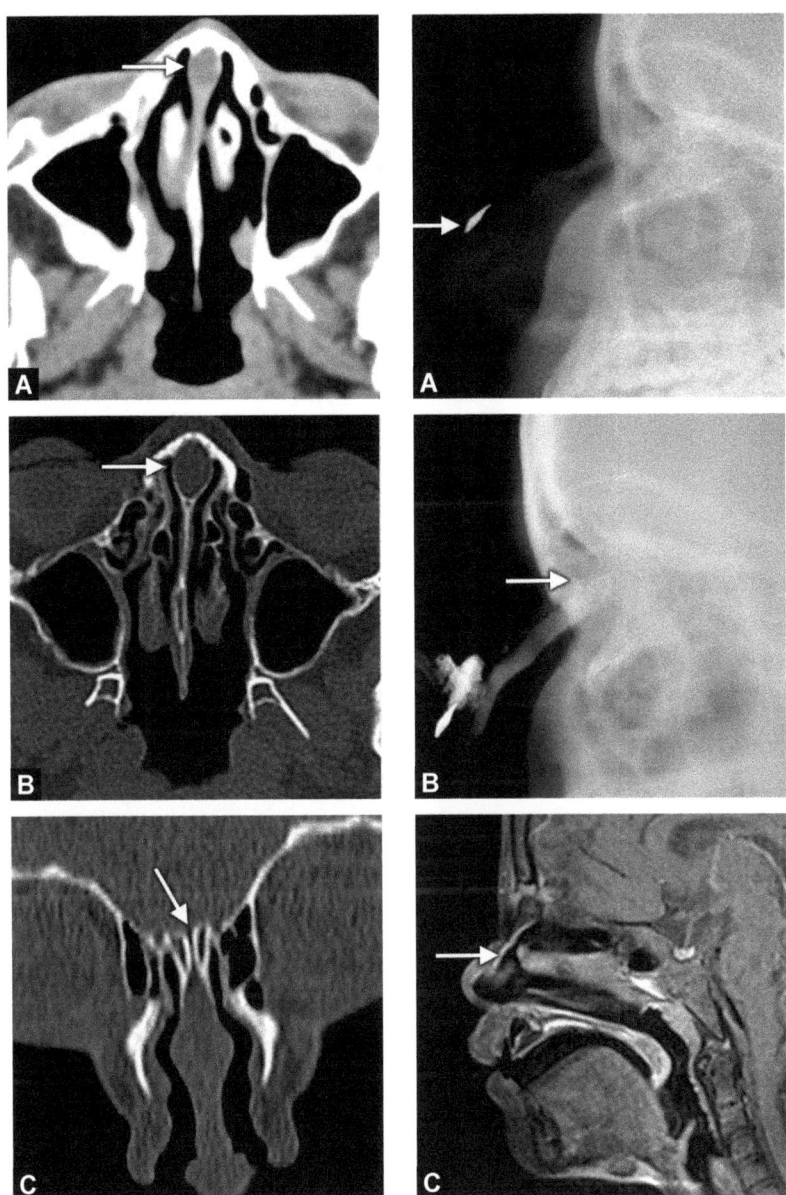

ILLUSTRATIVE CASES

Nasal Cavity Masses (Contd..)

Case 3: Intranasal Glioma

A. T1 postcontrast axial image shows a nonenhancing (arrow) soft tissue mass in the right nasal cavity.

B. Magnetic resonance imaging (MRI) T2 sagittal image shows T2 iso to hyperintense mass (arrow) with no intracranial communication. Intracranial attachment with a fibrous stalk is seen in up to 15% cases.

C. Computed tomography (CT) coronal image shows an intranasal hypodense mass with no fat, calcification or enhancement. Normal crista galli is noted (arrow).

> **Imaging pearl**
>
> Clinically nasal gliomas show telangiectatic overlying skin when presenting as root of nose mass.
>
> They are nonpulsatile, do not transilluminate and do not enlarge on valsalva maneuver/crying (negative Furstenberg test).

Case 4: Intranasal Encephalocele

A. Computed tomography (CT) sagittal image shows herniation of cranial content (predominantly cerebrospinal fluid) through a bony defect (arrow) in the anterior skull base into the nasal area.

B. Bone window shows the defect in the anterior part of cribriform plate (arrow).

C. Coronal CT image showing the intranasal mass in continuity with the anterior cranial fossa through the defect (arrow).

> **Imaging pearl**
>
> Clinically, these show positive Furstenberg test, are pulsatile and also transilluminate.
>
> They may be associated with hypertelorism and corpus callosum dysgenesis.

Chapter 20 Pediatric Sinonasal Disorders: Imaging 281

Case 3 (Figs. 20.18A to C)　　Case 4 (Figs. 20.19A to C)

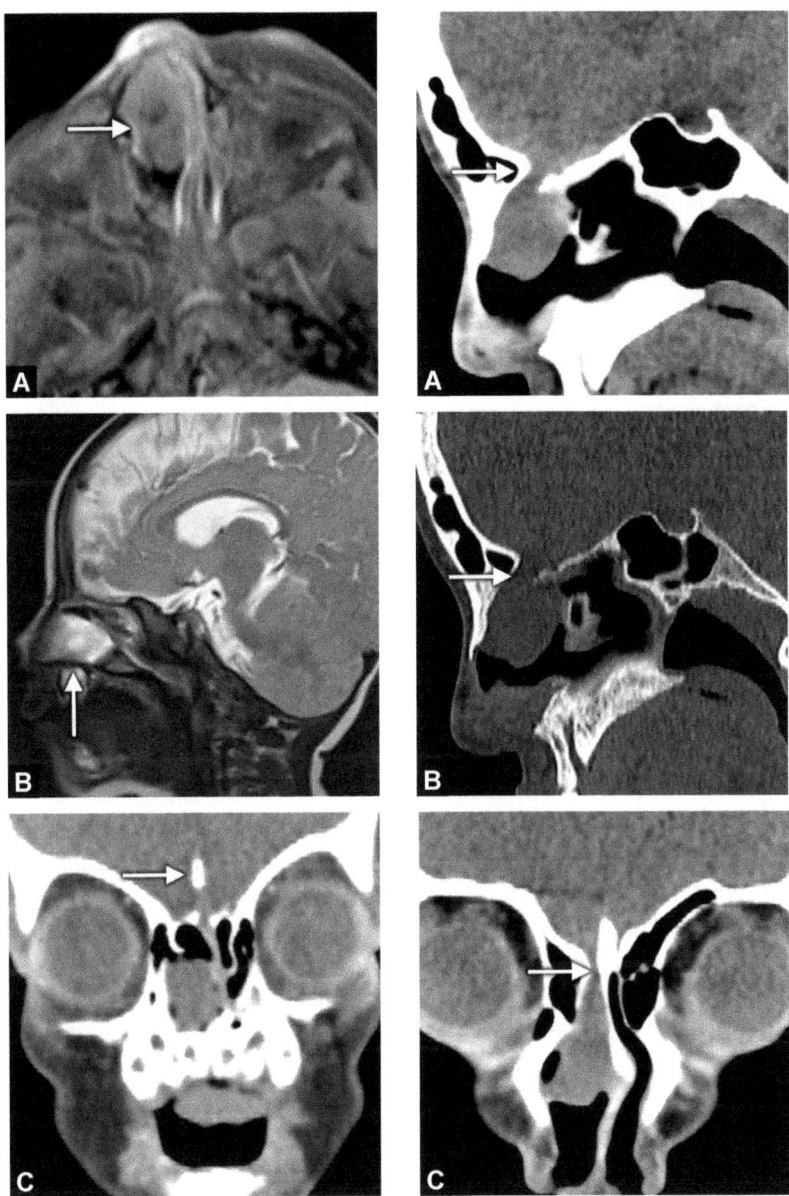

ILLUSTRATIVE CASES

Masses presenting in frontonasal region.

Case 1: Hemangioma Presenting as a Frontonasal Mass

A. Surface rendered computed tomography (CT) image shows a bulge in the frontonasal region (arrow) in a 6-year-old female.

B and *C.* CT shows well-circumscribed mass with arterial feeders and enhancement (arrows). No phleboliths were seen. There was no intranasal or intracranial extension.

> **Imaging pearl**
>
> Hemangiomas are vascular tumors and clinically present as bluish red mass. These are nonpulsatile and do not transilluminate and show negative Furstenberg test. On MRI, These are T2 hyperintense, show flow voids and intense enhancement.

Case. 2: Nasal Benign Nerve Sheath Tumor

A. Axial T2-weighted images show intermediate hyperintense mass in the nasal cavity with extension in the anterior ethmoid sinuses (arrow).

B. T1 coronal shows intracranial, extradural extension of the mass (arrows).

C. T1 post-contrast sagittal image shows the enhancing mass bulging in the frontonasal region and extension of the mass in the frontal sinus (arrow).

> **Imaging pearl**
>
> Sinonasal schwannoma is generally a well-defined soft-tissue mass most frequently occurring in the nasal cavity and ethmoid sinus and frequently associated with pressure remodeling of the adjacent bone. These tumors are isoattenuating on CT and show strong enhancement on MR images. Although sinonasal schwannomas are rare and their imaging findings are rather nonspecific, CT and MR imaging studies are helpful for preoperative diagnosis and surgical planning in patients with schwannoma of the sinonasal cavity.

Chapter 20 Pediatric Sinonasal Disorders: Imaging 283

Case 1 (Figs. 20.20A to C)   *Case 2 (Figs. 20.21A to C)*

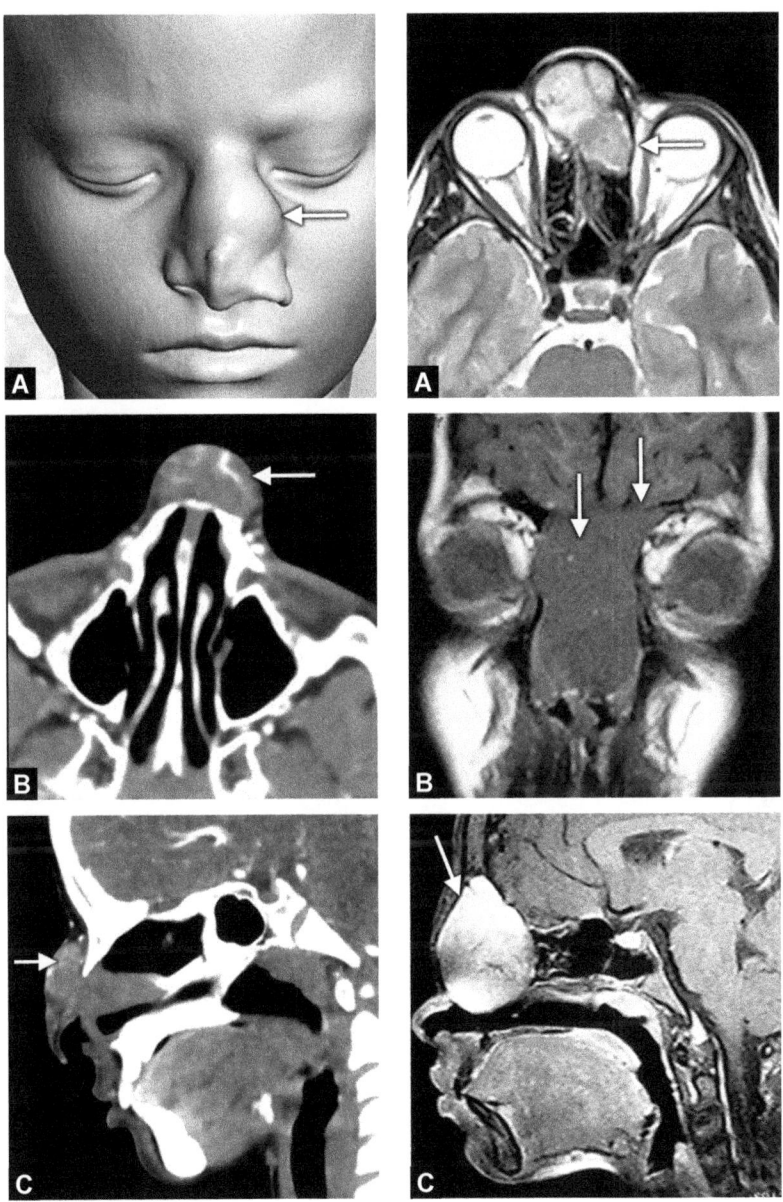

ILLUSTRATIVE CASES

Medial canthus masses (Figs. 20.22A to F).

Differential diagnosis of masses presenting in the region of medial canthus includes:
- NLD cyst/infection
- Dermoid
- Epidermoid
- Encephalocele
- Glioma
- Hemangioma.

A and *B.* Encephalocele presenting as bulge in right medial canthus region. Coronal computed tomography (CT) image shows the intracranial communication of the mass (arrows).

C. Dermoid/epidermoid cyst. A well-circumscribed high-attenuation mass seen on right side in medial canthus region (arrow).

D. Lipodermoid. A fat containing well-circumscribed mass (arrow) in right medial canthal region.

E. Dacryocystoceles. Dilated bilateral nasolacrimal sacs (arrow) seen in the region of medial canthus with peripheral enhancement due to secondary infection.

F. Dacryocystitis. Heterogeneous enhancement and inflammatory changes seen in the right medial canthus region in a case of unilateral dacryocystitis (arrow).

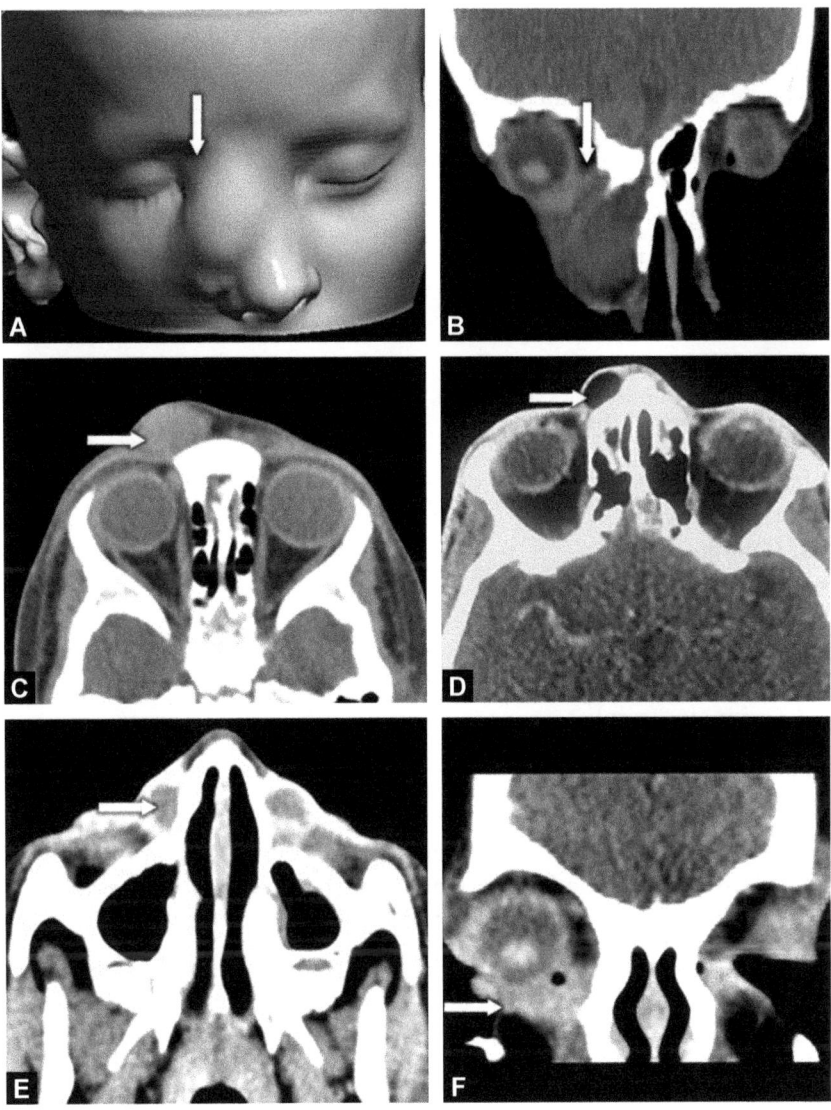

ILLUSTRATIVE CASES

Sinus Masses
Pediatric sinus masses can be benign or malignant.

Benign masses seen in children includes:
- Polyposis
- Mucocele
- Aneurysmal bone cyst
- Fibrous dysplasia
- Ossifying fibroma
- Osteoma.

Malignant masses includes:
- RMS
- JNA
- Lymphoma
- Chloroma
- Metastasis (Neuroblastoma)
- Aggressive hemangioma
- Ewings sarcoma
- Germ cell tumor
- Carcinoma (rare).

Benign:

Antrochoanal Polyp
A and *B*. Coronal computed tomography (CT) image shows homogenous hypodense mass in the left maxillary sinus projecting in the nasal cavity widening the osteomeatal unit (arrows).

C. Similar mass seen in another patient in right maxillary sinus obliterating the right nasal cavity (arrow). No bony destruction seen. No enhancement is seen within the mass s/o benign etiology.

Malignant:

Rhabdomyosarcoma
A to *C*. Computed tomography (CT) images of a 2-year-old boy shows large expansile heterogenously enhancing soft tissue mass in left maxillary sinus with surrounding aggressive type of bony destruction (arrow) and extension in the nasal cavity is noted s/o of a malignant etiology.

Chapter 20 Pediatric Sinonasal Disorders: Imaging 287

Benign
(Figs. 20.23A to C)

Malignant
(Figs. 20.24A to C)

ILLUSTRATIVE CASES

Sinus Masses (Contd..)

Nonaggressive benign sinus masses.

Ossifying Fibroma

A. Plain radiograph shows well-marginated, sclerotic epansile mass in left maxillary and ethmoid regions (arrows).

B and *C.* Computed tomography (CT) image shows mixed soft tissue mass with areas of bone density and thick bony walls in left maxillary and ethmoid sinuses obliterating the superior left nasal cavity (arrows). It also shows relatively well-defined margins.

Fibrous Dysplasia

A. Plain radiograph shows expansion and sclerosis of maxillary sinus with relatively maintained contour (arrow). Margins of the sclerotic region are merging with the surrounding bone in a patient of fibrous dysplasia (FD).

B and *C.* Computed tomography (CT) images show bony expansion of the left ethmoid and sphenoid sinuses which show ground glass matrix (arrows). Involvement of the left middle turbinate presented as an intranasal mass.

Chapter 20 Pediatric Sinonasal Disorders: Imaging 289

Ossifying Fibroma
(Figs. 20.25A to C)

Fibrous Dysplasia
(Figs. 20.26A to C)

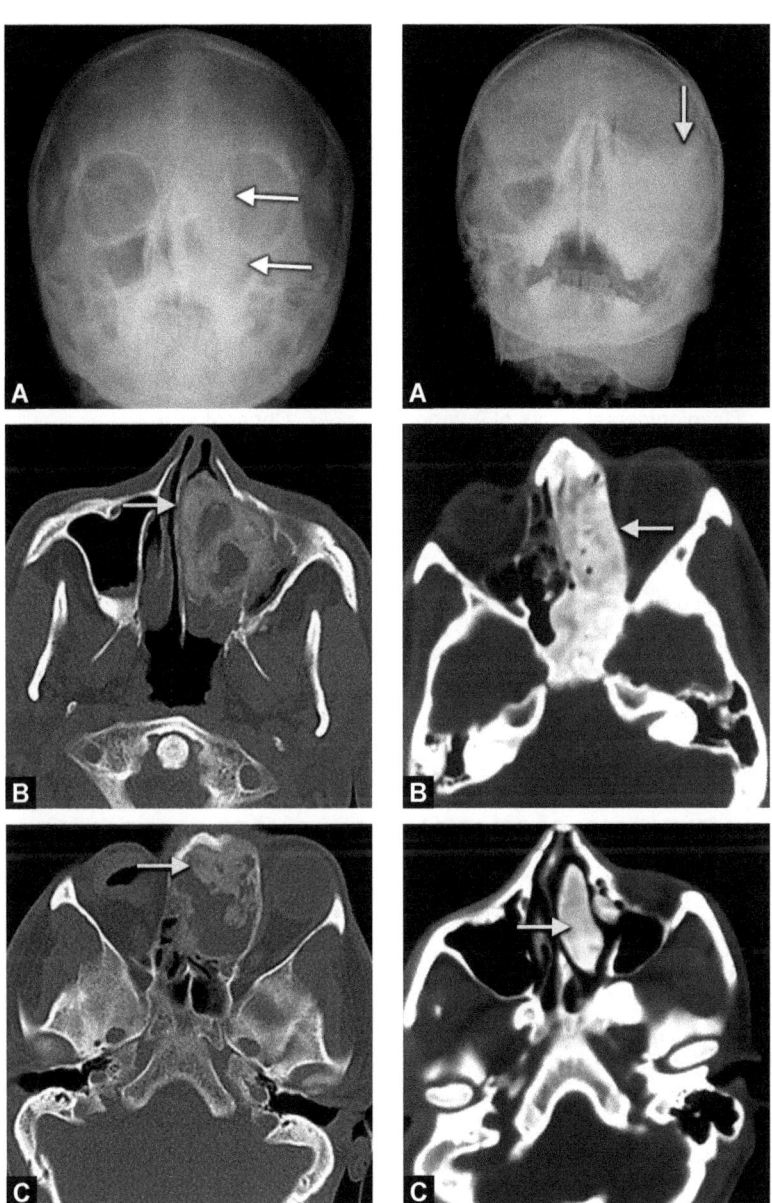

21
CHAPTER

Pediatric Sinonasal Disorders: Surgical Perspective

Prem Sagar, Shuchita Singh

- Congenital Malformations of the Nose
  - Developmental Errors of Anterior Neuropore
  - Developmental Errors of the Central Midface
    - Aplastic and Hypoplastic Anomalies
    - Atretic Anomalies
    - Hyperplastic and Duplication Anomalies
    - Craniofacial Clefts
  - Developmental Errors of the Nasobuccal Membrane
    - Choanal Atresia
- Rhinosinusitis
  - Acute Bacterial Rhinosinusitis
  - Chronic Bacterial Rhinosinusitis
- Chronic Adenoid Hypertrophy
- Specific Lesions

CONGENITAL MALFORMATIONS OF THE NOSE

Congenital malformations of the nose may be categorized as developmental errors of the anterior neuropore, errors of central midface, and errors of the nasobuccal membrane. Imaging features of these disorders are detailed in Chapters 20 and 23.

Developmental Errors of Anterior Neuropore

During first trimester, a dural projection extends through foramen cecum, prenasal space up to the ectoderm at the tip of the nasal bones. As the foramen cecum closes, this extension gets detached from the nasal bones and gets retracted into the cranium. Different type of errors in this developmental process leads to common congenital malformations as enumerated in Table 21.1.

- Encephaloceles may be meningoceles or meningoencephaloceles depending on the inclusion of meninges only or meninges along with brain tissue, respectively.
- Encephaloceles in sinonasal region may be sincipital (more common) or basal encephaloceles. Different types of sincipital and basal encephaloceles are summarized in Tables 21.2 and 21.3, respectively.

Table 21.1: Common developmental errors of the anterior neuropore.

Type of error	Pathophysiology	Schematic representation
Dermoid cyst/sinus/fistula	Posterosuperiorly retracted ectoderm through foramen cecum	Sinus opening on nasal dorsum; Dermoid cyst
Glioma	Premature closure of foramen cecum with entrapped glial tissue (without any patent communication with CNS)	Glioma with intracranial attachment
Encephalocele	Premature closure of foramen cecum with entrapped meninges ± brain parenchyma communicating with CNS	Dura mater; Anterior skull base defect; Encephalocele

Table 21.2: Characteristics of sincipital encephaloceles.

Type	Skull base defect	Clinical location of the encephalocele
Nasofrontal	Between orbits and nasal + frontal bones	Superficial to nasal bones as glabellar mass
Nasoethmoid	Foramen cecum, deep to nasal bones	Nasal dorsum
Naso-orbital	Deep to nasal and frontal bones through defect in medial orbital wall	Orbital mass

Table 21.3: Characteristics of basal encephaloceles.

Type	Skull base defect	Clinical location of the encephalocele
Transethmoidal	Cribriform plate	Nasal cavity
Sphenoethmoidal	Between posterior ethmoid cells and sphenoid sinus	Nasal cavity
Transsphenoidal	Craniopharyngeal canal	Nasopharynx
Spheno-orbital	Superior orbital fissure	Orbit

- The clinical presentation and treatment of these three types of anterior neuropore errors are summarized in Table 21.4 (Fig. 21.1).

Table 21.4: Clinical presentation and treatment protocol of different types of anterior neuropore errors.

Type of error	Symptoms	Signs	Treatment
Dermoids	Midline pit or swelling at the rhinion (Fig. 21.1), which may have intermittent caseous discharge or infections	Cysts are firm, lobulated and noncompressible, do not enlarge on coughing or crying and do not transilluminate	Complete surgical excision
Gliomas	Extranasal mass (most commonly at the glabella), intranasal mass arising from middle turbinate or septum or as both extra- and intranasal mass	Nonpulsatile, do not increase in size with coughing or crying and do not transilluminate	Early surgical excision
Encephaloceles	Mass lesion at locations as described previously	Pulsatile, bluish, compressible masses, which expand on crying or coughing and transilluminate brilliantly	Surgery

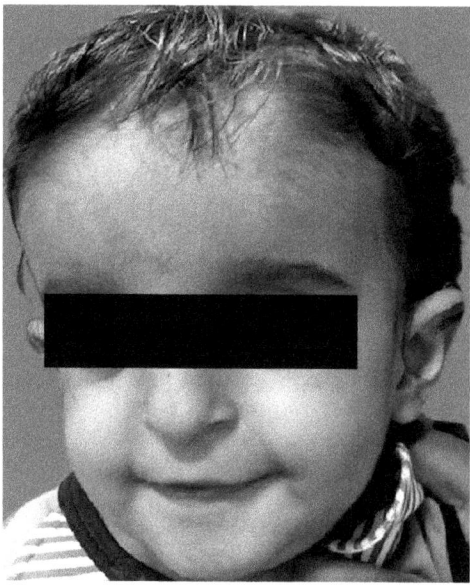

Fig. 21.1: Classical clinical picture of **nasal dermoid,** note the hair follicle coming out of the midnasal lesion along with the broad nasal bridge.

- Nasal dermoids may present along with aural atresia or deformities, hydrocephalous, cleft lip and palate, hypertelorism, hemifacial microsomia, branchial arch anomalies, and mental retardation.
- Dermoids with intracranial extension is not uncommon and is detected by computed tomography (CT) and magnetic resonance imaging (MRI).

Developmental Errors of the Central Midface

Aplastic and Hypoplastic Anomalies

- *Arhinia* is congenital absence of external nose and airway, along with paranasal sinuses and olfactory bulbs.
  - Distinctive "dish-face" deformity with hypertelorism or hypotelorism and normal labial as well as philtrum development.
  - May be associated with anophthalmia or hypoplasia of the eye and a high-arched palate.
  - Surgery involves reconstruction of the external nose and correction of the high-arched palate.
- *Heminasal aplasia* is the agenesis of unilateral nostril (Fig. 21.2).
  - Occurs in isolation or in combination with ipsilateral facial anomalies.
  - Radiology may show associated absence of cribriform plate.
  - Staged surgical correction.
- *Hypoplastic conditions* include columellar agenesis, complete or partial nasal bone agenesis, hypoplastic anterior nasal spine, nasomaxillary hypoplasia, underdeveloped nasal dorsum, and hypoplastic nares.

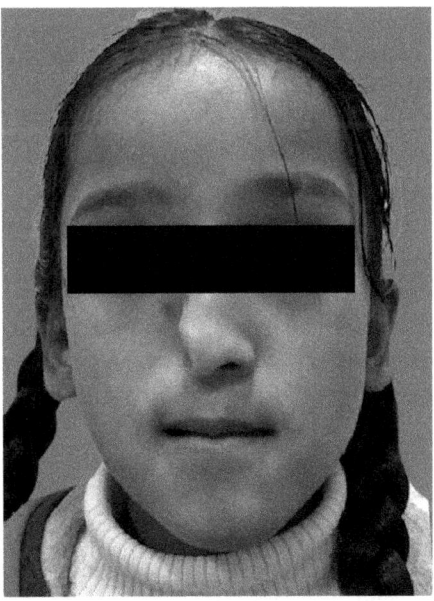

Fig. 21.2: Clinical picture of a patient with **heminasal aplasia** with absence of right half of the nose.

Atretic Anomalies

- Patients present with nasal obstruction, respiratory distress, and feeding difficulties along with cyanotic spells, which are temporarily relieved on crying.
- Inability to pass a nasal suction catheter is a reliable test to detect nasal stenosis, but nasal endoscopy confirms the diagnosis.
- The CT scan provides information about the site, extent, and nature (membranous or bony) of the stenosis, which is crucial prior to surgical correction.
- Mild forms may be managed conservatively using saline nasal drops, topical decongestants, humidification, and frequent suctioning.
- *Nasal pyriform aperture stenosis* results due to bony overgrowth of the nasal process of maxilla causing narrowed nasal inlet.
  - Clinical examination reveals narrow anterior nasal passage with bony thickening medially.
  - Patients may also have hypotelorism and a flat nasal bridge along with a central mega-incisor.
- *Midnasal stenosis* occurs either due to unequal growth of the lateral nasal walls or excessive folding of the nasal septum.

Hyperplastic and Duplication Anomalies

- *Polyrhinia* is the presence of two external noses, which arise from two pairs of normally developing nasal placodes.
  - May be associated with bilateral choanal atresia.
  - Correction involves excision of medial portions of each external nose.
- *Supernumerary nostril* is an extra-nasal opening either lateral, medial, or superior to the normal nostril.
  - May be unilateral or bilateral and may or may not connect with the nasal cavity.
  - Surgically excised.
- *Proboscis lateralis* is a rare craniofacial malformation in which external nose fails to develop on one side and is replaced by a tubular structure emanating from the medial canthus.
  - May occur in isolation or in association with a wide spectrum of anomalies of ipsilateral paranasal sinuses and nasolacrimal system, absent olfactory nerve, olfactory lobe, and cribriform plate on the affected side.
  - Surgery is done after complete facial growth.

Craniofacial Clefts

- The craniofacial clefts are very rare and the hallmark features are ocular hypertelorism, broad-nasal root, ill-defined nasal tip, anterior cranium bifidum occultum, median clefting of the nose, lip and palate, and unilateral orbital clefting or notching of the nasal ala.

- Deformities in median nasal clefts may range from a simple median scar at the cephalic end of the nasal dorsum to a completely bifid nose with two different halves with separate median nasal walls.
- Lateral nasal clefts range from alar scar like lines to triangular defects from medial canthus up to ala and affecting the nasolacrimal apparatus.
- Multidisciplinary surgical correction is indicated.

Developmental Errors of the Nasobuccal Membrane

- Persistence of the embryonic nasobuccal membrane, which separates the nasal cavity from the buccal space, gives rise to choanal atresia.

Choanal Atresia

- Unilateral atresia is twice more common than bilateral and when unilateral, right-sided atresia is more frequent.
- Unilateral atresia may be missed during early childhood and present with persistent unilateral nasal discharge.
- Bilateral choanal atresia is an emergency.
- Complete physical examination is done to assess for other congenital anomalies.
- Apart from diagnosis, radiology in the form of CT helps in differentiating it from deviated nasal septum, septal hematoma, turbinate hypertrophy, mid nasal stenosis, encephalocele, dermoid, hamartoma, chordoma, and teratomas.
- After initial maintenance of airway (by a simple nipple or endotracheal intubation), endoscopic surgical correction is warranted.

RHINOSINUSITIS

- Rhinosinusitis is an inflammatory condition of the nose and paranasal sinuses.
- Common cold caused by viruses is the most common form of rhinosinusitis.
- Following viral respiratory infection, mucosal edema, and obstructed sinus ostia along with hypofunctioning of the sinus ciliary function leads to stasis of secretions in the sinuses.
- Symptoms and signs of sinusitis appear when these sinuses become secondarily infected by bacteria from the nose and nasopharynx.
- In pediatric population, approximately 0.5–10% of upper respiratory infections may evolve into bacterial sinusitis.[1,2]
- Other underlying factors associated with sinusitis are deviated nasal septum, adenoid hypertrophy, allergy, gastroesophageal reflux disease (GERD), passive smoking, and systemic illnesses like immune deficiency, primary ciliary dyskinesia, and cystic fibrosis and should be looked for in recurrent rhinosinusitis.
- Based on the duration of symptoms, pediatric rhinosinusitis is categorized as acute (between 1 weeks and 4 weeks), subacute (4–12 weeks), and chronic (more than 12 weeks).

Acute Bacterial Rhinosinusitis

- *Presentation*—fever, facial fullness or pain, nasal stuffiness, purulent nasal discharge, dental pain, cough, and ear pain or fullness persisting beyond 10 days.
- Severe headache, vomiting, seizures, focal neurological deficits, periorbital edema, proptosis, and diplopia due to restricted extraocular muscle movement mandates CT to evaluate the complications.[3]
- Orbital complications constitute approximately 90% of the complications of acute rhinosinusitis (ARS).
- Medical management is the mainstay of treatment of uncomplicated ARS, which includes antibiotic therapy for at least 10 days along with antihistamines, oral, and nasal decongestants, topical steroid, and nasal irrigation.
- Patients with orbital complications are managed with parenteral antibiotics and functional endoscopic sinus surgery (FESS) with abscess drainage.

Chronic Bacterial Rhinosinusitis

- *Presentation*—persistence of the above-mentioned symptomatology beyond 12 weeks.
- Young patients may be irritable and may show behavioral changes.
- Chronic rhinosinusitis (CRS) is treated with broad-spectrum antibiotics for 3-6 weeks and oral decongestants, topical steroids along with saline irrigation.
- Surgery is planned after failed medical management.
- Preoperative CT scan is performed to know about the disease extent for complete disease clearance and anatomical abnormalities to reduce the risk of surgical complications.
- Surgery consists of adenoidectomy ± FESS.
- In pediatric patients, FESS does not have clinically significant impact on facial growth.[4]

CHRONIC ADENOID HYPERTROPHY

- Adenoids are favorably situated in the nasopharynx to mediate immunological protection of the upper aerodigestive system against inhaled antigens. They are small at birth, grow till 5 years of age and gradually get atrophied by adolescence.
- Chronic bacterial infection, passive smoking, and gastroesophageal reflux may lead to adenoid hypertrophy, which may obstruct the nasopharynx to variable extent.
- Patients present with snoring, mouth breathing, sleep disturbances like restless sleep, night terrors, sleep walking, etc. hearing impairment, enuresis, and recurrent rhinosinusitis.

- When associated with tonsillar hypertrophy, patients might have features of obstructive sleep apnea.
- Diagnosis is made by endoscopic visualization of enlarged adenoids in older children and by lateral neck X-ray in young patients.
- Medical management consists of aqueous nasal steroid spray.
- Surgical removal of the adenoids is considered for significantly enlarged adenoids causing obstructive symptoms as well as for recurrent or chronic sinusitis.

SPECIFIC LESIONS

Antrochoanal Polyps

- Mostly seen in pediatric patients.
  - These are unilateral and arise from the maxillary sinus. Large polyp extents up to posterior choana through the maxillary ostium and nasal cavity.
  - Patients present with unilateral nasal stuffiness, nasal discharge, and hearing loss due to middle ear effusion. When the polyp extends to the nasopharynx, patients might have bilateral nasal obstruction, mouth breathing, and muffled voice.
  - The CT scan helps in diagnosis and is performed prior to endoscopic excision.

Allergic Fungal Sinusitis (AFS)

- Less frequently seen in pediatric patients than adults. The details of the symptomatology and management are like the adult patients.

REFERENCES

1. Aitken M, Taylor JA. Prevalence of clinical sinusitis in young children followed up by primary care pediatricians. Arch Pediatr Adolesc Med. 1998;152:244-8.
2. Revai K, Dobbs LA, Nair S, et al. Incidence of acute otitis media and sinusitis complicating upper respiratory tract infection: the effect of age. Pediatrics. 2007;119:e1408-12.
3. DeMuri GP, Wald ER. Clinical Practice. Acute bacterial sinusitis in children. N Eng J Med. 2012;367:1128-34.
4. Bothwell MR, Piccirillo JF, Lusk RP, et al. Long term outcome of facial growth after functional endoscopic sinus surgery. Otolaryngol Head Neck Surg. 2002;126;628-34.

Section 6

Systemic Disorders/Surrounding Structures Involving PNS

22. Systemic Disorders Affecting Sinonasal Cavity
23. Anterior Skull Base Lesions: Imaging
24. Imaging of Dental Lesions and Sinonasal Cavity
25. Imaging of Disorders Involving Sinonasal Cavity and Orbit

22
CHAPTER

Systemic Disorders Affecting Sinonasal Cavity

Surabhi Vyas, Ashu Seith Bhalla

- Introduction
- Infections
  - Tuberculosis
  - Leprosy
  - Invasive Fungal Infections
  - Syphilis (*Treponema Pallidum*) Infection
- Chronic Inflammatory Disorders
  - Granulomatosis with Polyangiitis
  - Sarcoidosis
  - Relapsing Polychondritis
  - Others
- Immunodeficiency
  - Primary Immunodeficiency
    - Structural Defects
    - Cystic Fibrosis
    - Primary Ciliary Dyskinesia
  - Acquired Immune Disorders
    - Acquired Immunodeficiency Syndrome
  - Bone Marrow Transplant Recipients
  - Solid Organ Transplant Recipient
- Disorders with Sinopulmonary Involvement
  - Allergic Bronchopulmonary Aspergillosis
  - Asthma
  - Samter's Triad
  - Inflammatory Bowel Disease
  - Amyloidosis
- Granulomatous Disorders
  - Immunoglobulin-4-Related Disease
  - Rhinoscleroma
  - Rhinosporidiosis
- Illustrative Case

INTRODUCTION

Although involvement of the sinonasal cavity by systemic disorders is uncommon, a gamut of inflammatory disorders may involve the sinonasal cavity (Flowchart 22.1).

Flowchart 22.1: Classification of systemic disorders affecting the sinonasal cavity.

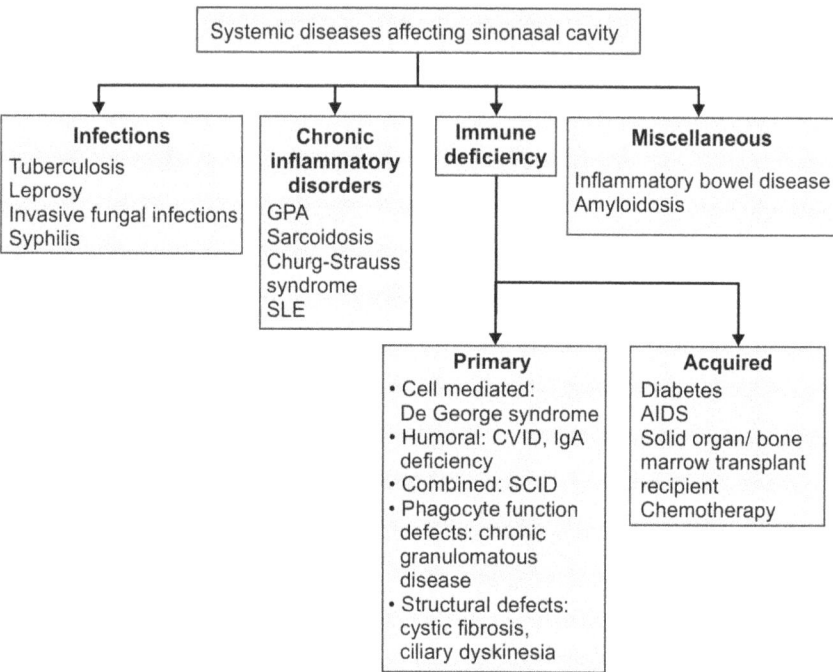

(AIDS: Acquired immunodeficiency syndrome; CVID: Common variable immunodeficiency; GPA: Granulomatosis with polyangiitis; IgA: Immunoglobulin A; SCID: Severe combined immunodeficiency; SLE: Systemic lupus erythematosus).

INFECTIONS

Tuberculosis

- Sinonasal cavity is an uncommon site of involvement.
- Clinical presentation is nonspecific with nasal obstruction or catarrh.
- Imaging findings include enlarged adenoids with enlarged nodes.
- Inflammatory polyps mainly in the region of inferior turbinate or septal perforation may also be seen.

Leprosy

- Nose may be involved in the lepromatous leprosy variant of the disease.
- Mucosal thickening and septal perforation are seen, later causing saddle nose (Fig. 22.1).
- Mucosal thickening in other sinuses has also been described.

Invasive Fungal Infections

- Invasive fungal infections in the immune-compromised host can involve multiple sites especially lungs and sinonasal cavity (Figs. 22.2A and B) and are covered elsewhere in the book.

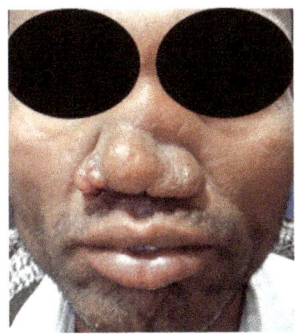

Fig. 22.1: Leprosy—Patient of leprosy showing depressed and deformed nasal bridge.

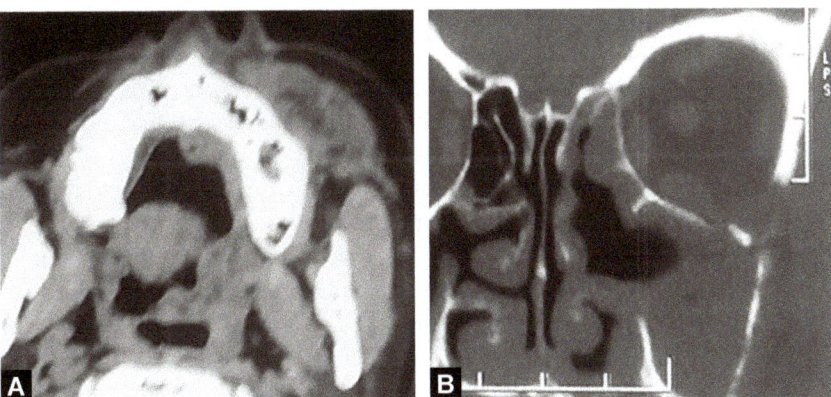

Figs. 22.2A and B: Mucormycosis in a poorly controlled diabetic lady. (A) Extrasinus soft tissue anterior to left maxillary sinus; and (B) Permeative bone destruction of left maxillary sinus lateral wall.

Syphilis (*Treponema pallidum*) Infection

- Nasal manifestations of syphilis are infrequently seen nowadays.
- While primary syphilis may have chancre of nasal vestibule, secondary form presents with copious nasal discharge, it is the tertiary form which has the most severe manifestations.
- Soft tissue thickening (gummata) seen resulting in septal perforation and eventually the typical "saddle nose deformity".
- Congenital syphilis also presents nasal discharge and may cause septal perforation.

CHRONIC INFLAMMATORY DISORDERS

Granulomatosis with Polyangiitis (GPA)

- Previously called Wegener granulomatosis.
- Multisystem auto-immune disease of unknown etiology, disorder characterized by necrotizing granulomas with small and medium vessel vasculitis.

- Characteristically involve the kidneys, sinonasal cavity, and lungs.
- *Laboratory investigations:* Elevated antineutrophil cytoplasmic antibodies (ANCAs), but these may not be elevated in a fourth of patients.
- Two forms: (1) Limited, and (2) Severe.
  1. *Limited:* Where no threat to life/vital organs function (earlier used for renal sparing forms).
  2. *Severe:* Severe forms need more aggressive management with cyclophosphamide or rituximab in addition to glucocorticoids.
- Head and neck region involvement includes the following sites: Nasal cavity, sinuses, orbits, anterior skull base, upper airway, and temporal bone.
- *Sinonasal involvement:*
  - Imaging findings in the sinonasal cavity primarily consist of nodular and mucosal thickening with bone erosion and sclerosis due to neo-osteogenesis.
  - Maxillary sinus is the predominant site of mucosal thickening. It is indistinguishable from chronic rhinosinusitis except that *nodularity is seen more often in GPA*
  - Bony erosions occur more frequently in the anterior ethmoid regions but other sinuses may also be involved
  - The destructive changes begin in the nasal septum, spreading laterally to the turbinates and then to the maxillary antra and subsequently to the other sinuses. Finally the sinonasal space appears as a single large cavity
  - The hard palate is usually spared, though it can be involved occasionally
  - Avascular necrosis due to vascular occlusion is the mechanism for bone destruction
  - Anterior skull base erosions may occur due to contiguous spread from the sinonasal disease process
  - On computed tomography (CT), sclerosis gives a layered appearance with less dense and more sclerotic bone seen parallel along the sinus wall (Figs. 22.3A and B)
  - On magnetic resonance imaging (MRI), while the more dense bone appears hypointense on T1-weighted images, the less dense bone may be hyperintense due to marrow in areas of neo-osteogenesis (vs periostitis) (Figs. 22.4A and B). MRI may reveal thickening and enhancement of the olfactory nerves in cases of olfactory nerve neuropathy with the patient developing anosmia.

Sarcoidosis

- Sinonasal cavity involvement is seen in less than 1% patients of sarcoidosis.
- Nodular mucosal thickening, or even polyposis may be seen, mainly involving inferior turbinates and nasal septum.

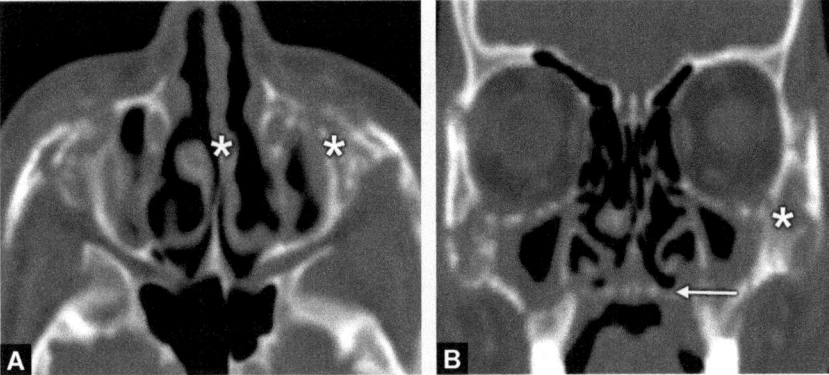

Figs. 22.3A and B: GPA, (A) Axial; and (B) Coronal CT images. Bony destruction, sclerosis with typical layered appearance of maxillary walls, zygoma, and nasal septum (*). Hard palate involvement (arrow) though seen in this patient is an unusual feature. (CT: Computed tomography; GPA: Granulomatosis with polyangiitis).

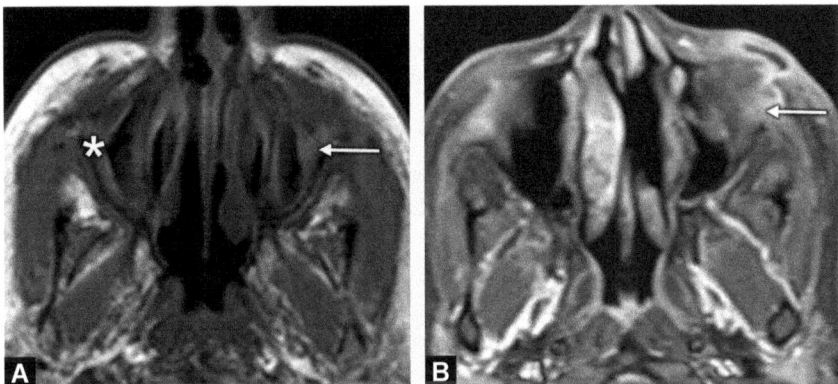

Figs. 22.4A and B: GPA, (A) Axial T1W; and (B) Postcontrast MR images. (A) T1W MRI showing hypointense sclerotic bone (*), and hyperintense marrow containing bone (arrow); and (B) CEMRI showing areas of enhancement in the involved bones (arrow). (GPA: Granulomatosis with polyangiitis; CEMRI: Contrast-enhanced magnetic resonance imaging; T1W: T1-weighted).

- Septal perforations and hard/soft palate erosions are rare. Neo-osteogenesis may be seen.

Relapsing Polychondritis

- *Synonym:* Relapsing perichondritis/chronic atrophic polychondritis.
- Chronic inflammatory disorders affecting cartilage of pinna, nose, airway with arthritis, and hearing loss.
- Nasal chondritis results in saddle nose deformity.
- There is no mucosal involvement hence no mucosal thickening/hypertrophy seen (vs GPA).

Others

- Recurrent acute sinusitis, chronic rhinosinusitis, polyposis, and even nasal perforations can be seen but less commonly in other vasculitis, such as Churg-Strauss syndrome, systemic lupus erythematosus, and polyarteritis nodosa. Nasal mucosal atrophy may be seen in Sjögren's syndrome.

IMMUNODEFICIENCY

Primary Immunodeficiency

- Inherited defects affecting cell-mediated/humoral immunity, phagocyte function, or mucociliary clearance can result in recurrent and persistent infections in the head and neck.
- These include rhinosinusitis, otitis media, oral cavity infections, and adenopathy.
- If a patient develops two or more episodes of severe sinusitis within a year, investigations for immunodeficiencies should be initiated.
- Therapy besides long-term antibiotics includes immunoglobulins and bone marrow transplantation, depending on the disorder.

Structural Defects

Dysfunctions affecting mucociliary clearance mechanism result in recurrent sinusitis and polyposis, in addition to frequent pulmonary infections.

Cystic Fibrosis

- Autosomal recessive inheritance.
- Sinonasal involvement seen in about 20% of patients.
- The various features of involvement include nasal polyposis and chronic rhinosinusitis. The mucopurulent secretions can lead to bulging of the lateral wall of the maxillary sinus simulating a mucocele, referred to as maxillary pseudomucoceles.

Primary Ciliary Dyskinesia

- Autosomal recessive disorder.
- About 50% of patients have Kartagener's syndrome comprising of bronchiectasis, situs inversus, and chronic sinusitis.
- Rhinitis, polyposis, maxillary, and ethmoid sinusitis are seen, while frontal sinuses are often hypoplastic (Figs. 22.5A to C).

Acquired Immune Disorders

Acquired Immunodeficiency Syndrome

- Nasopharyngeal mucosal inflammation and hypertrophy is seen.
- *Sinusitis:* It is usually recurrent, may be acute and chronic.
- *Rhinitis:* It may exacerbate allergic rhinitis.

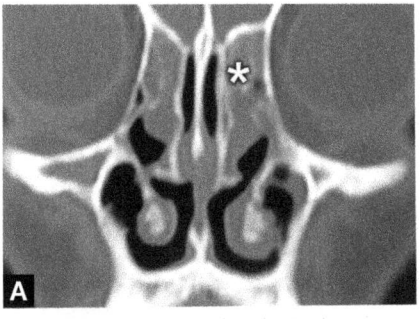
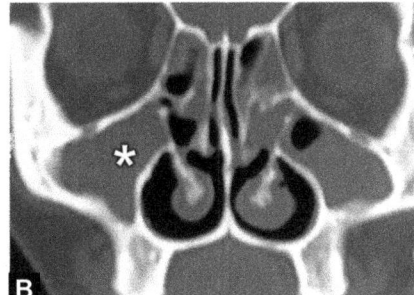
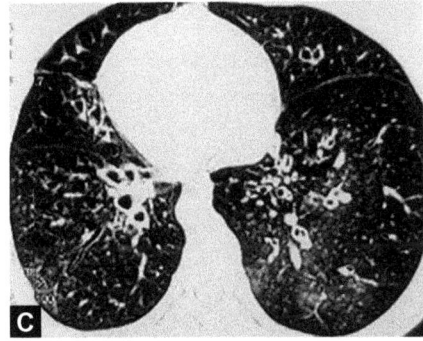

Figs. 22.5A to C: Primary ciliary dyskinesia. (A and B) Coronal computed tomography (CT)-paranasal sinus (PNS) showing maxillary and ethmoid sinusitis (*); and (C) Lung window CT showing extensive bronchiectasis, bronchial wall thickening with centrilobular nodules, and ground-glass opacities (*).

Bone marrow Transplant Recipients
- Increased predisposition to infections with Gram-negative bacteria and fungi.
- Sinusitis especially invasive fungal sinusitis is a real risk.

Solid Organ Transplant Recipient
- Similar increased risk of invasive fungal infections, especially aspergillosis.

DISORDERS WITH SINOPULMONARY INVOLVEMENT

Several disorders of varying etiology tend to involve the respiratory system, especially the airways and sinonasal apparatus (Flowchart 22.2).

Some of these have been discussed earlier in this chapter and elsewhere.

Allergic Bronchopulmonary Aspergillosis
- Allergic bronchopulmonary aspergillosis is a hypersensitivity response to *Aspergillus fumigatus* with bronchial and pulmonary manifestations, seen in asthmatics.
- It may be associated with allergic *Aspergillus* sinusitis with exacerbations parallel to the pulmonary symptoms.
- Imaging reveals chronic rhinosinusitis which is more often unilateral with central hyperdensities and sinus expansion (Figs. 22.6A and B).
- Seen in young asthmatics, patients give history of passage of brownish plugs/casts with nasal discharge.

Flowchart 22.2: Classification of disorders with sinopulmonary involvement.

```
                        Sinopulmonary involvement
        ┌───────────────────┬──────────────┬──────────────┐
        ▼                   ▼              ▼              ▼
    Allergic         Immunodeficiency    Chronic        Infectious
                                       inflammatory
   Bronchopulmonary   Cystic fibrosis    GPA           Invasive fungal
   aspergillosis      Primary ciliary    Sarcoidosis   infection
   Asthma             dyskinesia         CSS           Tuberculosis
   Samter's triad                        Relapsing     (uncommon)
                                         polychondritis
```

(GPA: Granulomatosis with polyangiitis; EGPA: Eosinophilic Granulomatosis with Polyangiitis also in the table also replace CSS with EGPA).

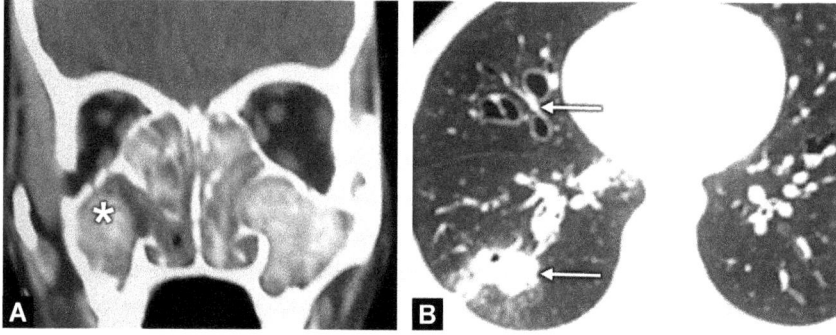

Figs. 22.6A and B: Allergic aspergillus sinusitis. (A) Coronal computed tomography (CT) image showing hyperdense contents distending the maxillary and ethmoid sinuses (*). Note that the edematous mucosa is hypodense; and (B) Lung window of same patient showing patchy area of consolidation in right lower lobe with central bronchiectasis (arrows).

Asthma

- It is logical that diseases of the upper and lower airway may coexist in the same patient. Hence, a large proportion (up to 80%) of patients with asthma has allergic rhinitis, while nasal polyposis can occur in 7%.
- Imaging reveals nonspecific findings of sinus opacification, air-fluid levels, mucosal thickening, or polyposis.

Samter's Triad

Aspirin-exacerbated respiratory disease (AERD), Widal's triad/aspirin sensitive asthma syndrome comprising of asthma and nasal polyposis related to aspirin/other nonsteroidal anti-inflammatory drugs (NSAIDs) intake.

Inflammatory Bowel Disease

Chronic mucosal inflammation may be present in up to 50% patients of ulcerative colitis, and rarely in Crohn's disease. Occasionally septal perforation may also be seen.

Amyloidosis
- Nasal or maxillary sinus mucosal thickening maybe seen in amyloidosis.
- It is mostly unilateral.

GRANULOMATOUS DISORDERS
- Granulomatous diseases are often multisystem disorders that result in formation of granulomas (macrophages or mononuclear inflammatory cells with or without giant cells surrounded by lymphocytes).
- In the head and neck, these essentially include the multisystem diseases that we have discussed earlier in the chapter.
- These disorders are of varying etiology, mainly autoimmune (GPA, Churg-Strauss syndrome, and Behcet disease), infectious (TB, fungal, leprosy, and rhinoscleroma), idiopathic (sarcoidosis), or hereditary (chronic granulomatous disease).
- As discussed earlier, in the head and neck region, malignancy is an important differential of these disorders (Figs. 22.7A and B).

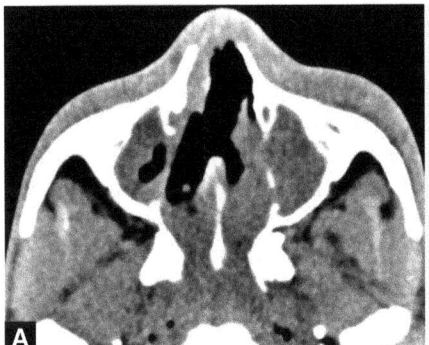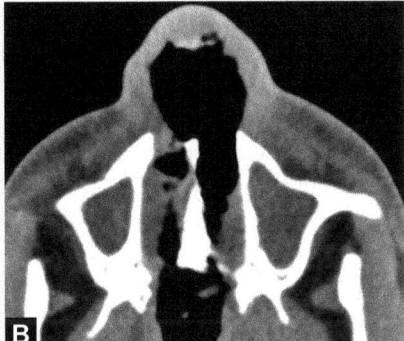

Figs. 22.7A and B: NK/T-cell lymphoma. (A) Axial CT soft tissue window; and (B) Coronal bone window CT showing destruction of the nasal septum and turbinates with heterogeneous soft tissue thickening. (CT: Computed tomography; NK: Natural killer).

Immunoglobulin-4-related Disease
- Relatively recently described entity, first reported in 2001.
- Multisystem disease, sinonasal involvement rare. Sinonasal involvement is part of multisystem disease isolated (more frequent).
- Nonspecific symptoms, epistaxis is common presenting symptom.
- *Imaging:* No specific feature.
  - *Site*—Maxillary sinus is most common, more often unilateral, and can be bilateral
  - Focal soft tissue mass with bony destruction. Perineural/marrow infiltration also seen
  - *Computed tomography*—Isoattenuating mass with bone expansion and remodeling. Bone sclerosis/erosion.
- *Magnetic resonance imaging*—Isointense to gray matter with homogenous enhancement (Figs. 22.8A and B).

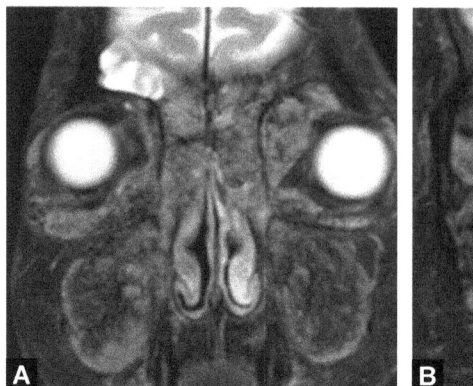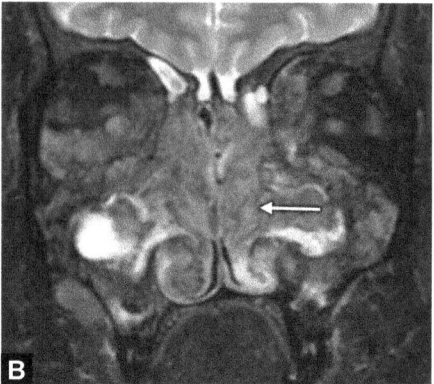

Figs. 22.8A and B: IgG4-related disease. (A) Coronal fat suppressed T2-weighted (T2W) images showing heterogeneously hypointense soft tissue filling bilateral maxillary, frontal, and ethmoid sinuses; and (B) Extension to extraconal compartment of both orbits and nasal cavities (arrow).

- Diagnostic criteria based on international consensus statement require presence of two out of three characteristic histopathological features which include a dense lymphoplasmacytic infiltrate (with more than 50 IgG4 plasma infiltration), fibrosis (characteristic storiform pattern), and obliterative phlebitis. Eosinophils are also seen within the infiltrate.
- Supportive evidence is elevation of serum IgG4 levels. It is, however, an insensitive marker and can be negative. Tissue biopsy is essential.
- Treated with steroids/surgery. In nonresponders rituximab has also been advocated.

Rhinoscleroma

- Chronic granulomatous disease of infectious etiology.
- *Organism:* Klebsiella rhinoscleromatis (Gram-negative bacteria).
- *Clinical features:* Nasal crusting, expansion of nasal cavity, and foetid odor.
- *Endemic areas:* Tropical and temperate regions including parts of India.
- *Sites:* Nasal cavity is involved in almost all patients with subsequent spread to the rest of upper airway, pharynx, nasopharynx, oropharynx, larynx, and less commonly trachea and even bronchi involved. Middle and inferior turbinate are involved first, then nasal septum. May extend through septum to maxillary sinus (40% cases). Sphenoid and ethmoid sinus involvement is uncommon.
- *Histopathology of scleroma:* Granulation tissue with plasma cells, Russell bodies (degenerated plasma cells), and Mikulicz cells (foamy histiocytes containing bacteria).
- *Treatment:* Antibiotics (broad spectrum), surgery, and laser for laryngeal lesions.

> **Box 22.1: Suspicion of granulomatous disorders on imaging.**
>
> When to suspect granulomatous disorders on imaging:
> - Chronic sinonasal inflammation (mucosal thickening and/or polyposis)
> - Osseous and cartilage erosion, perforation of nasal septum ± palate perforation
> - Nasal cavity is involved before the paranasal sinuses
> - Maxillary/ethmoid sinus involvement
> - Frontal sinuses usually spared
> - Orbital extension
> - Less commonly intracranial extension.

- *Imaging findings:*
  - Depend on the stage of the disease, there is expansion of the nasal cavity, scalloping of sinus wall (chronic disease unlike malignancy)
  - *Catarrhal stage:* Nonspecific mucosal thickening or soft tissue nodules
  - *Granulomatous (hypertrophic) stage:* Masses, bilateral asymmetrical in majority, and unilateral in one-third (Box 22.1).
  - *Computed tomography:* Scleromas are well-defined and homogenous in appearance.
  - *Magnetic resonance imaging:*
    - *T1-weighted image:* It may be hyperintense (increased protein in Mikulicz cells and Russell bodies)
    - *T2-weighted image:* Mildly hyperintense due to cellular component, with hypointense foci due to fibrotic component.
    - *Contrast-enhanced magnetic resonance imaging:* Homogenous enhancement.
    - *Diffusion-weighted imaging:* Restricted diffusion (high cellularity and fatty areas).
- *Sclerotic (fibrotic stage):*
  - Atrophy/destruction of turbinates
  - Nasal septum destruction
  - Vestibular, laryngeal stenosis.

Rhinosporidiosis

- Chronic granulomatous disease of infectious etiology.
- *Organism: Rhinosporidium seeberi*, fungus of class Mesomycetozoea.
- *Endemic areas:* Southern India, Sri Lanka, and Pakistan.
- Adult males commonly affected.
- *Predisposing factor:* Bathing in stagnant water ponds. Enters through skin and mucosal abrasions.
- *Sites of involvement:* Nasal cavity, nasopharynx, oropharynx, and nasolacrimal ducts (in decreasing order)
  - *Other systems reported:* Trachea, bones, central nervous system, and orbits.

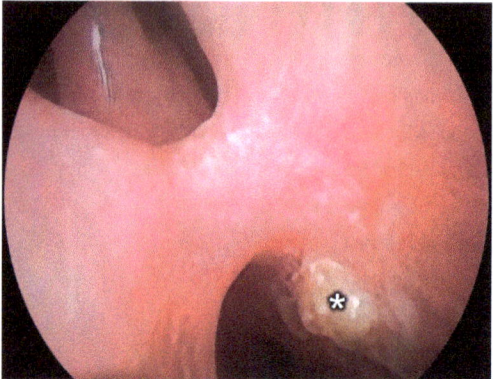

Fig. 22.9: Rhinosporidiosis. Clinical image showing vascular polyp of the nasal cavity (*).

- Imaging for atypical/recurrent cases and for extent of disease.
- *On clinical examination:* Vascular polyp with white dots classical in endemic areas (Fig. 22.9).
- *Computed tomography:* Nasal cavity with common sites including inferior turbinate, inferior meatus and floor
  - Well-defined polypoidal mass with moderate to intense enhancement
  - Foci or air and calcification within
  - Multiple dilated supplying vessels
  - Compared to nasal cavity and nasopharyngeal lesions, those in oropharynx or trachea show less enhancement
  - Nasolacrimal duct may be involved with spread to lacrimal sac
  - Adjoining bones involved with thinning/rarefaction or erosion. Marked erosion of inferior turbinate, septal erosion, and thinning of medial wall of the maxillary sinus
  - *Magnetic resonance imaging:* Heterogeneous appearance with flow voids. Intense enhancement on contrast-enhanced MRI (CEMRI). Imaging pattern may resemble the cribriform pattern of enhancement of inverted papilloma. However, site and spread is different.
- *Diagnosis:* Fine-needle aspiration cytology (FNAC) with examination under potassium hydroxide (KOH)/Papanicolaou smear. However, histopathology often required.
- *Treatment:* Surgical removal with high recurrence rates. Dapsone is also used.

ILLUSTRATIVE CASE

Demographics
A 40-year-old housewife.

Clinical Picture
- Chronic cough
- Nasal discharge
- Skin ulcers
- Microscopic hematuria
- Received oral prednisolone.

Baseline Imaging (Figs. 22.10A to C)
Axial CT paranasal sinus (Fig. 22.10A) and coronal reconstruction (Fig. 22.10B):
- Opacification of the left maxillary and ethmoid sinuses
- Rarefaction of the left maxillary wall
- Nasal septum intact
- Polypoidal soft tissue the right maxillary sinus.

Coronal reconstruction CT thorax (Fig. 22.10C):
- Cavitating lesions in right middle lobe and a nodule in left lower lobe.

6 Months Follow-up Imaging (Figs. 22.10D to F)
Axial CT paranasal sinus (Fig. 22.10D) and coronal reconstruction (Fig. 22.10E):
- Characteristic lateral progression of the destructive process to involve the septum and the maxillary walls.
- Note the final appearance is indistinguishable from primary atrophic rhinitis.
- Coronal CT lung window (Fig. 22.10F) showing increase in the size as well as the cavitation of both right and left side lesions.

Diagnosis
Granulomatosis with polyangiitis.

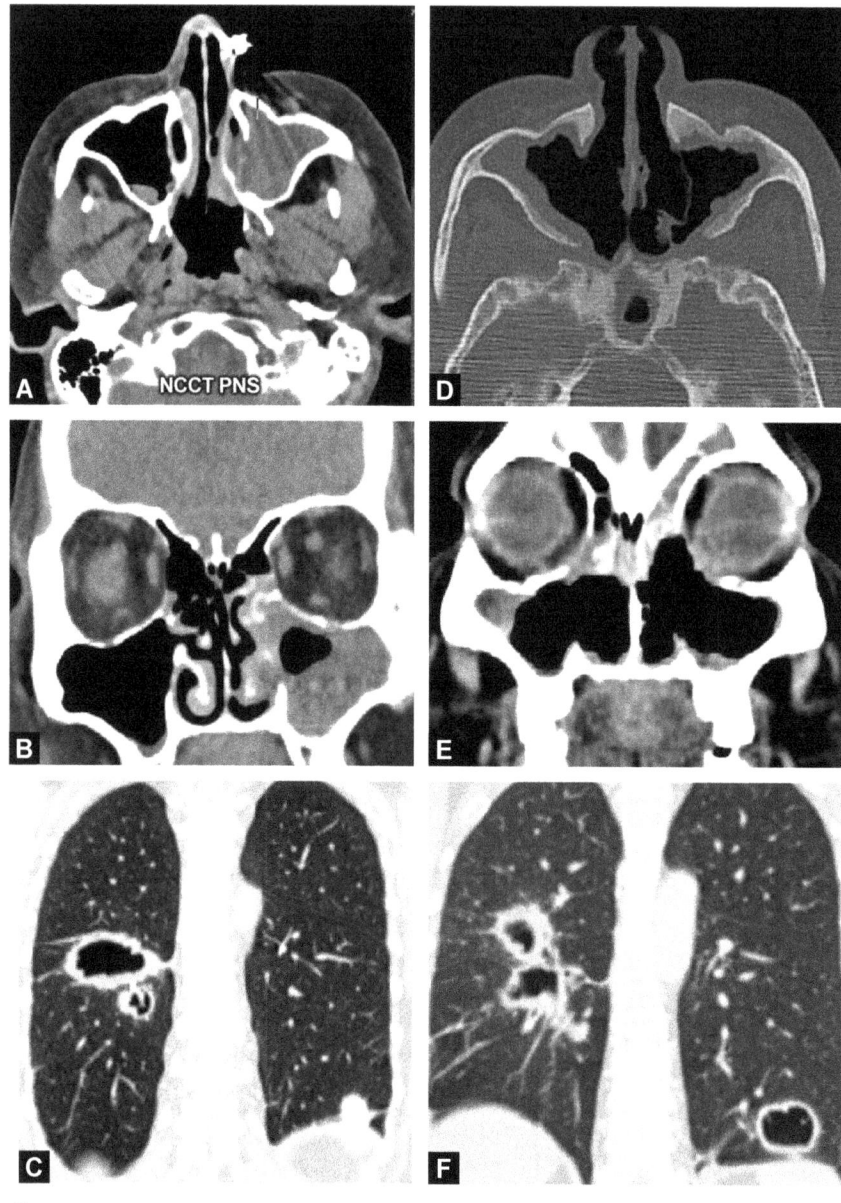

Figs. 22.10A to F

BIBLIOGRAPHY

1. Abdel Razek AA. Imaging of scleroma in the head and neck. Br J Radiol. 2012;85(1020):1551-5.
2. Alobid I, Guilemany JM, Mullol J. Nasal manifestations of systemic illnesses. Curr Allergy Asthma Rep. 2004;4(3):208-16.
3. Deshpande V. IgG4 related disease of the head and neck. Head Neck Pathol. 2015;9(1):24-31.
4. Nwawka OK, Nadgir R, Fujita A, et al. Granulomatous disease in the head and neck: developing a differential diagnosis. Radiographics. 2014;34(5):1240-56.
5. Pakalniskis MG, Berg AD, Policeni BA, et al. The Many Faces of Granulomatosis with Polyangiitis: A Review of the Head and Neck Imaging Manifestations. AJR Am J Roentgenol. 2015;205(6):W619-29.

23
CHAPTER

Anterior Skull Base Lesions: Imaging

Ajay Garg, Anuj Prabhakar

- Introduction
- Congenital Anterior Skull Base Lesions
  - Nasal Dermal Sinus, Dermoid Cyst, and Epidermoid Cyst
  - Nasal Glioma
  - Anterior Cephalocele
  - Kallmann Syndrome
- Trauma
  - Classification of Frontobasal Fractures
  - Complications
- Nontraumatic Cerebrospinal Fluid Rhinorrhea
  - Spontaneous Cerebrospinal Fluid Rhinorrhea
- Tumors
  - Meningioma
  - Hemangiopericytoma/Solitary Fibrous Tumors of the Dura
  - Pituitary Macroadenoma
  - Subfrontal Schwannomas
  - Metastasis

INTRODUCTION

Anterior skull base lesions can be classified based on etiology (Table 23.1).

CONGENITAL ANTERIOR SKULL BASE LESIONS (ALSO *SEE* CHAPTER 20)

- Nasal dermal sinus
- Anterior cephalocele
- Nasal glioma
- Kallmann syndrome.

Nasal Dermal Sinus, Dermoid Cyst, and Epidermoid Cyst

- These are congenital inclusion cysts.
- Incomplete dural separation from the skin and subcutaneous tissue during regression pulls dermal elements into the dural tract.
- Occur along the course of the dural tract.
- Seen in subcutaneous region of the nasal bridge from the glabella to tip of the nose, the nasal septum, prenasal space and at level of foramen cecum, adjacent to the crista galli, or anterior third ventricle margin.

Table 23.1: Classification of anterior skull base lesions based on etiology.

Congenital	• Nasal dermal sinus, epidermoid, and dermoid cyst • Nasal glioma • Anterior encephalocele • Kallmann syndrome
Trauma (anterior skull base fractures)	
Nontraumatic cerebrospinal fluid (CSF) rhinorrhea	
Infection/inflammatory	• Extension of sinonasal infection (osteomyelitis) • Pseudotumor

Tumors	• Tumors arising from above:
	  – Meningioma
	  – Pituitary adenoma
	  – Hemangiopericytoma
	  – Anterior skull base schwannoma
	• Tumors from below:
	  – Metastases
	  – Paget's disease

- Rarely sinus tract may extend up to philtrum.
- Intracranial extension may be seen in 20%; while 80% are extracranial.
- These are associated with third ventricle colloid cysts, craniofacial anomalies in 15%.
- Present as broadened nasal root, nasoglabellar mass with pit on nasal bridge with/without hair, and sebaceous discharge. Recurrent meningitis may be seen, if tract is patent throughout.
- *Computed tomography:*
  - Large foramen cecum, bifid crista galli, and deformity of cribriform plate on bone window.
  - Focal mass along nasal bridge or in the sinus tract.
- *Magnetic resonance imaging (Figs. 23.1A to F):*
  - *Dermal sinus tract:* Appears as a midline, subcutaneous, linear T1 hypointensity within the nasal bridge and coursing toward the prenasal space.
  - *Epidermoid cyst:* Low signal on T1, bright signal on T2 with diffusion restriction.
  - *Dermoid cysts:* Fat containing lesion showing T1 and T2 hyperintensity and variable diffusion-weighted imaging (DWI) signal.

Nasal Glioma

- *Synonyms:* Benign congenital nasal neuroectodermal tumor/nasal cerebral heterotopia/glial heterotopia.
- Fibrous stalk representing the rudimentary intracranial connection can be found in 15%.

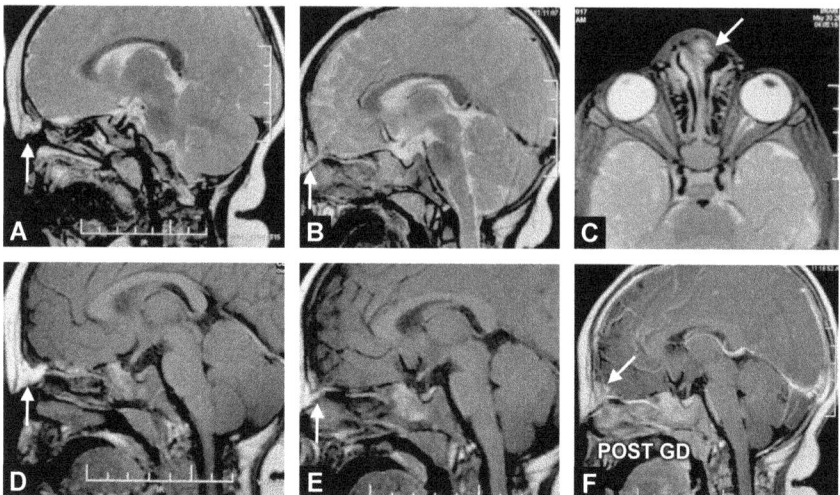

Figs. 23.1A to F: Nasal sinus with dermoid. T1, T2 hyperintense lesion (arrows in A, B, D, and E) extending from the subcutaneous planes in the bridge of the nose up to the intracranial compartment across the foramen cecum (arrow in E). Partial fat suppression (arrow in C). Subtle enhancement along the intracranial margin (arrow in F).

- Detected at birth or in infancy and grow with the child.
- Composed of dysplastic, neuroglial tissue, and fibrovascular tissue.
- The mass may be seen along the nasal dorsum in the region of glabella (most common) or slightly off midline as a medial canthal lesion.
- The tumor might also be intranasal (30%), arising from the lateral nasal wall, middle turbinate, or nasal septum or mixed intra and extranasal masses (10%).
- Often misdiagnosed initially as capillary hemangiomas.
- Present with nasal airway obstruction.
- Appears as a solid soft tissue mass in the nasal dorsum or cavity without intracranial extension.
- *Computed tomography:*
  - Thinning of nasal bones
  - Midline fibrous pedicle showing an intracranial connection
  - Defect in cribriform plate
  - Nonenhancing heterogeneous soft tissue density mass
  - Cisternography does not reveal any communication between the lesion and the brain.
- *Magnetic resonance imaging:*
  - Well-circumscribed, rounded, or polypoid in shape that is iso to hypointense on T1W and hyperintense on T2W
  - Areas of cysts and myxoid degeneration
  - Peripheral enhancement of the surrounding nasal mucosa is seen
  - The mass itself does not enhance.

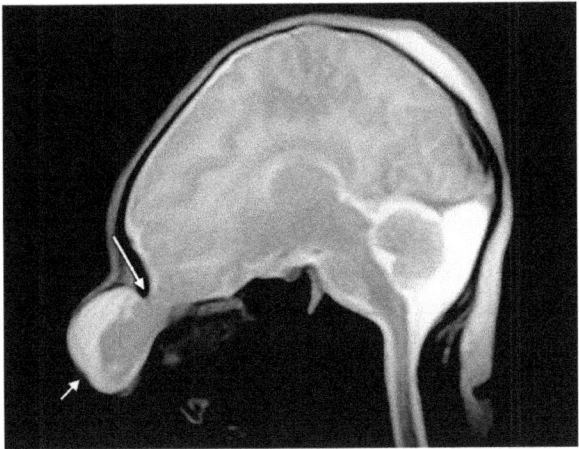

Fig. 23.2: Nasofrontal encephalocele. Herniation of the brain parenchyma with meninges (small arrow) through a midline defect between the frontal and nasal bones (large white arrow).

- Can be differentiated from hemangioma using magnetic resonance imaging (MRI) or Doppler, which shows low diastolic flow in nasal gliomas.

Anterior Cephalocele

- Due to incomplete separation of neural and surface ectoderm at the site of closure of the rostral neuropore in the 4th week of gestation resulting in a midline mesodermal defect.
- *Classification based on location:*
  - *Nasofrontal cephalocele:* It projects out via fonticulus frontalis. Present as glabellar mass (Fig. 23.2).
  - *Nasoethmoidal cephalocele:* It projects via foramen cecum into the prenasal space. Present with lesion at the nasal root/intranasally (Figs. 23.3A and B).
  - *Naso-orbital encephalocele:* It projects via foramen cecum, behind the frontal processes of the maxillary bones into both orbits, and displacing globes laterally. Present with a medial canthal region mass.
  - Basal encephaloceles including spheno-orbital, transethmoidal, sphenoethmoidal, sphenomaxillary, and transsphenoidal encephaloceles (Fig. 23.4).
- *Classification based on content:*
  - Meninges only (meningocele)
  - Cerebrospinal fluid (CSF), meninges, and brain (meningo-encephalocele)
  - Dura, dysplastic neural tissue, and fibrous tissue (atretic cephalocele)
  - Glial-lined cysts containing CSF (glioceles).
- These are not linked to neural tube defects.

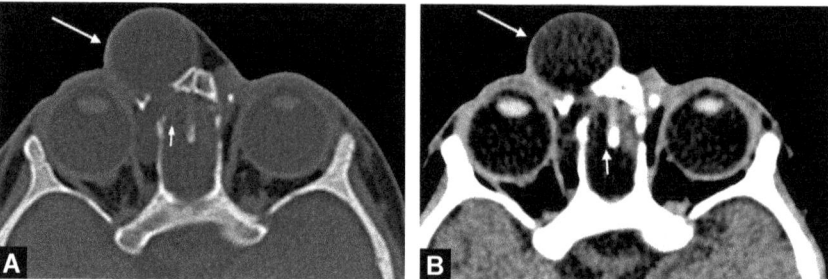

Figs. 23.3A and B: Nasoethmoidal encephalocele. Hypodense lesion (large arrows) extending across a defect in the right cribriform plate (small arrows) below the nasal bone.

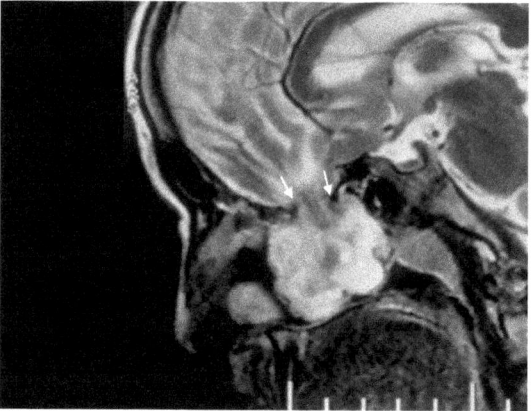

Fig. 23.4: Transsphenoidal encephalocele. Well-defined T2 hyperintense lesion with central hypointensity, in the nasal cavity. Extension across the sphenoid bone (arrows) anterior to the dorsum sellae. Herniating gliotic brain parenchyma is seen at the site of intracranial communication and within the lesion.

- Broadening of the nasal bridge, hypertelorism, and enlargement with crying/jugular compression (positive Furstenberg sign) are seen.
- Associated anomalies include: Anophthalmia, arrhinencephaly, microphthalmos, corpus callosum anomalies, interhemispheric lipomas, arachnoid cysts, colloid cyst, cerebral cortical malformations, and hydrocephalus.
- Mass with intracranial extension across a bony defect is seen on imaging.
- *Computed tomography:*
  - Widening of the foramen cecum
  - Deformity or absence of the normal crista galli and cribriform plate.
- *Magnetic resonance imaging:*
  - *T1:* Variable hypointense CSF with isointense tissue
  - *T2:* Bright CSF signal and gliosis within the herniated tissue
  - Meningeal enhancement may be seen in case of inflammation/infection. No enhancement within the herniated tissue.

Table 23.2: Differences between dermoid cyst and encephalocele.

Dermoid cyst	Encephalocele
This is a congenital inclusion cyst formed due to incomplete separation of the dural and dermal elements	This is an extracranial herniation of meninges with/without brain across a bony defect
No enlargement with crying/jugular compression	Enlargement with crying/jugular compression is seen
Hair and sebaceous discharge with sinus opening are seen on the surface	No hair/sebaceous discharge/sinus opening seen
Intracranial extension may or may not be seen	Mass with intracranial extension across a bony defect
Fat containing lesion showing T1 and T2 hyperintensity on imaging	Bright CSF signal with gliotic tissue seen within the lesion on MRI

(CSF: Cerebrospinal fluid; MRI: Magnetic resonance imaging).

Table 23.2 describes the differences between dermoid cyst and encephalocele.

Kallmann Syndrome

- Hypogonadotropic hypogonadism and anosmia/hyposmia.
- Due to abnormal development of olfactory axon ending and gonadotropin-releasing hormone (GnRH) neuron migration.
- All modes of inheritance have been described. X-linked is the most common.
- Associated anomalies include: Cardiovascular abnormalities, renal agenesis, cryptorchidism, midline defects, sensorineural deafness, small anterior lobe of the pituitary gland, short fourth metacarpal and facial anomalies, and septo-optic dysplasia.
- Low levels of the gonadotropin hormones are seen.
- *Computed tomography:*
  - Ethmoid bone abnormalities in the form of reduction in the height, width, and surface area of olfactory fossa.
  - Flattening of the ethmoid floor with loss of normal gull wing appearance of the ethmoid.
- *Magnetic resonance imaging of the olfactory region:*
  - Unilateral or bilateral hypoplasia or aplasia of the olfactory bulbs
  - Hypoplastic olfactory sulci
  - Hypoplastic anterior pituitary
  - Abnormalities of the olfactory tracts.

TRAUMA (ALSO REFER TO CHAPTER 17)

- Direct frontal trauma results in frontobasal injuries, involving the upper facial third (frontal bone/sinus and superior orbital rim), and anterior skull base (cribriform plate, ethmoid roofs, and planum sphenoidale).

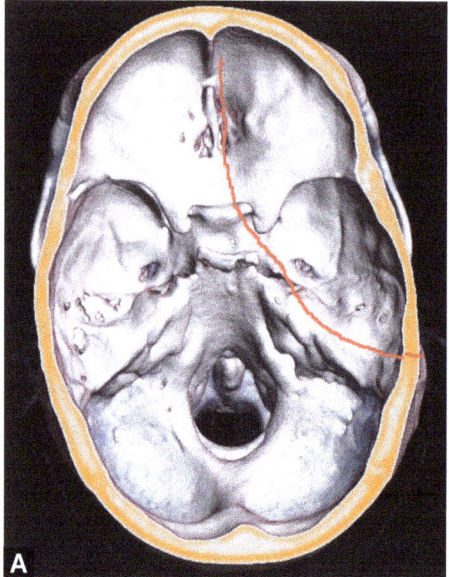 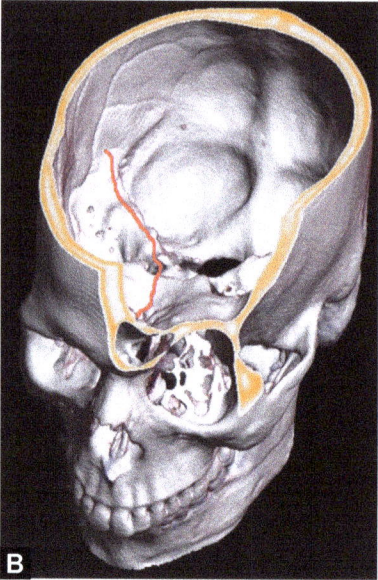

Figs. 23.5A and B: Frontobasal fracture type 1. Pictorial representations (A) and (B) show a longitudinal fracture (red line) of the cranial base that is parallel to the cribriform plate. Fracture line subsequently extends posteriorly to separate the anterior and middle fossa from the posterior fossa.

Classification of Frontobasal Fractures[8]

- *Type I frontobasal fractures (Figs. 23.5A and B):*
  - Generally associated with a relatively lower impact frontal injury
  - Linear fractures that initially parallel the cribriform plate
  - May extend posteriorly along the sella and petrous ridge to separate the anterior and middle cranial fossa from the posterior cranial fossa
  - Medially located, involving the medial third of the supraorbital rim
  - Less frequently associated with complications.
- *Type II fractures (Figs. 23.6A and B):*
  - Lateral vertical linear fractures of the frontal calvarium and anterior skull base
  - Involve the lateral two-thirds of the supraorbital rim, squamous portion of the temporal bone, orbital roof, lateral orbital wall, or orbital apex
  - Occur due to higher velocity impact
  - Frequently associated with CSF leak and intracranial injury
  - Associated with midface injuries.
- *Type III fractures (Fig. 23.7):*
  - Combined central and lateral frontobasilar fractures
  - Comminution of the entire frontal bone, orbital roof, and lateral cranial vault may be seen

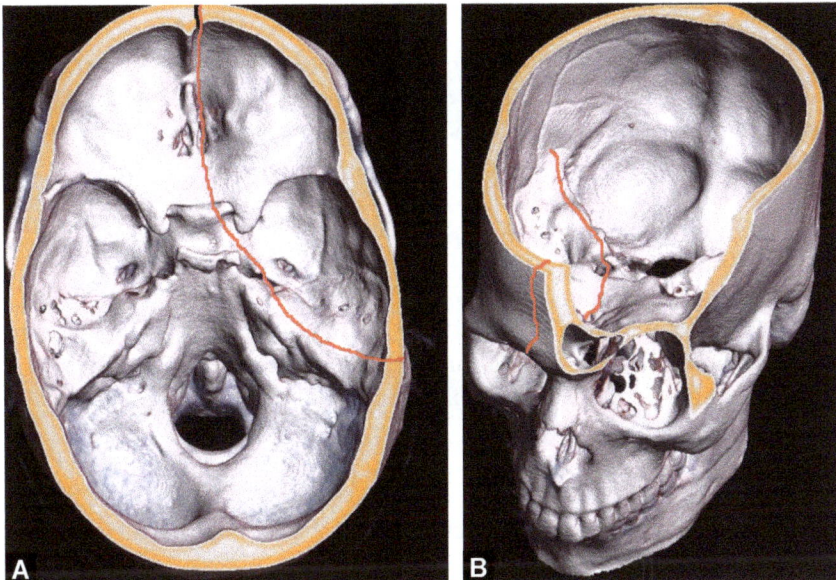

Figs. 23.6A and B: Frontobasal fracture type 2. Pictorial representations (A) and (B) show a linear fracture (red line) involving the frontal bone in addition to extension into the skull base.

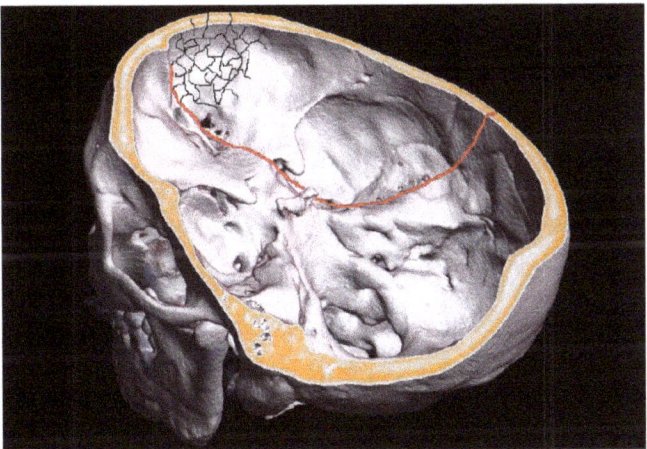

Fig. 23.7: Frontobasal fracture type 3. Pictorial representation shows a comminuted fracture (black lines) of the frontal bone involving a lateral and a central area, associated with comminuted fracture of the orbital roof also. A linear fracture (red line) extends into the middle and posterior cranial fossa.

- Associated with midface injuries
- Related to a higher velocity impact from lateral/inferior frontal/supraorbital direction
- Most often associated with complications such as intracranial injury and CSF leak (25% of cases).

Complications

- Skull base fractures often require repair only if there is associated intracranial injury requiring decompression, persistent CSF leak or significant cranial nerve, vascular injury, or to prevent mucocele formation.
- Associated complications are:
  - Cerebrospinal fluid leak
  - Olfactory nerve injury
  - Frontal lobe contusion
  - Intraorbital injuries.
- Post-traumatic CSF leak is a complication of anterior skull base fracture. It has been described in detail in Chapter 18.
- *Olfactory nerve injury:*
  - Anosmia occurs
  - Incidence is 7%
  - Increased risk in medial fractures along the cribriform plates
  - Associated with traumatic CSF leak
  - Only 10% of all patients with traumatic anosmia are estimated to recover sense of smell, months to years after the injury.

NONTRAUMATIC CEREBROSPINAL FLUID RHINORRHEA

- May be spontaneous or secondary leaks.

Spontaneous Cerebrospinal Fluid Rhinorrhea (also *See* Chapter 18)

- Occur in the absence of congenital abnormality, underlying lesion, previous trauma, or surgery.
- Spontaneous leaks may be more common than was previously considered, ranging from 20.8% to 40% of CSF leaks.
- Clinically leak should be confirmed with beta-2 transferrin testing.
- Mostly caused by underlying idiopathic intracranial hypertension (IIH) (discussed in Chapter 18).

TUMORS

Meningioma

- It is the most common intracranial lesion affecting the anterior skull base.
- Are more common in females.
- Classified into olfactory groove meningioma, planum sphenoidale meningioma, or tuberculum sellae meningioma based on the site of the dural attachment.
- Olfactory groove meningiomas may extend through the cribriform plate into the ethmoid sinuses and nasal cavity.
- Symptoms may occur late in the course of the disease as the frontal lobes are able to tolerate more compression.

- Behavioral changes, personality changes, headache, and anosmia may be seen.
- Visual symptoms and seizures may also occur.
- Planum sphenoidale and tuberculum sellae meningiomas may present with headache, visual field defects, and endocrinopathies secondary to pituitary stalk compression.

Imaging
- Appear as well circumscribed, smooth, or lobulated lesions with variable amount of perilesional edema.
- *Computed tomography:*
  - Isoattenuating to hyperattenuating mass
  - Intratumoral calcifications may be present
  - Hyperostosis may be seen in the adjacent bone.
- *Magnetic resonance imaging (Figs. 23.8A to C):*
  - Well-circumscribed lesions that are isointense to brain on both T1W and T2W images.
  - Show intense and homogeneous gadolinium enhancement with an adjacent linear dural tail in 58–72% of cases.

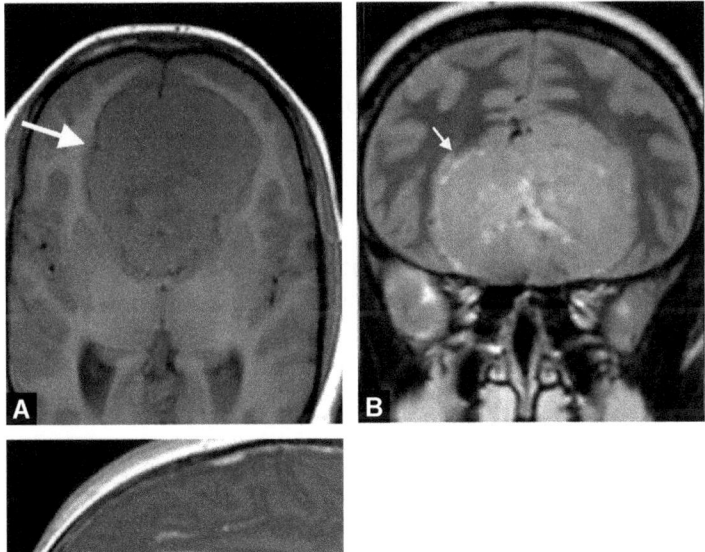

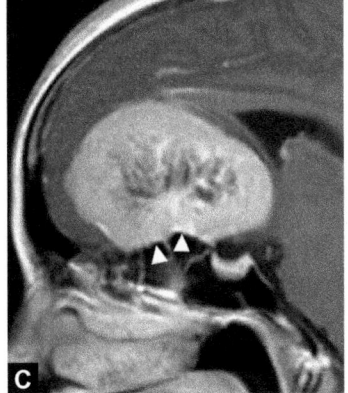

Figs. 23.8A to C: Planum sphenoidale meningioma. Well-defined extra-axial T1 isointense to mildly hyperintense lesion in the midline (arrow). The lesion is isointense to gray matter on T2 with areas of central hyperintensity. Cerebrospinal fluid (CSF) cleft is seen along the margin of the lesion (small arrow). Intense enhancement with few nonenhancing areas within. Attachment to the planum sphenoidale (arrowheads).

Hemangiopericytoma/Solitary Fibrous Tumors of the Dura

- Are rare malignant lesions that arise from pericytes within the meninges.
- Are considered to be aggressive grade 2/grade 3 lesions.
- These tumors account for less than 1% of intracranial lesions.
- Mean age ranges from 37 years to 44 years.
- They are aggressive lesions that occur at an earlier age as compared to meningiomas.
- There are higher chances of recurrence and distant metastasis in hemangiopericytomas.
- The most common presenting complaint is headache.
- May have a narrow dural attachment.

Imaging

- *Computed tomography:*
  - Hyperdense dural-based extra-axial mass with lobulated margins
  - Intratumoral calcifications and hyperostosis are not seen
  - Bone erosion may occur
  - Peritumoral edema is less common
  - Show heterogeneous enhancement.
- *Magnetic resonance imaging:*
  - Heterogeneous isointensity on T1-weighted imaging
  - Iso to mild hyperintensity on T2-weighted images
  - Prominent internal flow voids is common
  - Show heterogeneous enhancement.

Pituitary Macroadenoma

- Pituitary tumors larger than 1 cm is referred to as "macroadenomas".
- These are slow growing, benign tumor.
- They usually arise within the sella and may rarely originate from the pituitary stalk also.
- Other ectopic sites include sphenoid sinus, cavernous sinuses, nasopharynx, or sphenoid bone.
- Pituitary macroadenomas are mostly nonsecreting.
- Macroadenomas present with vision disturbances or cranial neuropathy due to infiltration of the surrounding region and mass effect by the lesion.
- Macroadenomas may spread in any direction. Superiorly they extend into the suprasellar cistern. Inferiorly, infiltration into the clivus and nasopharynx may occur. Bilaterally, the lesion may extend into the cavernous sinuses.
- Tumor cysts, necrosis, or hemorrhage may develop within the tumor.

Imaging

- Magnetic resonance imaging is the modality of choice in imaging macroadenomas.

- *Magnetic resonance imaging:*
  - Heterogeneous signal is seen within the tumor on both T1, T2-weighted images.
  - Moderate to intense enhancement is seen within the lesion.
  - The normal pituitary gland is compressed.
  - The posterior pituitary bright spot may be compressed, displaced, or absent.
  - Pituitary apoplexy, due to acute hemorrhage within the tumor, may cause enlargement of the lesion leading to compression of parasellar structures, including the optic nerves and chiasm. Sudden rapid vision loss or acute cranial neuropathy may occur.
  - Magnetic resonance imaging appearance depends upon the age of the hematoma. Fluid-fluid levels may be seen. Susceptibility-weighted imaging (SWI) may demonstrate areas of signal loss around areas of hemorrhage.

Subfrontal Schwannomas

- Are rare neoplasms of unclear origin.
- "Developmental theory of origin"—These lesions may arise from aberrant Schwann cells. Multipotent mesenchymal cells or displaced neural crest cells which may form abnormal intraparenchymal foci of Schwann cells have also been implicated in the pathogenesis of these lesions.
- "Nondevelopmental theory of origin"—Schwann cells are normally found in the perivascular region of the nerve plexuses and in adrenergic nerve fibers that supply the cerebral vessels. These may lead to formation of schwannomas.
- Arise from the olfactory nerves or from a meningeal branch of fifth cranial nerve.
- Mean age of presentation is 33 years. They are seen in an older age group as compared to intracranial schwannomas.
- They are benign, slow growing lesions.
- Nasal obstruction, anosmia, and epistaxis may occur.
- Remodel adjacent bone.
- Grow into the subfrontal region and into the nasal vault.

Imaging (Figs. 23.9A to D)

- *Computed tomography:*
  - Well-defined lesion causing scalloping of the surrounding bone with mild enhancement.
- *Magnetic resonance imaging:*
  - The lesion is hyperintense on T2, hypointense on T1 with moderate postcontrast enhancement.

Table 23.3 describes the differences between various primary anterior skull base tumors.

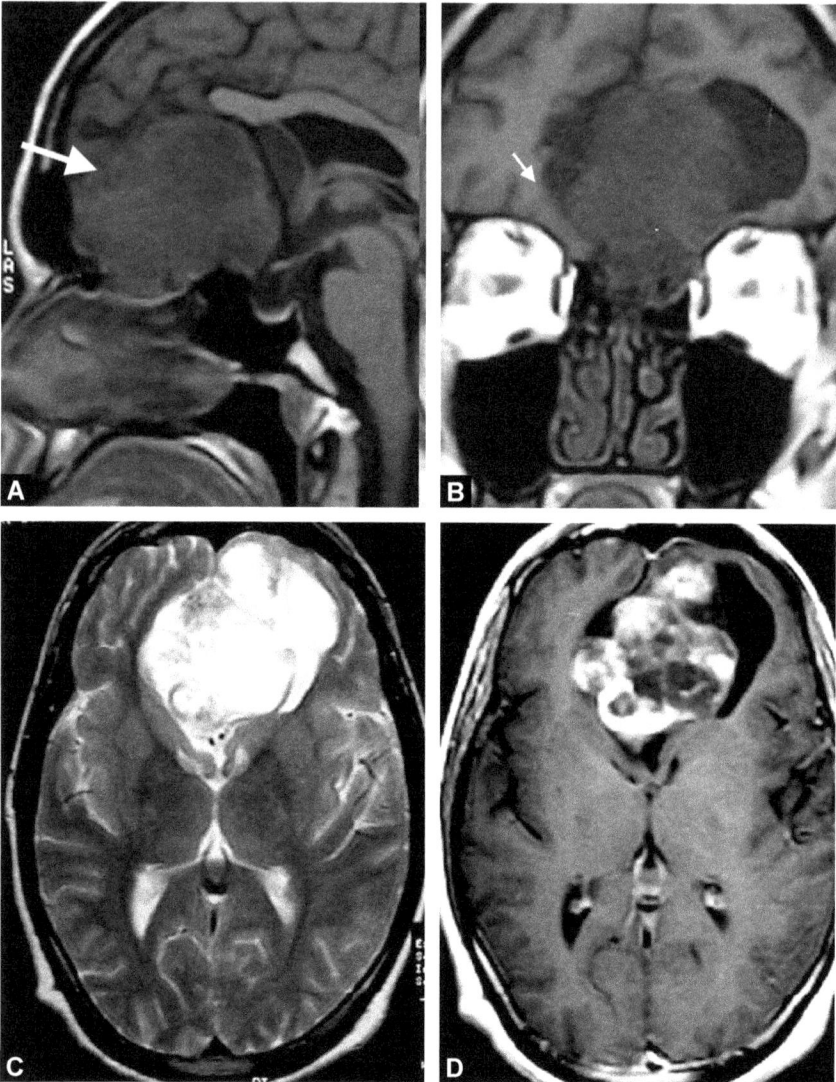

Figs. 23.9A to D: Olfactory schwannoma. Extra-axial T1 iso to hypointense, T2 hyperintense lesion involving the olfactory groove and the anterior cranial fossa. Heterogeneous post-contrast enhancement.

Metastasis

- Skull base Metastases are lesions that are usually diagnosed in patients who are known to suffer from metastatic cancer.
- The common primary tumors include breast, lung, prostate cancer, and lymphoma.
- Metastasis may spread via hematogenous seeding, retrograde venous seeding, or direct spread.

Table 23.3: Main imaging characteristics of primary intracranial tumors that may extend into the anterior skull base.

Lesion	Site of origin	CT	MRI
Meningioma	Meningocytes/arachnoid cap cells	<ul><li>Iso to hyperattenuating lesion</li><li>Intratumoral calcifications and hyperostosis of the adjacent bone may be present</li></ul>	<ul><li>Well-circumscribed T1 and T2 isointense lesions to brain</li><li>With intense homogeneous enhancement</li><li>Adjacent linear dural tail in 58–72% of cases</li></ul>
Hemangiopericytoma/solitary fibrous tumor	Pericytes in the meninges	<ul><li>Hyperdense dural-based lobulated mass</li><li>Intratumoral calcifications, hyperostosis are not seen</li><li>Bone erosion may occur</li><li>Peritumoral edema is less common</li><li>Show heterogeneous enhancement</li></ul>	<ul><li>Isointense on T1 and iso to mildly hyperintense on T2</li><li>Prominent internal flow voids are seen</li><li>Show heterogeneous enhancement</li></ul>
Pituitary macroadenoma	Pituitary gland	<ul><li>Enlarged sella</li><li>Heterogeneously enhancing sellar mass</li><li>Erosion of the sella floor is seen</li></ul>	<ul><li>Heterogeneous signal within the tumor on both T1, T2 images</li><li>Moderate to intense enhancement</li><li>The normal pituitary gland is compressed</li><li>Pituitary apoplexy, due to acute hemorrhage may cause a variable MRI imaging appearance depending upon the age of the hematoma</li><li>Invasion into the adjacent structures is seen</li></ul>
Subfrontal schwannoma	Schwann cells in olfactory nerve or the meningeal branch of fifth cranial nerve	Well-defined lesion causing scalloping of the surrounding bone with mild enhancement	<ul><li>Hyperintense on T2, and hypointense on T1</li><li>Moderate postcontrast enhancement</li></ul>

- These may be asymptomatic or may present with features of cranial neuropathies and craniofacial pain.
- Orbital lesions present with pain, swelling, local tenderness, and palpable mass in the involved orbit.
- Frontal headache, diplopia, proptosis, and blurred vision also occur.

Imaging

- Imaging findings are nonspecific.
- Computed tomography may show lytic lesions in the skull base.
- *Magnetic resonance imaging:*
  - Replacement of the normal fatty marrow is seen on T1-weighted imaging
  - High signal intensity on T2 weighted images
  - Diffusion-weighted imaging shows restricted diffusion
  - Enhancement is seen on postcontrast imaging.

BIBLIOGRAPHY

1. Abbassy M, Woodard TD, Sindwani R, et al. An overview of anterior skull base meningiomas and the endoscopic endonasal approach. Otolaryngol Clin North Am. 2016;49:141-52.
2. Barkovich AJ, Vandermarck P, Edwards MS, et al. Congenital nasal masses: CT and MR imaging features in 16 cases. AJNR. 1991;12:105-16.
3. Baugnon KL, Hudgins PA. Skull base fractures and their complications. Neuroimag Clin N Am. 2014;24:439-65.
4. Chiechi MV, Smirniotopoulos JG, Mena H. Intracranial hemangiopericytomas: MR and CT features. AJNR Am J Neuroradiol. 1996;17:1365-71.
5. Hedlund G. Congenital frontonasal masses: developmental anatomy, malformations, and MR imaging. Pediatr Radiol. 2006;36:647-62.
6. Louis DN, Perry A, Reifenberger G, et al. The 2016 World Health Organization Classification of Tumors of the Central Nervous System: a summary. Acta Neuropathol (Berl). 2016;131(6):803-20.
7. Maione L, Benadjaoud S, Eloit C, et al. Computed tomography of the anterior skull base in Kallmann syndrome reveals specific ethmoid bone abnormalities associated with olfactory bulb defects. J Clin Endocrinol Metab. 2013;98(3):E537-46.
8. Manson PN, Stanwix MG, Yaremchuk MJ, et al. Frontobasal fractures: anatomical classification and clinical significance. Plast Reconstr Surg. 2009;124:2096-106.
9. Mitsuya K, Nakasu Y, Horiguchi S, et al. Metastatic skull tumors: MRI features and a new conventional classification. J Neuro Oncol. 2011;104(1):239-45.
10. Parmar H, Gujar S, Shah G, et al. Imaging of the anterior skull base. Neuroimag Clin N Am. 2009;19:427-39.
11. Policeni BA, Smoker WR. Imaging of the skull base: anatomy and pathology. Radiol Clin North Am. 2015;53:1-14.

12. Prasad D, Jalali R, Shet T. Intracranial subfrontal schwannoma treated with surgery and 3D conformal radiotherapy. Neurol India. 2004;52:248-50.
13. Schirmer CM, Heilman CB. Hemangiopericytomas of the Skull Base. Neurosurg Focus. 2011;30:E10.
14. Smith SE, Murphey MD, Motamedi K, et al. From the archives of the AFIP. Radiologic spectrum of Paget disease of bone and its complications with pathologic correlation. Radiographics. 2002;22:1191-216.
15. Yuen A, Trost N, McKelvie P, et al. Subfrontal schwannoma: a case report and literature review. J Clin Neurosci. 2004;11:663-5.
16. Zaghouani H, Slim I, Zina NB, et al. Kallmann syndrome: MRI findings. IJEM. 2013;17(Suppl 1):S142-5.

CHAPTER 24

Imaging of Dental Lesions and Sinonasal Cavity

Smita Manchanda, Ashu Seith Bhalla

- Introduction
- Congenital Lesions
- Dental Infections and Maxillary Sinusitis
  - Complications Following Dental Procedures
- Odontogenic Cysts/Masses
  - Dentigerous Cysts
  - Keratocystic Odontogenic Tumor
  - Ameloblastoma
  - Odontogenic Myxoma
- Nonodontogenic Osseous Lesions
  - Giant Cell Reparative Granuloma
  - Ossifying Fibroma
  - Fibrous Dysplasia
- Mucosal Lesions
- Osteonecrosis of Maxilla

INTRODUCTION

- Pathologies of the maxillary alveolus frequently involve the nasal cavity and maxillary sinuses.[1] Failure to recognize dental etiology as the source of persistent sinonasal disease may lead to inadequate or delayed treatment in such cases. The spectrum of these disorders is enlisted in Table 24.1.
- Odontogenic cysts protrude into maxillary sinus elevating its floor.
- The elevated floor is convex upwards and thinned out.
- The thin bone forming the superior margin of the lesion helps to differentiate these from other expansile intrasinus lesions, such as mucoceles.
- If isolated, persistent unilateral maxillary sinus opacification is seen, a dental cause must always be excluded.

CONGENITAL LESIONS

- These include cleft lip, cleft palate and midface anomalies (Crouzon's syndrome and Apert's syndrome).
- Detailed discussion of these entities is beyond the purview of this book.

Table 24.1: Disorders involving maxillary alveolus and sinonasal cavity.	
Congenital	• Cleft lip and palate • Midface anomalies, e.g. Crouzon syndrome, Apert syndrome
Infections	• Secondary infection of odontogenic lesions • Osteomyelitis
Odontogenic lesions	• Periapical cyst • Dentigerous cyst • Keratocystic odontogenic tumor (KOT) • Ameloblastoma • Odontogenic myxoma

Nonodontogenic lesions	• *Miscellaneous lesions:*
	  – Central giant cell granuloma
	  – Simple bone cyst
	  – Aneurysmal bone cyst
	• *Fibro-osseous lesions:*
	  – Fibrous dysplasia
	  – Ossifying fibroma
	  – Osteosarcoma

Mucosal lesions	Carcinoma buccal mucosa
Miscellaneous	Osteonecrosis of maxilla

DENTAL INFECTIONS AND MAXILLARY SINUSITIS

- Persistent opacification of unilateral maxillary sinus necessitates the exclusion of an odontogenic source of infection, which may be responsible in up to 20% cases with isolated unilateral maxillary sinus involvement.[2]
- Spread of infection from carious tooth is the cause, and there may be a history of dental extraction (Figs. 24.1A and B).
- The roots of upper molars and premolars are closely related to the floor of the maxillary sinuses. Hence, chronic infection in the periapical region can result in reactive mucosal thickening. This thickening happens even without any breach of the sinus floor. Two patterns of dental infection are seen:
    1. *Dental caries:* Dental caries results in the formation of periapical cysts/abscess/granuloma which are seen as a lucent lesion around the root of the affected tooth. This can result in mucosal hyperplasia in the overlying maxillary sinus.
    2. *Periodonitis:* In those with chronic gingivitis and in the elderly, there is chronic inflammation of periodontal ligament causing resorption of the supporting bone located around the roots of the teeth. This is referred to as periodontitis, and it also results in eventual involvement of roots of teeth and resultant mucosal response in the sinus.
- Patients may present with persistent oral discharge due to oroantral or oronasal fistula (Figs. 24.2A and B).

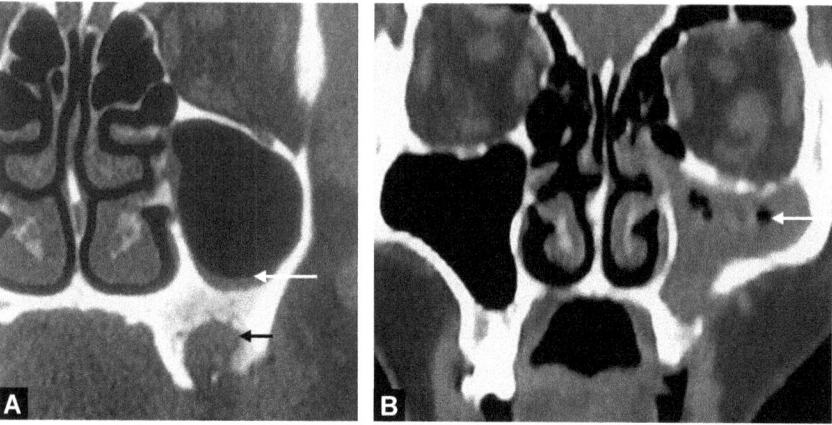

Figs. 24.1A and B: Dental infection and maxillary sinusitis. (A) Reactive mucosal thickening (white arrow) of left maxillary sinus in periapical cyst of left upper alveolus (black arrow); (B) Chronic sinusitis and silent sinus (white arrow) post-tooth extraction with breach in sinus floor.

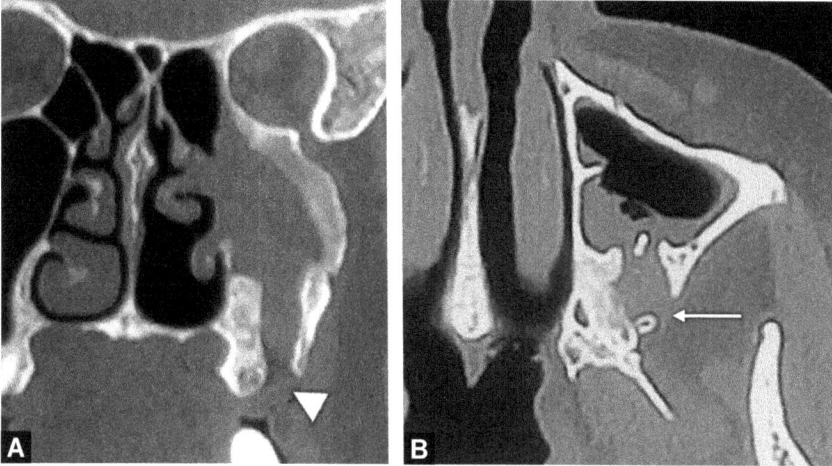

Figs. 24.2A and B: Oroantral fistula post-tooth extraction. (A) Oroantral fistula (arrowhead) post-tooth extraction; (B) Chronic left maxillary sinusitis with mucoperiosteal thickening (arrow).

- Eventual breach/osteomyelitis of the intervening bone leads to more florid sinusitis with/without fistulae formation.

Complications Following Dental Procedures

- Maxillary sinusitis may develop following dental procedures especially tooth extraction. Chronic sinusitis may be followed by development of silent sinus (Figs. 24.1A and B).
- There may be breach of the sinus floor or less commonly, displacement of a tooth fragment into the sinus.

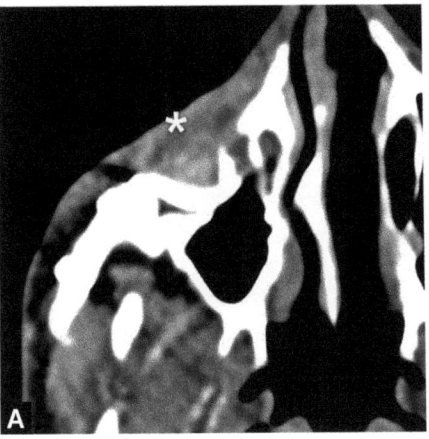 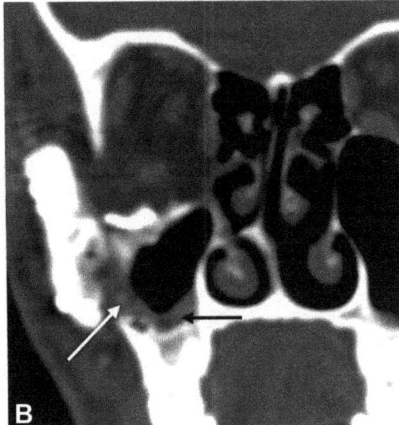

Figs. 24.3A and B: Postoperative (plate reconstruction post-trauma) infection. (A) Premaxillary soft tissue (asterisk); and (B) Mixed lytic sclerotic appearance of right maxilla and zygomatic bone (white arrow), mucosal thickening of right maxillary sinus (black arrow).

- Even without direct injury to the floor, if severe infection/osteomyelitis develops following extraction sinusitis will develop, besides spread into surrounding soft tissues (Figs. 24.3A and B).

ODONTOGENIC CYSTS/MASSES

- When a dental cause is suspected it is essential to review the orthopantogram (OPG) or the dental panoramic reconstructions of the multidetector computed tomography (MDCT). Essential to diagnosing these lesions is the demonstration of their relationship to the roots/crown of teeth which cannot be adequately evaluated on routine coronal/axial planes.
- The most frequent among these is the *periapical cyst*[3] related to dental caries (as detailed previously).
- The other common lesions encountered include dentigerous cyst, keratocystic odontogenic tumor (KOT), ameloblastoma, and odontogenic myxoma.

Dentigerous Cysts

- Most common developmental cyst of odontogenic origin.
- Majority are solitary and more common in mandible than maxilla.
- Presents as a unilocular cystic lesion that is pericoronal (around the crown of the tooth) in location as it arises from the crown-root junction.
- Associated with an unerupted tooth (often a molar/canine). The unerupted molar (Fig. 24.4) is often visualized high within the maxillary sinus.

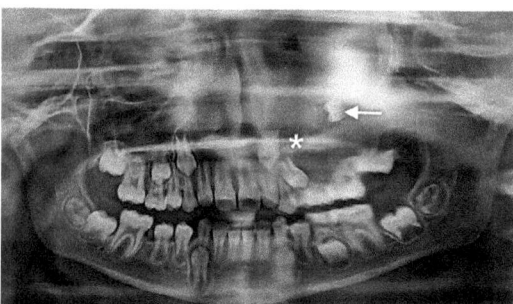

Fig. 24.4: Dentigerous cyst. Panoramic radiograph. Unilocular expansile lytic lesion within left upper alveolus (asterisk). Unerupted left upper molar tooth (arrow). Left maxillary sinus is not seen separately, right maxillary sinus is normal.

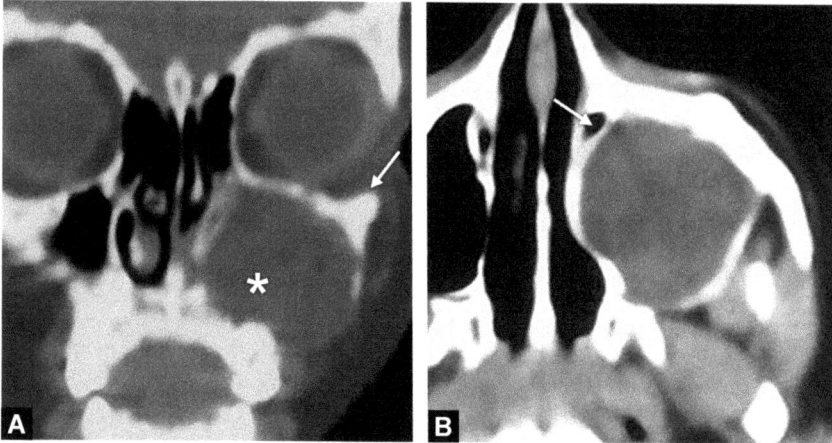

Figs. 24.5A and B: Dentigerous cyst (same patient as in Fig. 24.4). (A) Unilocular expansile cystic lesion within left upper alveolus (asterisk). Unerupted left upper molar tooth (arrow); (B) Well-defined margins of the lesion. Left maxillary sinus is displaced anteriorly (arrow).

- *Imaging (Figs. 24.4 and 24.5):*
  - Cystic, unilocular, and expansile lesion
  - Well-defined border, may be sclerotic
  - Ill-defined margin with spread beyond the lesion suggests secondary infection
  - Solid component with or without bony erosion suggests an intramural ameloblastoma.

Keratocystic Odontogenic Tumor

- Previously referred to as odontogenic keratocyst, it is now recognized and classified as a tumor.
- *Imaging:*
  - Unilocular/multilocular, lucent (on OPG) and high-density cyst (on CT) lesion (Figs. 24.6A and B).

- Due to the presence of keratin it is intermediate SI/hyperintense on T1-weighted images (WIs), shows hyperintensity on T2WI, and restricted diffusion. Characteristic low signal intensity—"T_2 fall out" is seen at the center of the lesion in few cases (Figs. 24.7A to D).
- It is locally aggressive and may show solid component.

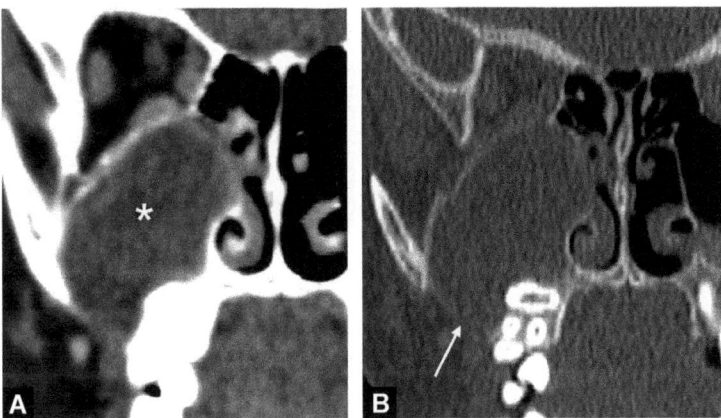

Figs. 24.6A and B: Keratocystic odontogenic tumor (KOT). NCCT. (A) Unilocular expansile high density cystic lesion within right upper alveolus (asterisk); (B) Thinning of inferior margin with bone erosion (arrow). Difficult to differentiate from dentigerous cyst, though KOT is associated with root resorption and bone erosion with milky fluid on aspiration.

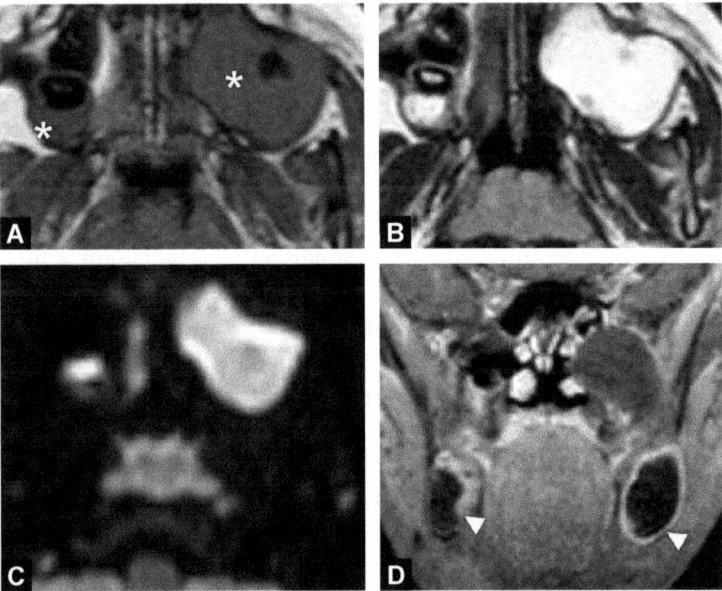

Figs. 24.7A to D: Keratocystic odontogenic tumor (KOT) magnetic resonance imaging (MRI). Multiple unilocular cystic lesions, bilateral maxilla (asterisks in A), and angle of mandibles (arrowheads in D). (A) Intermediate signal intensity on T1WI; (B) Hyperintense on T2WI; (C) Restricted diffusion; and (D) Minimal peripheral enhancement. Restricted diffusion and T1 hyperintensity is characteristic for this lesion.

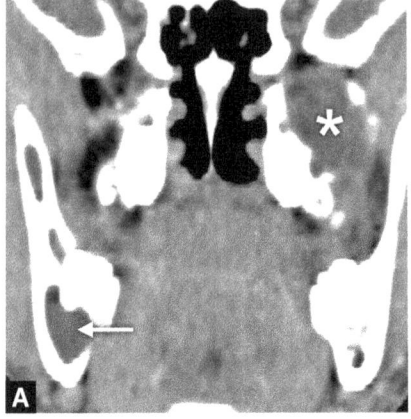
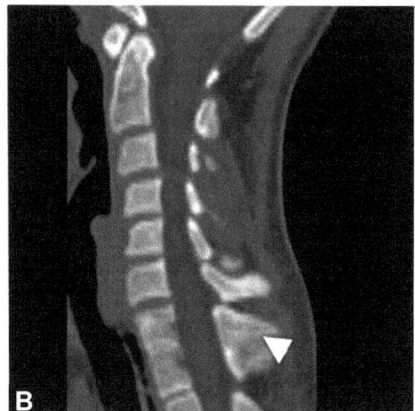
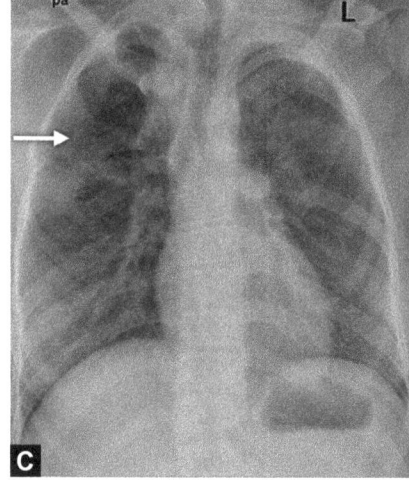

Figs. 24.8A to C: Multiple keratocystic odontogenic tumor (KOT) (Gorlin-Goltz syndrome). (A) Multiple unilocular cystic lesions, left maxilla (asterisk), and right mandible (arrow) s/o multiple KOT; (B) Fusion of C7 and D1 vertebral bodies and posterior elements (arrowhead); and (C) Bifid ribs with fusion anomalies of right 2–6 ribs (arrow) and left 5–7 ribs.

- The tumor may also exist with squamous cell carcinoma in up to one-fourth of cases.
- In view of high recurrence rates postsurgery follow-up with CT is required.
- *Gorlin-Goltz syndrome:*
  - Rare autosomal dominant inherited disorder
  - Multiple odontogenic keratocysts and basal cell carcinomas, skeletal (bifid ribs, Sprengel's deformity, vertebral anomalies), ophthalmic, and neurological abnormalities (Figs. 24.8A to C).

Ameloblastoma

- Ameloblastoma is the most common odontogenic tumor.
- It is a benign epithelial tumor but shows locally aggressive behavior, metastases are rare.[3,4]

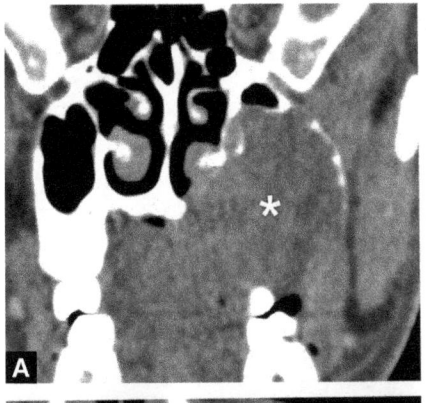
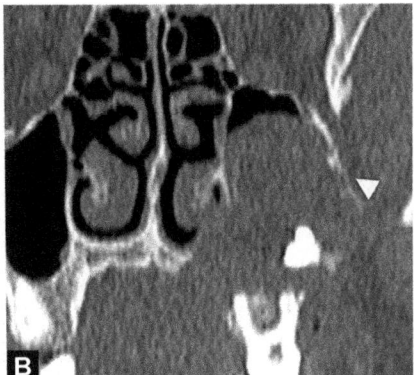
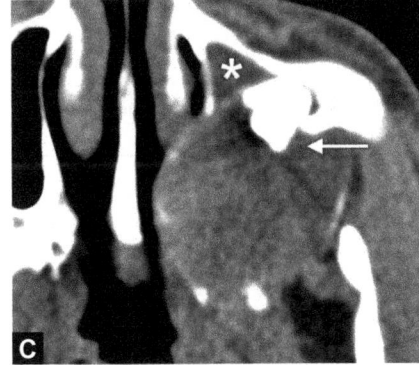

Figs. 24.9A to C: Ameloblastoma. (A) Pericoronal mixed solid-cystic (asterisk) expansile lesion; (B) Thinning of cortex (arrowhead) and bone erosion (posterior, inferior and lateral margins); (C) Lesion in relation to left upper 4 tooth (arrow) and retained secretions in left maxillary sinus (asterisk).

- *Imaging:* More frequent in the mandible. Common site in maxilla-premolar/first molar.
  - *Orthopantogram:*
    - Unilocular/multilocular, expansile lytic lesion causes root resorption.
    - It may be pericoronal or may replace a tooth.
  - *Computed tomography:*
    - Mixed solid cystic lesion, either component may predominate. Thinning of cortex with scalloped margins (Figs. 24.9A to C).
    - Multilocular lesions have a honeycomb/bubbly appearance.
    - Solid component is enhancing and may cause bone erosion and soft tissue extension (Figs. 24.10A and B).
  - *Magnetic resonance imaging:*
    - *T1-weighted image:* Isointense, T2WI—hyperintense signal intensity.
    - *Contrast-enhanced magnetic resonance imaging:* Heterogeneous enhancement, nonenhancing foci seen within.
    - *Diffusion-weighted imaging:* Cystic component shows free diffusion while solid component may show restriction.

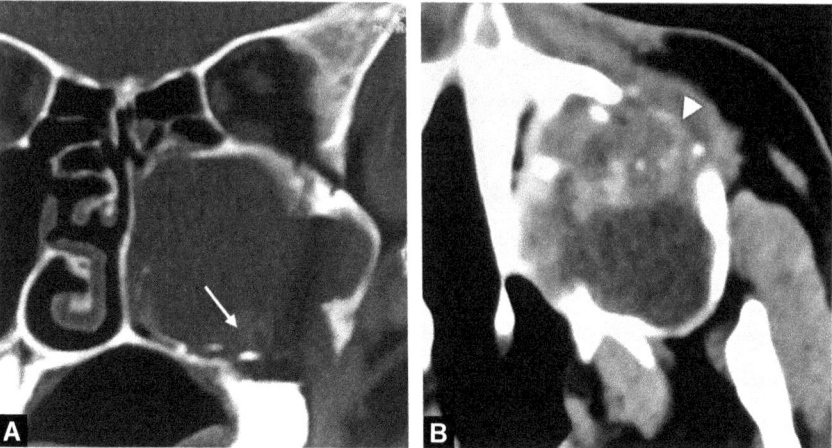

Figs. 24.10A and B: Ameloblastoma. (A) Large expansile (arrow) lesion with bone erosion; (B) Mixed solid cystic lesion (arrowhead). Solid component and erosions is more common in ameloblastoma.

- *Differential diagnosis:*
  - *Dentigerous cyst:*
    - The closest differential diagnosis.
    - In fact it is thought that about half of ameloblastomas arise from the lining of a dentigerous cyst.
    - Both are more frequent in the mandible than maxilla.
  - *Keratocystic odontogenic tumor:*
    - It is the other close differential diagnosis.
    - Characteristically cystic lesion, hyperintense on T1WI.

Odontogenic Myxoma

- Uncommon benign but locally aggressive odontogenic tumor.[5]
- *Pathology:* Nonencapsulated tumor with spindle cells/collagen fibers within a mucoid matrix.
- Occurs in young patients, in 2nd or 3rd decade of life, and is more frequent in females.
- The predominant site in the maxilla (or mandible) is in the posterior aspects. Can grow as a large, painless mass in the maxillary sinus.
- *Imaging:*
  - *Plain radiographs:* Expansile radiolucent tumors. Often with expansion. Thinning of the cortex and perforation at places. Teeth displacement is frequent, while resorption is infrequent.
  - Internal architecture is variable ranging from no trabeculation to fine to thick trabeculations within. Variants with thin and straight septa gives the characteristic "tennis racket" appearance, curved or coarse

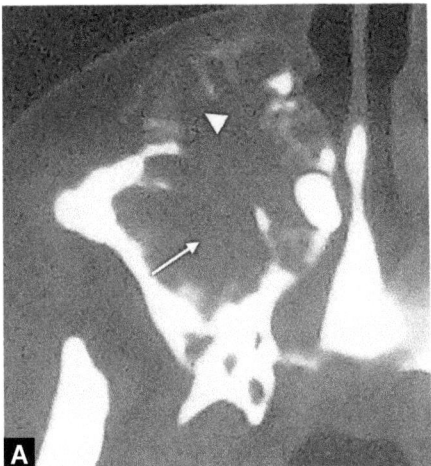 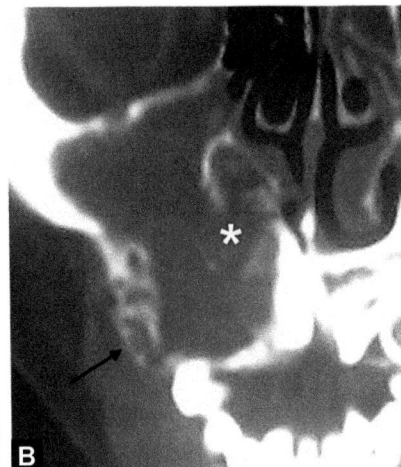

Figs. 24.11A and B: Odontogenic myxoma. (A) Expansile lytic lesion right maxilla with few thin septations (arrow) and erosion of the anterior cortex (arrowhead); (B) Erosion of the lateral (black arrow) cortex and thin, lace like trabeculations (asterisk).

septae give a "soap bubble" or "honeycomb pattern", while fine septae produce a "fish net" appearance.
- *Computed tomography (Figs. 24.11A and B):* The density compared to muscle is hypodense/isodense. Presence of thin lace-like trabeculations is characteristic. Cortical thinning/perforation is often seen but tumor margins are well-defined, not infiltrative.
- *Magnetic resonance imaging:* Tumors show variable signal intensity and contrast enhancement.

NONODONTOGENIC OSSEOUS LESIONS

- Nonodontogenic lesions which involve the maxillary alveolus and expand the bone or are associated with a soft tissue component can also protrude into/involve the maxillary sinus.
- These include lesions, such as central giant cell granuloma, simple bone cyst, aneurysmal bone cyst, and fibro-osseous lesions like ossifying fibroma and dysplasia. These lesions are frequent in the maxilla/mandible but can less commonly arise within the sinonasal cavity (*see* Chapter 12).

Giant Cell Reparative Granuloma

- Common sites are mandible/maxilla, infrequently seen involving sinonasal cavity.
- *Age:* Young adults, females more than males.[6]
- *Imaging findings (also see Chapter 12):*

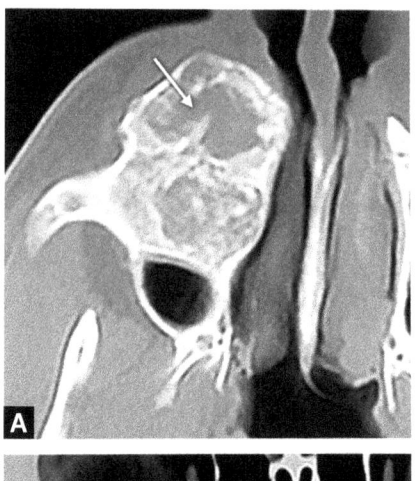
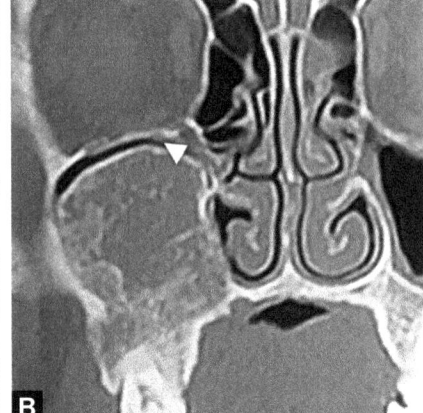
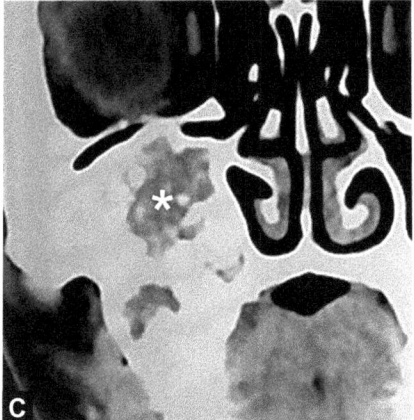

Figs. 24.12A to C: Giant cell reparative granuloma. (A) Large, heterogeneous, expansile mixed density mass in right upper alveolus (arrow); (B) Maxillary sinus displaced posterosuperiorly (arrowhead); and (C) Heterogeneous postcontrast enhancement (asterisk).

- Expansile lesions with bone erosion (Figs. 24.12A to C)
- Cystic/hemorrhagic foci may be seen within with heterogeneous signal intensity on magnetic resonance imaging (MRI).

Ossifying Fibroma

- Ossifying fibroma (OF) is a relatively common lesion in the mandible/maxilla.[3,7]
- It is classified under the *benign odontogenic and maxillofacial bone tumors.*
- *Imaging findings:*
  - *Computed tomography (Figs. 24.13A and B):* Well-defined mixed density lesion with soft tissue component, matrix mineralization, and calcification along the periphery. The amount of soft tissue versus mineralized matrix is variable.
  - Expansile lesion, occasionally bone erosion seen.
  - Well-defined margins of the lesion aids in its distinction from fibrous dysplasia.

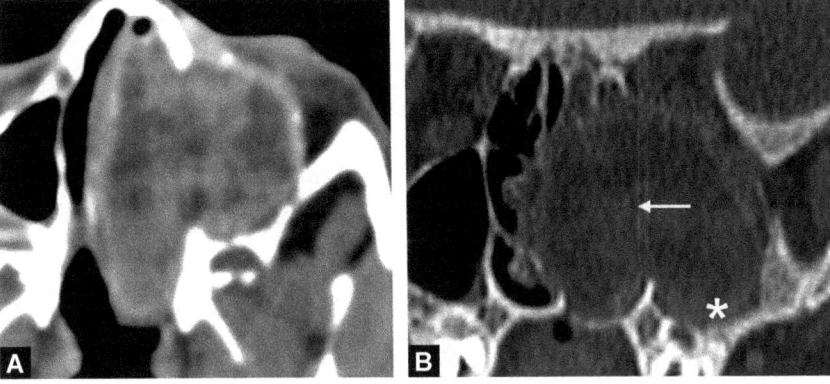

Figs. 24.13A and B: Ossifying fibroma. (A) Large well-defined mixed density expansile mass lesion in left nasal cavity and maxillary sinus; and (B) Thinning of bony margins and extension into upper alveolus (asterisk). Erosion of turbinates and medial maxillary wall (arrow).

- *Magnetic resonance imaging:* The soft tissue component of the lesion shows heterogeneous enhancement, while the mineralized matrix/rim appear as signal voids.

Fibrous Dysplasia

- Fibrous dysplasia is not a neoplastic disorder, but a benign disorder involving multiple bones wherein the medulla is replaced by immature fibrous tissue and eventually osseous tissue.
- Craniofacial bones are a frequent site of involvement, may be part of the polyostotic form.[3,7]
- *Imaging findings (Figs. 24.14A and B):*

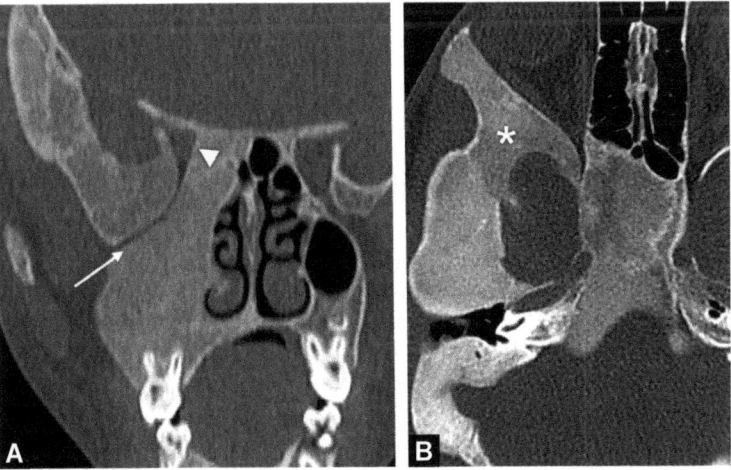

Figs. 24.14A and B: Fibrous dysplasia. (A) Narrowing of right optic canal (arrowhead) and inferior orbital fissure (arrow); and (B) Expanded left frontal, maxillary, zygomatic, and sphenoid bones with intact contour. Ground-glass density (asterisk).

- *CT:* Involved bone is expanded but basic shape and contour intact.
- Its margins with the adjoining bone are ill defined, i.e. it merges imperceptibly.
- Matrix may initially appear lucent, then assume a "cotton wool" appearance, and finally evolves into "ground glass" density.
- *MRI:* Intermediate signal on T1WI, intermediate or low signal intensity on T2WI with significant contrast enhancement in fibrous tissues.

MUCOSAL LESIONS

- Primary mucosal malignancies such as carcinoma buccal mucosa or carcinoma palate can erode into the maxillary sinus.
- *Imaging findings (Figs. 24.15A and B):*
  - Enhancing soft tissue mass causing permeative bone destruction and erosion with extension into the maxillary sinus.

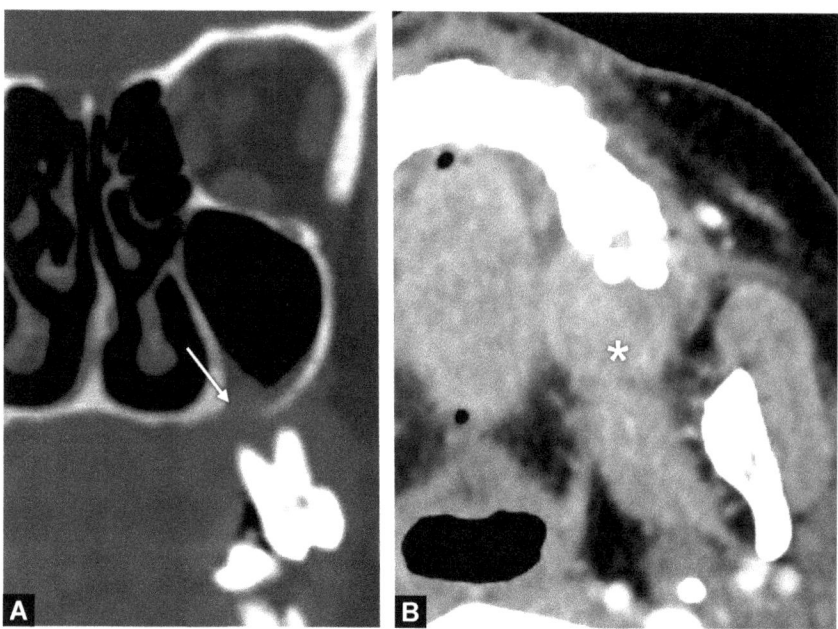

Figs. 24.15A and B: Carcinoma palate eroding into maxillary sinus. (A) Erosion of floor of left maxillary sinus with soft tissue extension (arrow); and (B) Enhancing soft tissue density mass palate (squamous cell carcinoma) (asterisk).

OSTEONECROSIS OF MAXILLA

- Osteonecrosis is characterized by bone destruction of the maxillary alveolus.[8]
- In an immunocompromised patient, the cause is usually osteomyelitis (bacterial/fungal). The infection can have a dental origin and spread along the sinus walls, pterygoid plates, and skull base (*see* Chapter 7).

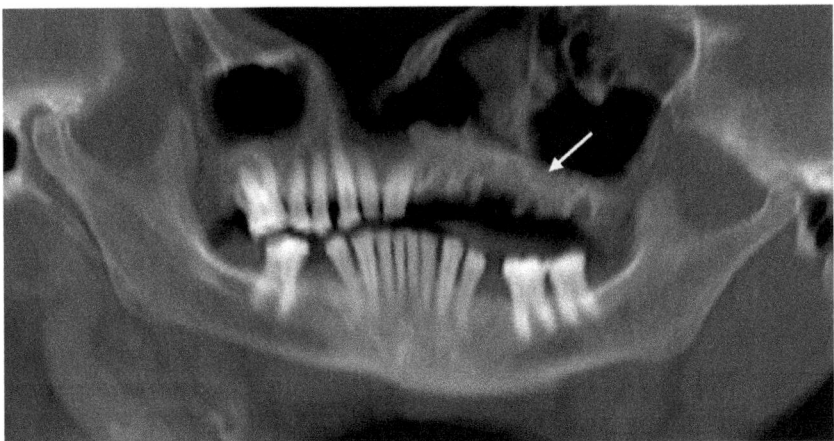

Fig. 24.16: Osteonecrosis of maxilla. Panoramic computed tomography (CT) reconstructed image. Osteolysis of left half of maxilla with absent teeth (arrow). Unilateral involvement in herpes zoster.

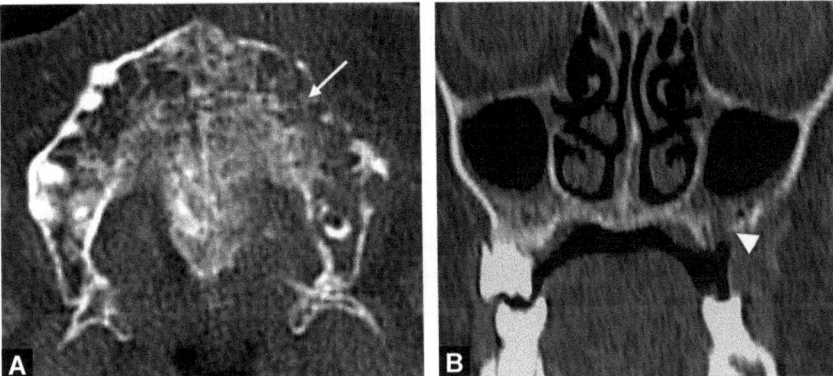

Figs. 24.17A and B: Osteonecrosis of maxilla (unilateral involvement in herpes zoster). (A) Irregular lysis of left alveolar arch (arrow); and (B) Osteolysis of left half of maxilla with absent teeth (arrowhead) and adjacent soft tissue.

- In an immunocompetent patient, aseptic necrosis occurs with an appearance similar to osteomyelitis. This is reported to be due to small vessel occlusion. Causes include radiotherapy, bisphosphonate use, sickle cell anemia, hemoglobinopathies, postviral infection, and electric shock.
- Unilateral involvement is seen in cases of herpes zoster infection with distribution along the same dermatome of the nerve (Fig. 24.16).
- Clinical presentation is with pain, mucosal swelling, and progressive loosening of teeth.

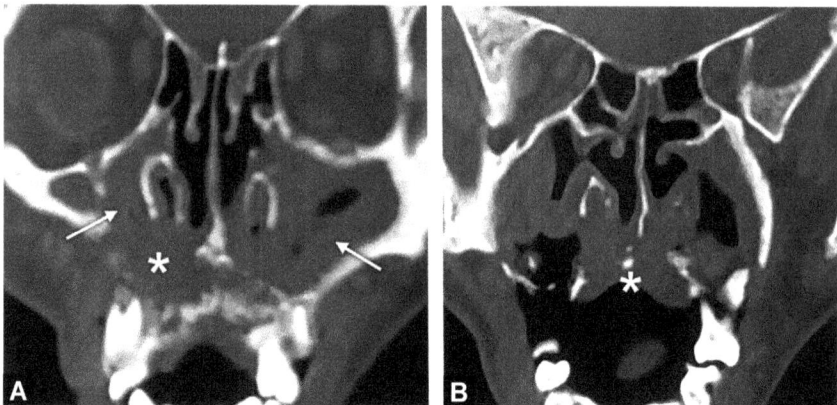

Figs. 24.18A and B: Osteonecrosis of maxilla (postradiotherapy). (A) Bilateral maxillary sinusitis (arrows); and (B) Osteolysis of maxilla with absent teeth (asterisks). Missing maxilla appearance.

- *Imaging:*
  - *Panoramic radiography:* Osteolysis of maxilla with floating teeth—"missing maxilla appearance".
  - *Noncontrast computed tomography (Figs. 24.17 and 24.18):* Osteolysis with periosteal reaction, and sequestrum formation. Mixed lytic sclerotic appearance may be seen especially in bisphosphonate-induced osteoradionecrosis.

CONCLUSION

Dental lesions are an important differential of unilateral sinus disease or infrequently even bilateral maxillary sinus diseases.

REFERENCES

1. Broderick DF. The opacified paranasal sinus: approach and differential. Appl Radiol. 2015;44:9-17.
2. Mafee MF, Tran BH, Chapa AR. Imaging of rhinosinusitis and its complications: plain film, CT, and MRI. Clin Rev Allergy Immunol. 2006;30(3):165-86.
3. Sen S, Chandra A, Mukhopadhyay S, et al. Sinonasal tumors: computed Tomography and MR imaging features. Neuroimaging Clin N Am. 2015;25(4):595-618.
4. Whyte A, Chapeikin G. Opaque maxillary antrum: a pictorial review. Australas Radiol. 2005;49(3):203-13.
5. Kheir E, Stephen L, Nortje C, et al. The imaging characteristics of odontogenic myxoma and a comparison of three different imaging modalities. Oral Surg Oral Med Oral Pathol Oral Radiol. 2013;116(4):492-502.

6. Desai SM, Dubey RB, Tara NP. Giant cell tumor of sinonasal cavity an uncommon location for a common bone tumor. Indian J Radiol Imaging. 2003;13(1):134.
7. Connor SE. The skull base in the evaluation of sinonasal disease: role of computed tomography and MR Imaging. Neuroimaging Clin N Am. 2015;25(4):619-51.
8. Smith J, Birkeland AC, McHugh JB, et al. Maxilla Osteonecrosis: a differential diagnosis in patients with metastatic cancer on bisphosphonates. J Case Rep Med. 2016;5:235969.

25
CHAPTER

Imaging of Disorders Involving Sinonasal Cavity and Orbit

Ashu Seith Bhalla, Smita Manchanda

- Introduction
- Infections
  - Complicated Acute Sinusitis
  - Invasive Fungal Sinusitis
- Inflammatory Disorders
  - Orbital Pseudotumor
- Tumors
  - Direct Extension
  - Extension through Inferior Orbital Fissure
  - Spread through Nasolacrimal Duct
  - Perineural Spread
- Trauma

INTRODUCTION

Pathologies of the nasal cavity and paranasal sinuses frequently involve the orbits and vice-versa. These include infections and tumors with the spread of disease from paranasal sinuses to orbit being much more common. The spectrum of these disorders is enlisted in Table 25.1.

Table 25.1: Disorders involving sinonasal cavity and orbit.	
Infections	• Complicated acute sinusitis • Invasive fungal sinusitis
Inflammatory disorders	• Orbital pseudotumor
Tumors	• Direct extension • Extension through inferior orbital fissure • Spread through nasolacrimal duct (NLD) • Perineural spread
Trauma	• Component of complex facial fractures

INFECTIONS

Complicated Acute Sinusitis

- About two-thirds of significant orbital infection results from adjoining sinusitis, the rest being due to foreign bodies.

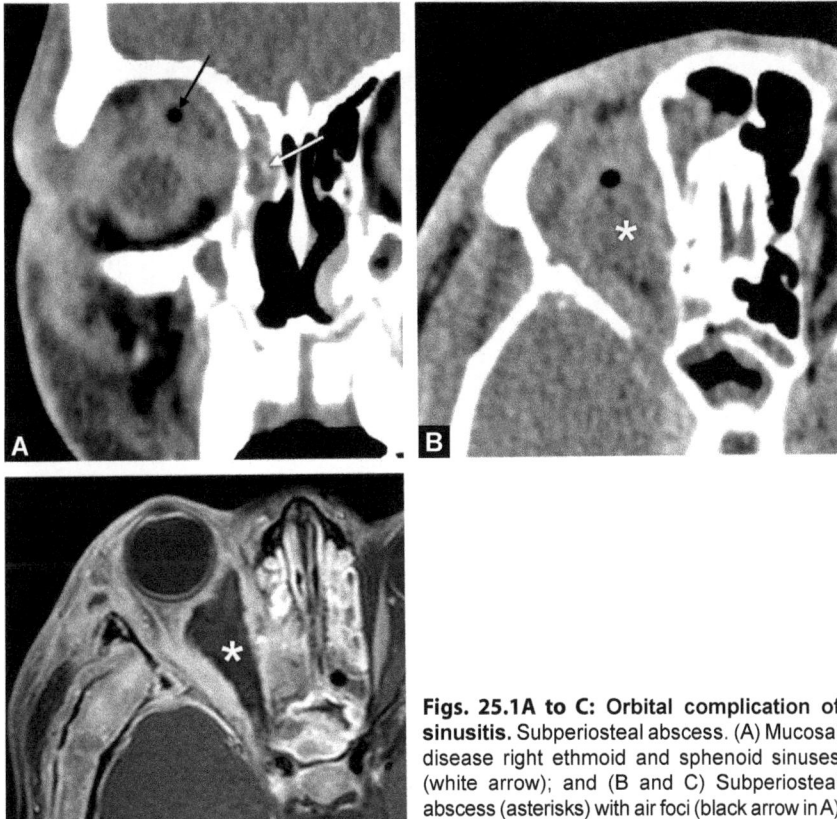

Figs. 25.1A to C: Orbital complication of sinusitis. Subperiosteal abscess. (A) Mucosal disease right ethmoid and sphenoid sinuses (white arrow); and (B and C) Subperiosteal abscess (asterisks) with air foci (black arrow in A) along roof and medial wall of right orbit.

- Orbital cellulitis may be the first presenting symptom of sinusitis in children.[1,2]
- On imaging, it is important to differentiate preseptal (periorbital) cellulitis from postseptal (orbital) cellulitis as clinical presentation can be similar. The demarcation between the two is the fibrous orbital septum.
- Orbital cellulitis requires aggressive management as it is a threat to vision of the patient.
- *Orbital abscess:* Rim-enhancing collection with central part showing restricted diffusion (Figs. 25.1A to C).
- Inflammation from orbit can extend along nasolacrimal duct (NLD) till inferior meatus (Figs. 25.2A and B).
- Severe infection can occasionally result in the orbital compartment syndrome (OCS). This is a serious emergency requiring immediate decompression. On imaging, it is recognized by the presence of proptosis with periorbital edema, tenting of the posterior wall of the globe, retrobulbar fat stranding, and a stretched optic nerve.

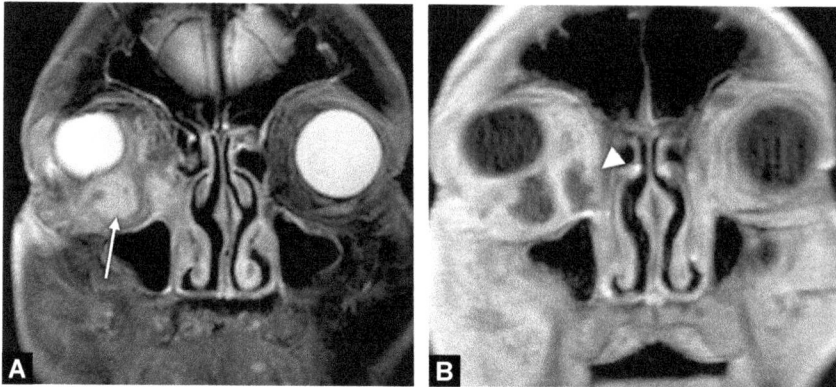

Figs. 25.2A and B: Right orbital cellulitis and nasolacrimal duct (NLD) inflammation. (A) Right orbital and periorbital cellulitis with abscess formation (arrow); and (B) Inflammation extending along right NLD till lower end (arrowhead).

Flowchart 25.1: Evolution of orbital complications.

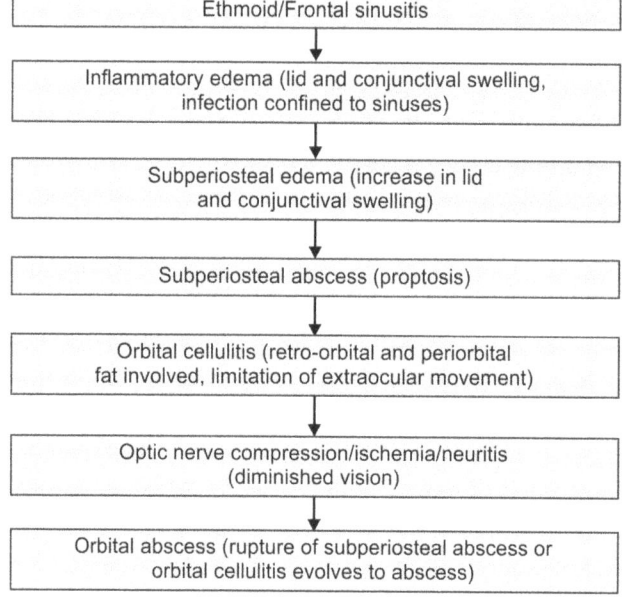

- Inflammatory edema results in swelling of eyelid. However, in early stages when the term inflammatory edema is used, there is only soft tissue swelling but there is no spread of infection into the orbit. Computed tomography (CT)/magnetic resonance imaging (MRI) reveals secretions confined to the sinuses.
- Further evolution of orbital complications, especially if untreated is detailed in the algorithm (Flowchart 25.1).

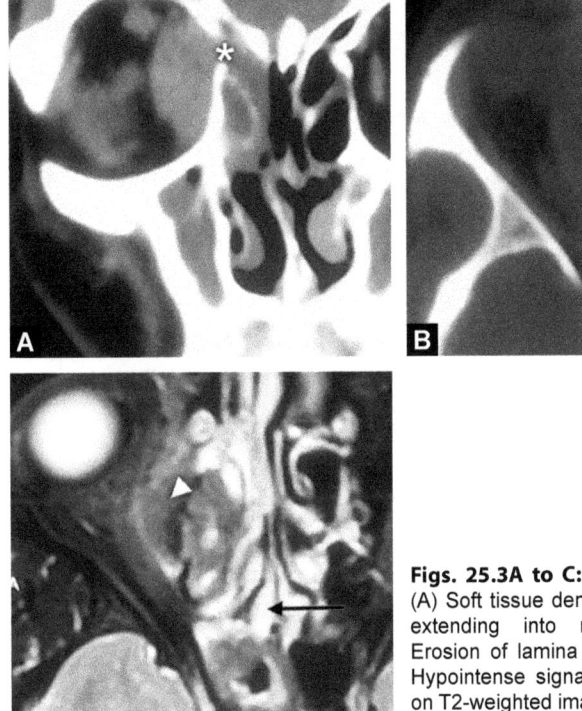

Figs. 25.3A to C: Invasive fungal sinusitis. (A) Soft tissue density in right ethmoid sinuses extending into right orbit (asterisk); (B) Erosion of lamina papyracea (arrow); and (C) Hypointense signal of soft tissue (arrowhead) on T2-weighted image (T2WI) with hyperintense mucosal thickening (black arrow).

Invasive Fungal Sinusitis

- Acute invasive fungal sinusitis is indistinguishable from bacterial cellulitis.
- Proptosis and periorbital inflammation can be seen.
- Optic nerve appears stretched with ill-defined outline.
- Magnetic resonance signs include necrosis with variable or nonenhancement of affected extraocular muscles.
- Globe may show deformity with tenting of the posterior wall—"Guitarpick sign".
- Increase signal intensity of vitreous on inversion recovery [fluid-attenuated inversion recovery (FLAIR)] sequences indicates invasion of the globe (endophthalmitis).
- In cases of endophthalmitis thickening and enhancement of the wall of the globe is also seen. This is an ocular emergency.[2,3]
- Chronic invasive fungal sinusitis (Figs. 25.3A to C) is seen as soft tissue in sinuses with bone erosion and extension into orbital cavity. Resembles locally invasive diseases like pseudotumor.

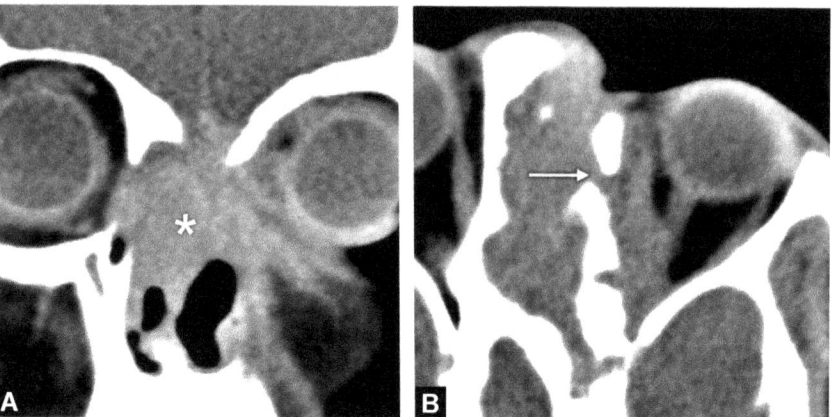

Figs. 25.4A and B: Pseudotumor. (A) Soft tissue (asterisk) in nasal cavity and bilateral orbits; and (B) Erosion of left lamina papyracea (arrow).

INFLAMMATORY DISORDERS

Orbital Pseudotumor

- It is a nongranulomatous inflammatory lesion involving multiple orbital compartments. Lesion is usually confined to orbit, may occasionally spread to adjoining sinuses.
- Characteristic painful and bilateral in up to a fourth of patients.
- Soft tissue density on noncontrast CT (NCCT) (Figs. 25.4A and B) and shows low signal intensity on T2W fat suppressed images.
- D/D: Chronic invasive fungal sinusitis, lymphoma, and immunoglobulin G-4 (IgG4)-related disorders (see Chapter 22).

TUMORS

As in inflammatory conditions, spread of tumors from paranasal sinuses to orbit is far more frequent than the reverse spread from orbit to sinuses.[4,5]

Direct Extension

- Contiguous extension of maxillary sinus tumors and ethmoid sinus tumors can occur by erosion of the intervening orbital floor and lamina papyracea, respectively (Figs. 25.5 and 25.6).
- Earliest sign of orbital infiltration is the elevation of periorbita with loss of interface between the tumors and periorbita. "Periorbita" refers to the periosteum of the bony orbital walls, and provides a barrier to spread of tumor. On MRI, it appears hypointense (similar to cortical bone), and loss of this hypointensity is seen once periorbita is breached.
- Subsequently there is involvement of the extraocular muscles which may be displaced or thickened with abnormal enhancement.
- Orbital fat stranding is seen.
- Direct sign is disruption of the bony orbital wall (Figs. 25.6A to C).

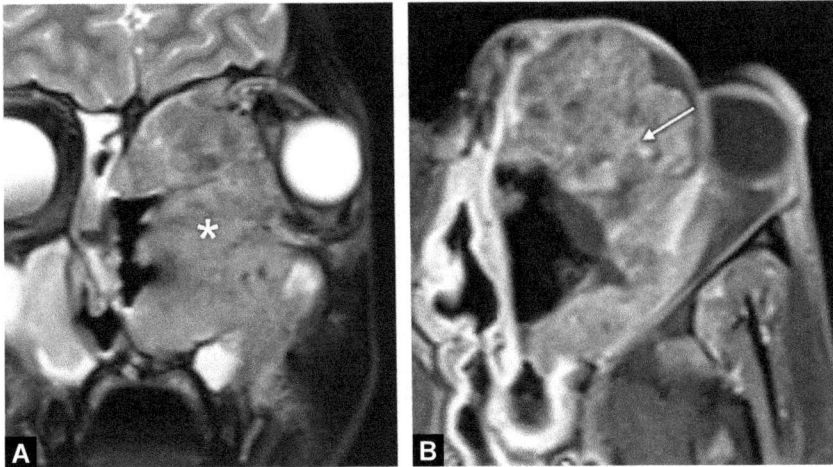

Figs. 25.5A and B: Direct tumor extension into orbit (squamous cell carcinoma). (A) Large intermediate signal intensity mass left in maxillary and ethmoid sinuses (asterisk); and (B) Orbital extension by erosion of orbital floor and lamina papyracea (arrow) deforming the globe.

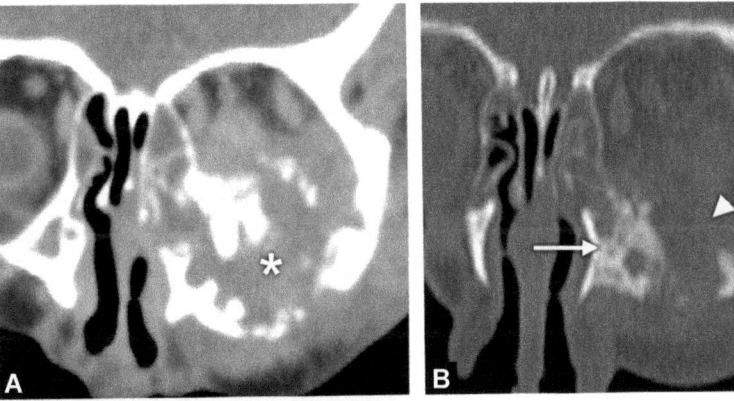

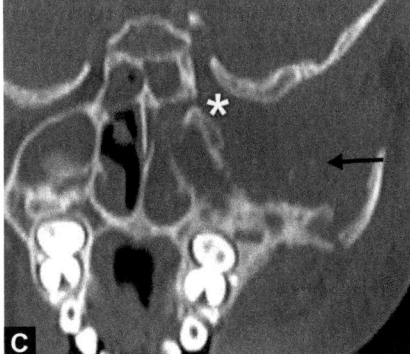

Figs. 25.6A to C: Direct tumor extension into orbit [primitive neuroectodermal tumor (PNET) maxilla]. (A) Large expansile mildly enhancing mass left in maxilla (asterisk); (B) Mixed lytic sclerotic pattern of bone destruction (arrow). Orbital extension by erosion of orbital floor (arrowhead); and (C) Widening of inferior orbital fissure (asterisk), pterygomaxillary fissure, and extension into infratemporal fossa (arrow).

Extension through Inferior Orbital Fissure

- Tumors extending to pterygopalatine fossa and infratemporal fossa may spread to the orbit through inferior orbital fissure (Figs. 25.7A and B).

Spread through Nasolacrimal Duct

- Primary tumors (e.g. adenoid cystic carcinoma) of NLD show soft tissue and enlargement of NLD canal (Figs. 25.8A and B).

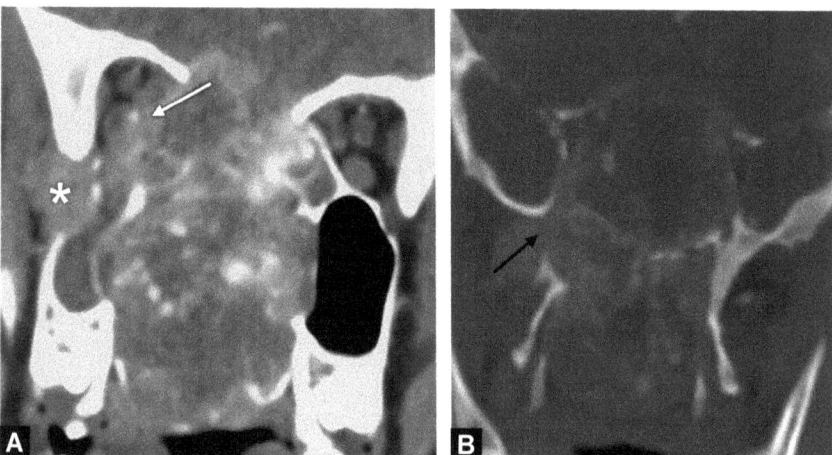

Figs. 25.7A and B: Extension through inferior orbital fissure (juvenile nasopharyngeal angiofibroma-atypical aggressive form with bone erosion). (A) Intensely enhancing heterogeneous mass lesion in nasal cavity, nasopharynx laterally extending into the pterygomaxillary fissure (asterisk); and (B) Extension into orbit through direct extension/bone erosion (white arrow in A) and widened inferior orbital fissure (black arrow in B).

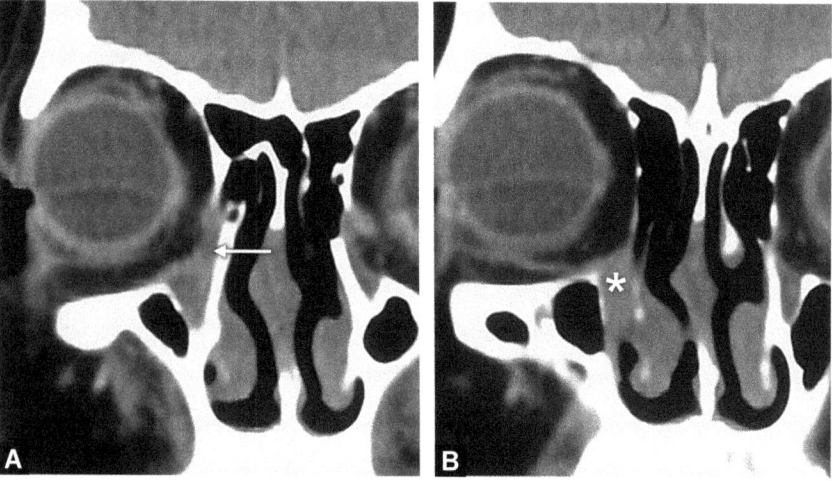

Figs. 25.8A and B: Adenoid cystic carcinoma in nasolacrimal duct. (A) Mildly enhancing soft tissue seen along the right nasolacrimal duct (arrow); and (B) Widened canal on right side (asterisk).

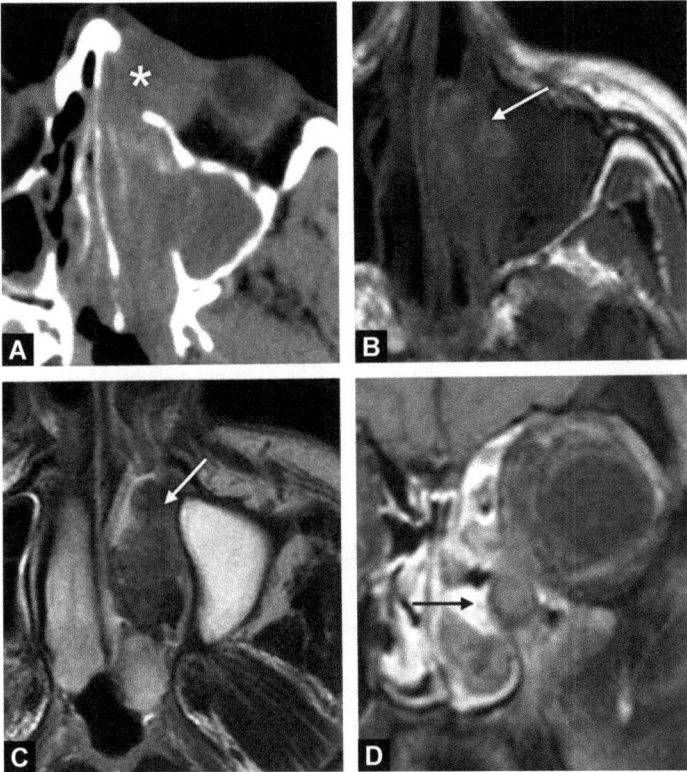

Figs. 25.9A to D: Nasolacrimal duct melanoma. (A) Soft tissue density mass along left lacrimal sac and nasolacrimal duct (asterisk); (B and C) Mildly hyperintense on T1-weighted image (T1WI) (arrow in B), hypointense on T2WI (arrow in C); and (D) Heterogenous postcontrast enhancement (arrow in D).

- Tumors involving the nasal cavity can spread to orbit through the NLD. Similarly, tumors originating in the lacrimal sac may spread downward along the NLD (Figs. 25.9A to D).

Perineural Spread

- Once maxillary sinus tumors invade the premaxillary soft tissue these may spread along the infraorbital nerve and then through infraorbital foramen to the orbit.

TRAUMA

Orbit fractures (Table 25.2) are often a component of more complex facial fractures (also *see* Chapter 17).
- Fractures involving optic canal result in traumatic optic neuropathy. In orbit trauma, optic traumatic neuropathy may occur even in absence of direct impingement of the optic nerve.[6]
- Imaging findings including presence of soft tissue/fat stranding around the optic nerve in the optic canal.

Table 25.2: Orbital involvement in facial fractures.

Type of fractures	Orbital structure involved	Special consideration
Le Fort II	• Medial wall • Floor	
Le Fort III	• Medial wall • Lateral wall	
Naso-orbito-ethmoidal (NOE) complex fractures (Figs. 25.10A and B)	• Medial wall	• Medial canthus tendon avulsion • Nasolacrimal duct (NLD) injury → Blockage
Zygomaticomaxillary complex (ZMC) fractures	• Lateral wall • Floor	• Increased orbital volume (enophthalmos)
Blow out fractures (Figs. 25.11A and B)	• Floor • Medial wall	• Increased volume • Extraocular muscle entrapment

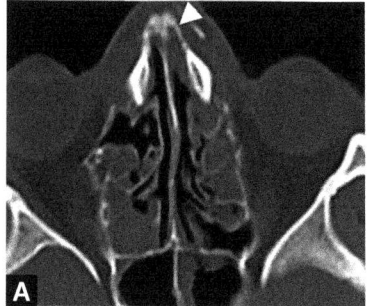 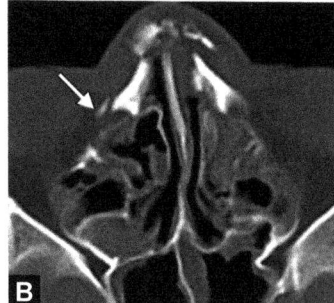

Figs. 25.10A and B: NOE fracture with medial canthal tendon avulsion. (A) Comminuted naso-orbital-ethmoidal fracture (arrowhead); and (B) Disrupted medial canthal attachment site (arrow).

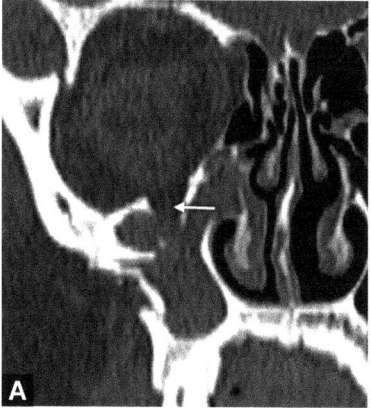 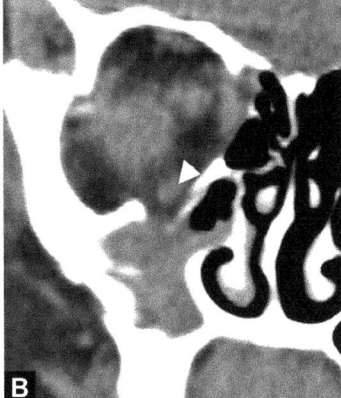

Figs. 25.11A and B: Blow out fracture with entrapment of inferior rectus. (A) Herniation of intraorbital fat (arrow); and (B) Likely entrapment of inferior rectus muscle (arrowhead).

CONCLUSION

Due to the anatomic proximity lesions originating in the orbit/sinonasal cavity often involve the other compartment.

REFERENCES

1. Mafee MF, Tran BH, Chapa AR. Imaging of rhinosinusitis and its complications: plain film, CT, and MRI. Clin Rev Allergy Immunol. 2006;30(3):165-86.
2. Joshi VM, Sansi R. Imaging in sinonasal inflammatory disease. Neuroimaging Clin N Am. 2015;25(4):549-68.
3. Nguyen VD, Singh AK, Altmeyer WB, et al. Demystifying orbital emergencies: a pictorial review. Radiographics. 2017;37(3):947-62.
4. Sen S, Chandra A, Mukhopadhyay S, et al. Imaging approach to sinonasal neoplasms. Neuroimaging Clin N Am. 2015;25(4):577-93.
5. Sen S, Chandra A, Mukhopadhyay S, et al. Sinonasal tumors: computed tomography and MR imaging features. Neuroimaging Clin N Am. 2015;25(4):595-618.
6. Winegar BA, Murillo H, Tantiwongkosi B. Spectrum of critical imaging findings in complex facial skeletal trauma. Radiographics. 2013;33(1):3-19.

Section 7

Clinico-Radiological Approach

26. Approach to Nasal Obstruction
27. Approach to Epistaxis
28. Imaging Approach to Sinus Lesions

26
CHAPTER

Approach to Nasal Obstruction

Rakesh Kumar, Ashu Seith Bhalla, Manisha Jana

- Introduction
- Clinical Presentation
  - Important Points in History
- Clinical Examination
  - Local Examination
    - Nose
    - Nasopharynx
- Diagnostic Imaging
- Imaging Findings
  - Nasoethmoidal Lesions
  - Nasal Cavity/Lateral Wall Lesion
  - Nasal Septal Lesions
  - External Nose and Vestibular Lesion
- Management

INTRODUCTION

- Nasal obstruction is a sensation of blockage or difficulty in breathing out of one or both nostrils. This can be seen with diseases like rhinitis, sinusitis, septal deviation, and adenoid hypertrophy. There is also a physiological nasal cycle—cyclical pattern of turbinate mucosal swelling alternating between sides at intervals of 2-5 hours.
- Nasal obstruction may also be divided into mucosal and structural causes:
  - *Mucosal causes:* The obstruction tends to fluctuate. The common causes are rhinitis, sinusitis, nasal polyp, and soft tissue turbinate hypertrophy.
  - *Structural causes:* It is progressive. The causes are septal deviation (cartilaginous or bony), concha bullosa (air cell in the middle turbinate), tumors (benign and malignant), and choanal atresia/stenosis.
- Etiological classification of the causes of nasal obstruction is listed in Table 26.1.

CLINICAL PRESENTATION

Important Points in History

- Unilateral (structural causes) or bilateral (mucosal causes)
- *Trauma:* Nasal trauma/surgery

Table 26.1: Causes of nasal obstruction.	
Infective/inflammatory	• Rhinitis (infective/allergic) • Fungal infections • Polyp • Atypical retention cyst • Granulomatosis with polyangiitis (GPA)
Neoplastic—Benign	• Papilloma • Pleomorphic adenoma • Osteoma • Juvenile nasopharyngeal angiofibroma (JNA) • Schwannoma • Hemangioma
Neoplastic—Malignant	• Squamous cell carcinoma • Adenocarcinoma • Adenoid cystic carcinoma • Lymphoma • Esthesioneuroblastoma • Malignant melanoma • Mesenchymal tumors
Neoplastic—Secondary	• Metastases • Lymphoma
Contiguous extension from surrounding structures	• Meningioma • Chordoma • Lacrimal sac tumors [through nasolacrimal duct (NLD)] • Sinus tumors
Congenital	• Encephalocele • Hamartoma (glioma) • Dermoid/epidermoid cysts • Teratoma • Hemangioma

- *Diurnal and seasonal variation:* Allergies
- *Precipitating factors:* Allergic stimuli and airborne exposures
- *Rhinosinusitis:* Facial pain/or pressure, congestion, headache, and purulent nasal discharge
- *Malignancy:* Facial deformity, cranial nerve involvement (facial numbness), and epistaxis
- *Drugs:*
  - Oral contraceptives, antithyroid medication, antihypertensive, antidepressants, and benzodiazepines
  - *Local:* Prolong use of nasal drops (rhinitis medicamentosa).
- *Part of systemic illness:* Wegener's granulomatosis, cystic fibrosis, sarcoidosis, and syphilis.

CLINICAL EXAMINATION

Local Examination

Examine neck for cervical lymphadenopathy if nasal malignancy is suspected.

Nose

- Occluded nasal passage by boggy, red nasal mucosa (allergies, nonallergic rhinitis, or overuse of nasal decongestants)
- Septal deviation
- Glistening, smooth, pale single (AC polyp), or multiple (ethmoidal) nasal mass at the level of the middle turbinate or midnasal cavity (polyp)
- Purulent nasal discharge (rhinosinusitis)
- Ulcerated, friable mucosa bleeds on touch (granulomatous disease or malignancies).
  - *Granulomas:*
    - *Syphilis:* Granular lesion on septum with history and biopsy plus serology clinches diagnosis.
    - *Lupus vulgaris/tuberculosis:* It involves nasal vestibule and slowly destructive. Granulation tissue/ulceration and mucopurulent discharge.
    - *Sarcoid:* Systemic disease. Lesion involves septum or lateral wall and secondarily infection causing serosanguineous discharge. Patient complain of general ill health and disfigurement.
    - *Wegener's granulomatosis:* Systemic condition affecting lungs and kidney. Any unusual appearance in the nose and unexplained septal perforation need further investigation.
- *Fungi:*
  - *Aspergillosis:* Acute form in immune-compromise patients can be very aggressive and potentially fatal. It can extend from nose to sinuses and cranial cavity as well as into the soft tissue of face. Chronic form is not life threatening.
  - *Mucormycosis:* Fulminant infection and rapidly fatal. Nasal blockage discharge and presence of black turbinate are typical.
- *Nose benign tumors/granulomas:*
  - *Papilloma:*
    - *Squamous:* Wart-like growth arising from vestibular skin if trauma can bleed.
    - *Inverted:* Considered as intermediate tumors. Arises from lateral nasal wall and involve maxillary and ethmoid sinuses. Tumor is soft, friable, and bleed with hard nose blowing.
  - *Angioma:*
    - *Fibroangioma of septum:* Pedunculated friable red lesion arising from septum, bleed on touch. Seen in adults.
    - *Angioma of sinuses:* Maxillary and ethmoids in early childhood and presents with frightening epistaxis.

- *Fibroma:* Rare soft pedunculated lesions
- *Ossifying fibroma:* Frequent in 2nd and 3rd decades. Usually involve maxillary and ethmoid sinuses. It causes local discomfort and expansion, present with firm cheek swelling, and unilateral obstruction.
- *Osteomas:* Common in 2nd–4th decades and mostly incidental findings. 70% are in frontal, 25% in ethmoid, and 5% are in maxillary and sphenoid sinuses.
- *Fibrous dysplasia:* Fibro-osseous thickening of facial bones. Present as swelling around orbit, cheek, or alveolus. Present in 1st and 2nd decades of life. It can be monostotic or polyostotic.
- *Miscellaneous:*
  - *Rhinosporidiosis:* It presents as bleeding polypus. Typical appearance is strawberry like.
  - *Rhinolith:* Calcareous mass in the nose. Rough hard object in the nose.

Nasopharynx

- *Carcinoma:* It mostly arises in lateral wall of nasopharynx (fossa of Rosenmuller) and present as mucosa covered mass or ulcerative lesion. These patients have multiple neck metastases.
- *Angiofibroma:* Mucosa covered mass in the nasopharynx, nose with bleeding in a adolescent male is typical feature.

DIAGNOSTIC IMAGING

Only indicated if diagnosis is not clear based upon the history and physical examination.
- Computed tomography (CT) scan of the nose and paranasal sinuses is the primary diagnostic imaging modality.
- *Magnetic resonance imaging:* Generally a secondary study and is indicated for better characterization of nasal tumors.

IMAGING FINDINGS

- While interpreting imaging findings as elsewhere clinical details should be taken into consideration including age, symptom, duration of illness, and any systemic comorbidities/symptoms.
- Multiple factors guide the radiological differential diagnosis such as—location, bone expansion, bone destruction, soft tissue signal, and calcification. Some of the factors are common to sinus masses and discussed in Chapter 4. In the nasal cavity the location is an important determinant and the lesions have been classified accordingly (Table 26.2).

Table 26.2: Lesions according to the region of origin.	
Nasoethmoidal	• Encephalocele (frontoethmoidal) • Meningioma • Esthesioneuroblastoma • Chordoma
Lateral nasal wall, turbinates, and nasal cavity	• Rhinosinusitis • Inverted papilloma • AC polyp • Melanoma • Rhinolith • Rhinoscleroma • Rhinosporidiosis
Nasal septum (vide infra)	• Granulomatosis with polyangiitis (GPA) • Midline lethal granuloma (now recognized as a form of NHL) • Metastasis • Melanoma
External nose and vestibule	• Congenital lesions • Basal cell carcinoma, squamous cell carcinoma, and melanoma • Cellulitis, vestibulitis, and abscess • Nasoalveolar cyst
From surrounding structures	From posterior nasal cavity: Juvenile nasopharyngeal angiofibroma (from sphenopalatine foramen, pterygopalatine fossa involved)

Nasoethmoidal Lesions (Figs. 26.1 to 26.3)

Most of the lesions are described in detail in Chapter 23.

Due to close proximity of the nasal roof and the anterior ethmoid cells the lesions affecting them are often considered together.

- *Lesions in this region:*
  - May arise intracranially and extend downward
  - May arise from within the sinonasal cavity
  - Also there are lesions which may arise on either side of the skull base (i.e. intracranial or sinonasal), e.g. schwannoma.
- This is because olfactory nerves pass through the pores of the cribriform plate to the olfactory bulbs intracranially, and the tumors can arise anywhere along this path.
- Osseous lesions (primary or secondary) may arise from the anterior skull base (ASB) or from the osseous structures within the sinonasal cavity/its walls.
- Lesions from the orbit can spread into the ethmoid cells.
- *Some critical points* are highlighted and are further covered in detail in relevant chapters.

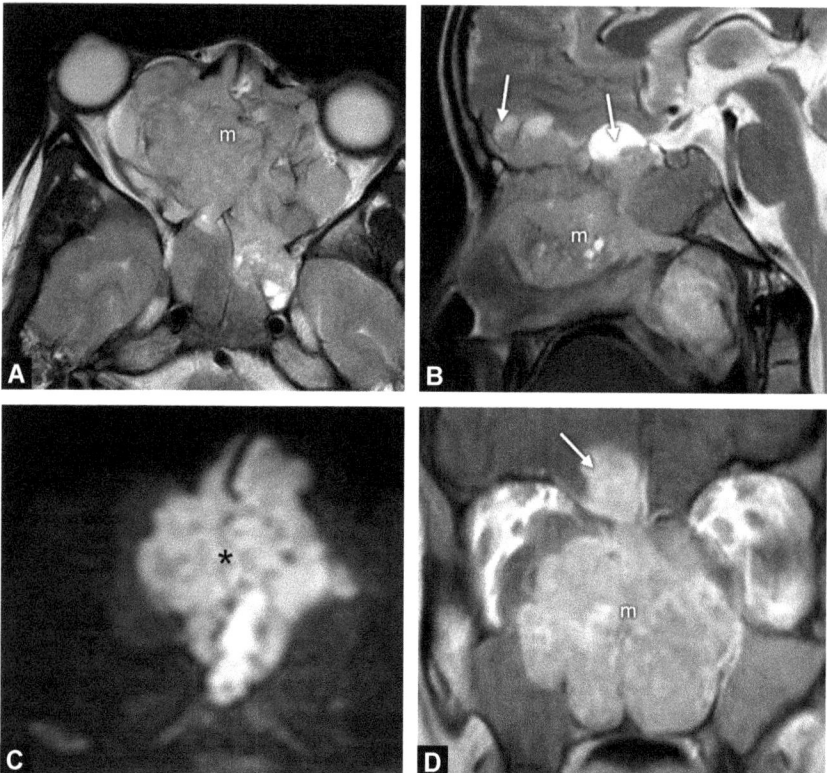

Figs. 26.1A to D: Esthesioneuroblastoma. (A) Large mass (m) with epicenter at superior nasal cavity. Hypointense signal on T2WI; (B) Cysts (arrows) in the tumor-CSF interface; (C) Restricted diffusion in the mass 9 (asterisk); and (D) Intense contrast enhancement. Intracranial extension of the mass also shows contrast enhancement (arrow).
(CSF: Cerebrospinal fluid; T2WI: T2-weighted image).

- The close proximity of this region to the ASB result in spread of diseases intracranially, and similarly to the orbit.
- Disease spread may be direct (with bone erosion), through valveless diploic veins that traverse the fovea ethmoidalis (roof of ethmoid) or along olfactory nerves that traverse the cribriform plate (roof of nose).
- Variant anatomy of ASB always to be borne in mind when endoscopic surgery planned in this region.
- Cerebrospinal fluid (CSF) rhinorrhea can occur in fractures affecting the lesion. Small defects in cribriform plate/lateral lamella can be normal and are confusing when imaging for site of leak.
- The nasal roof is the part of the nose fulfilling its "smell function". Olfactory bulb abnormalities may be seen in those with smell disorders.
- Postnatally the opacification of midline ASB is very variable. Awareness of normal variants versus abnormal defects of cribriform plate, crista galli, and foramen cecum is critical when imaging congenital sinonasal lesions.

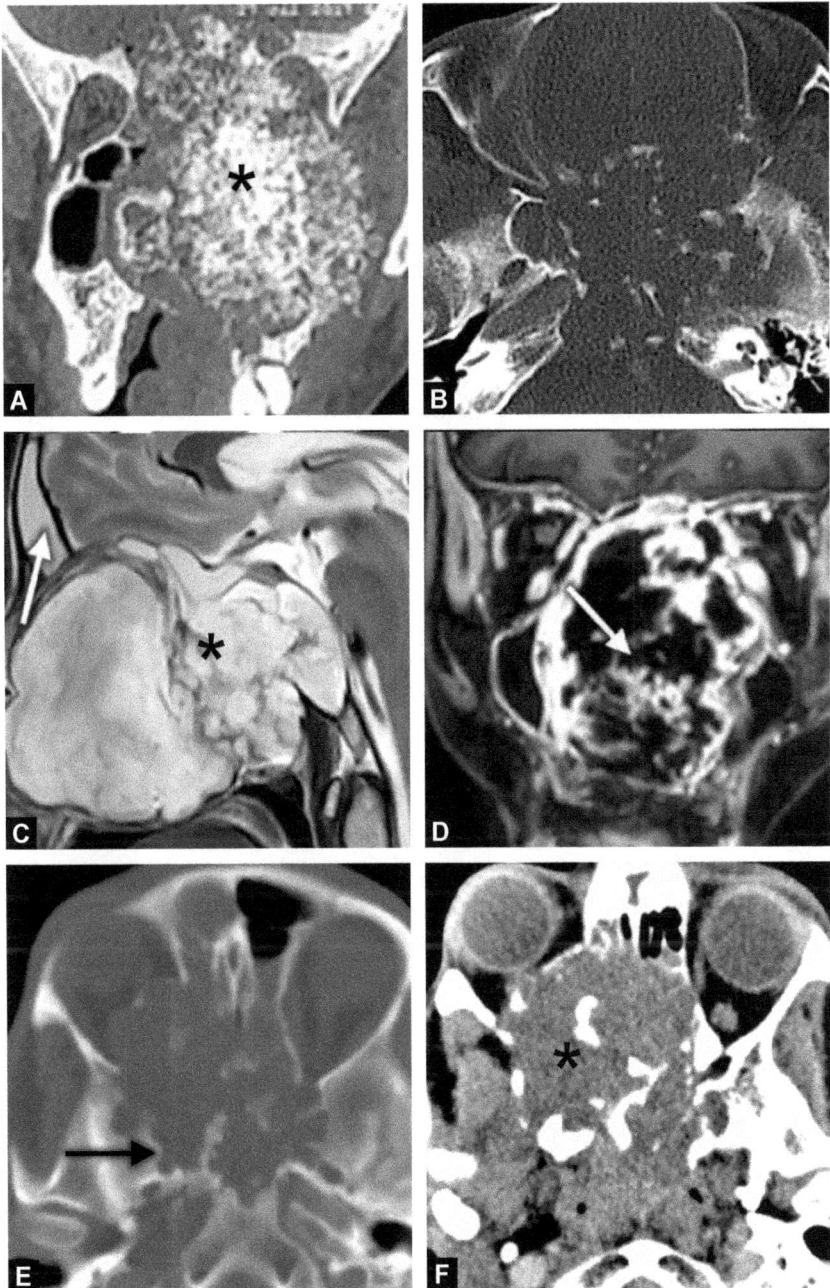

Figs. 26.2A to F: Nasoethmoidal masses of bony origin. (A) Chondrosarcoma. Extensive chondroid matrix mineralization (asterisk); (B) Chondroid matrix mineralization (ring and arc-shaped); (C) T2W hyperintense signal of the mass (asterisk) and retained secretion in frontal sinus (arrow); (D) Lobular contrast enhancement of septae (arrow); (E) Chordoma. Midline expansile lytic lesion with bone destruction (arrow); and (F) No contrast enhancement of the mass (asterisk).

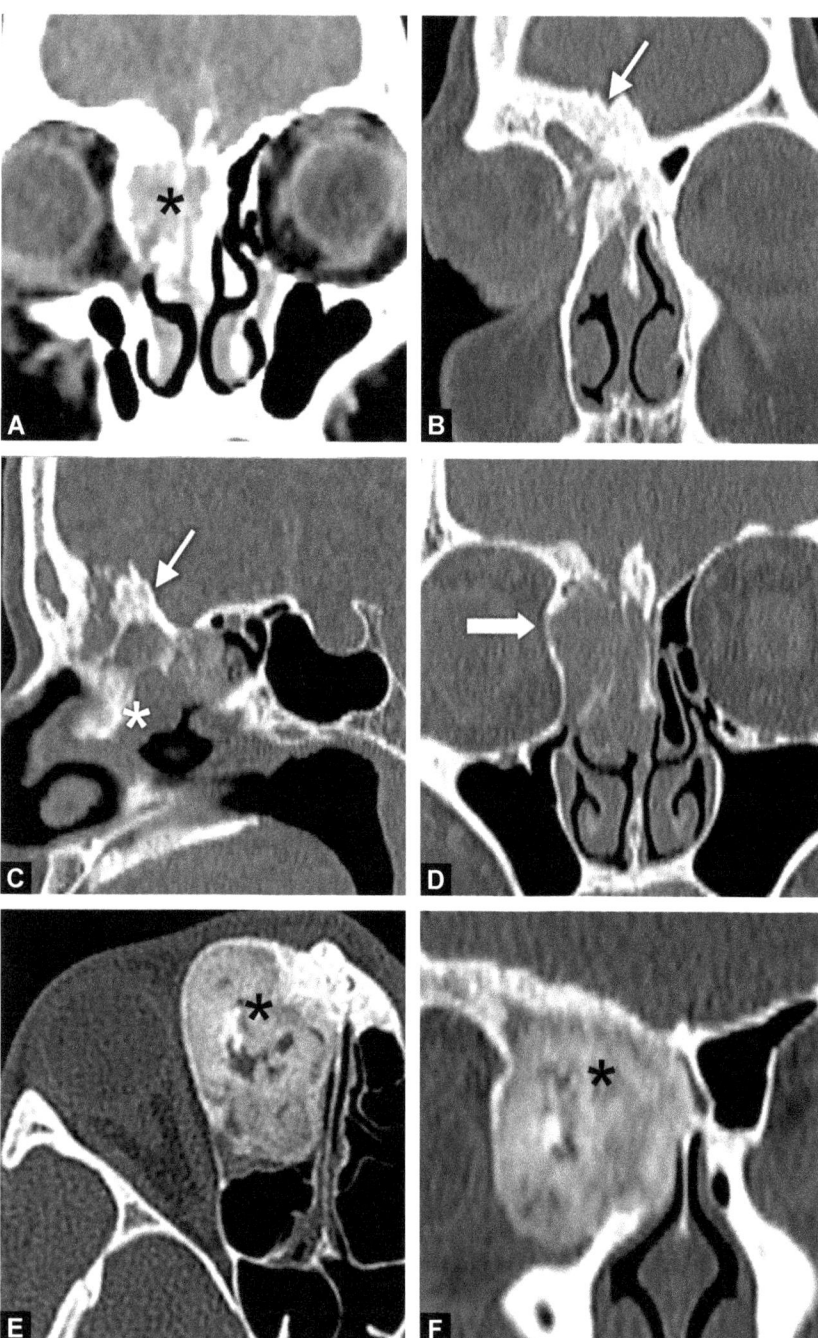

Figs. 26.3A to F: Nasoethmoidal masses with bony sclerosis. (A) Olfactory groove meningioma. Superior nasal cavity mass (asterisk) with intense enhancement on contrast-enhanced computed tomography (CECT); (B and C) Hyperostosis of the frontal bone (arrows); (D) Bony expansion of the nasal cavity (block arrow); (E) Ossifying fibroma. Expansile bony mass arising from right anterior ethmoid air cells (asterisk); and (F) Ground-glass matrix (asterisk).

Table 26.3: Nasoethmoidal masses and their key imaging points (see Figs. 26.1 to 26.3).	
Masses	Key imaging points
Esthesioneuroblastoma	• Soft tissue mass at superior nasal cavity with cribriform plate erosion • *T2-weighted magnetic resonance imaging:* Heterogeneously hyperintense • Intense contrast enhancement on CT/MRI • T2WI bright areas (cyst) at the apical part of the tumor (tumor/brain interface)
Chondrosarcoma	• Soft tissue mass with bone destruction • Matrix shows ring and arc-shaped calcification • Soft tissue mass with T2WI bright signal, lobular contrast enhancement
Chordoma	• Rare tumor, usually involves the spheno-occipital synchondrosis • Expansile lytic bone lesion • Lobular soft tissue mass with foci of calcification • Heterogeneous T2W hyperintense signal • Heterogeneous contrast enhancement
Meningioma	• Unusual tumors • Variable T2W signal on MRI (T2W hypointense) • Intense contrast enhancement • Bony hyperostosis
Schwannoma	• Heterogeneous hyperintense T2W signal intensity • Variable contrast enhancement • Bony remodeling, lack of frank bone destruction

(CT: Computed tomography; MRI: Magnetic resonance imaging; T2WI: T2-weighted image).

Pediatric nasoethmoidal masses are covered in Chapters 20 and 23. Adult nasoethmoidal masses are described in Table 26.3.

Congenital lesions are described in Chapter 20.

Nasal Cavity/Lateral Wall Lesion (Figs. 26.4 to 26.6)

Nasal cavity/lateral wall lesions are listed in Table 26.4.

Causes of masses arising from lateral wall of the nasal cavity are diverse including mostly infective/ neoplastic lesions (Table 26.4).

Several of these tumors are benign and difficult to differentiate from common inflammatory pathologies such as polyps.

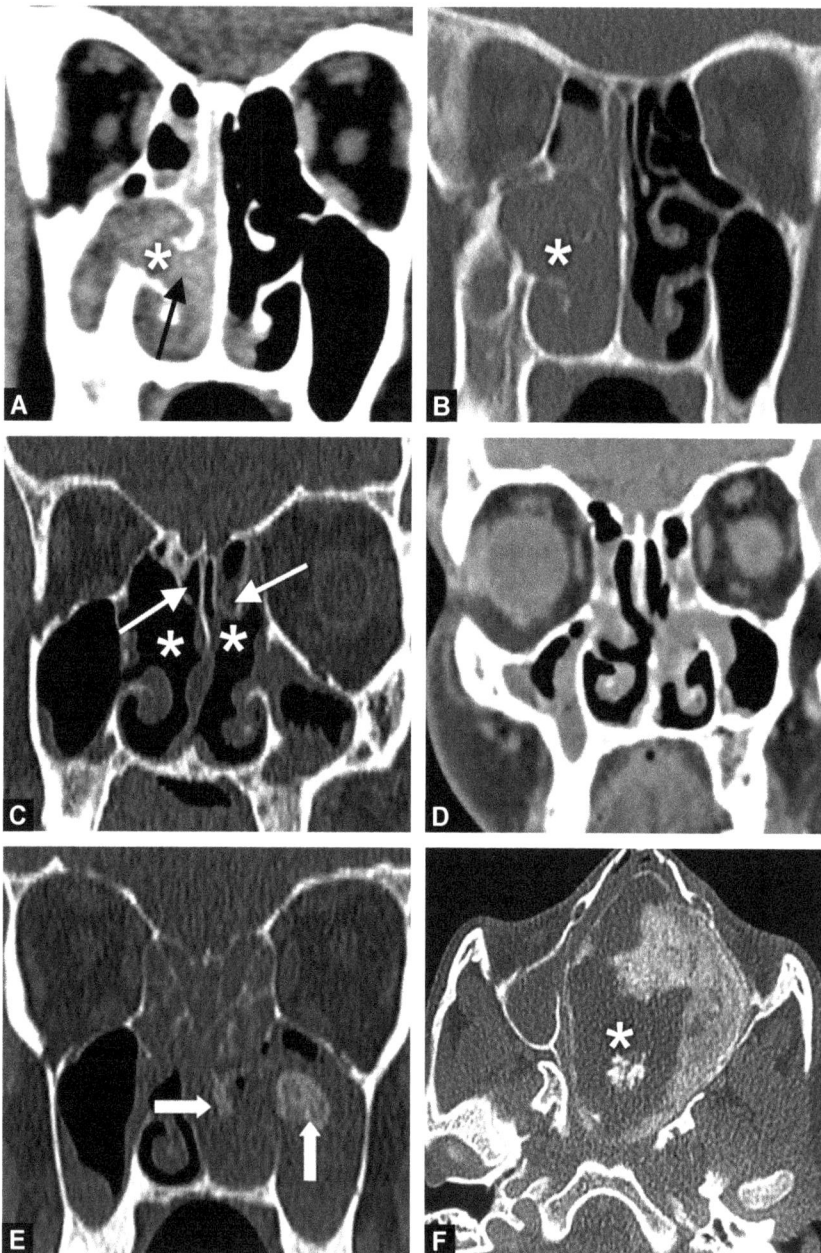

Figs. 26.4A to F: Nasal cavity lesions causing obstruction. (A) Chronic rhinosinusitis with polyposis. Soft tissue opacification of right nasal cavity. Enhancing mucosa (arrow); (B) Widened and blocked OMC (asterisk); (C and D) Atrophic rhinitis. Mucoperiosteal thickening of nasal cavity and maxillary sinuses. Destruction of turbinates (arrows), missing middle turbinates (asterisks); (E) Rhinolith. Chronic rhinosinusitis with mucosal thickening and calcified areas within (block arrows) suggestive of rhinoliths; and (F) Ossifying fibroma of the nasal cavity causing nasal obstruction. Peripheral ossification of the mass (asterisk), with central hypodense area.

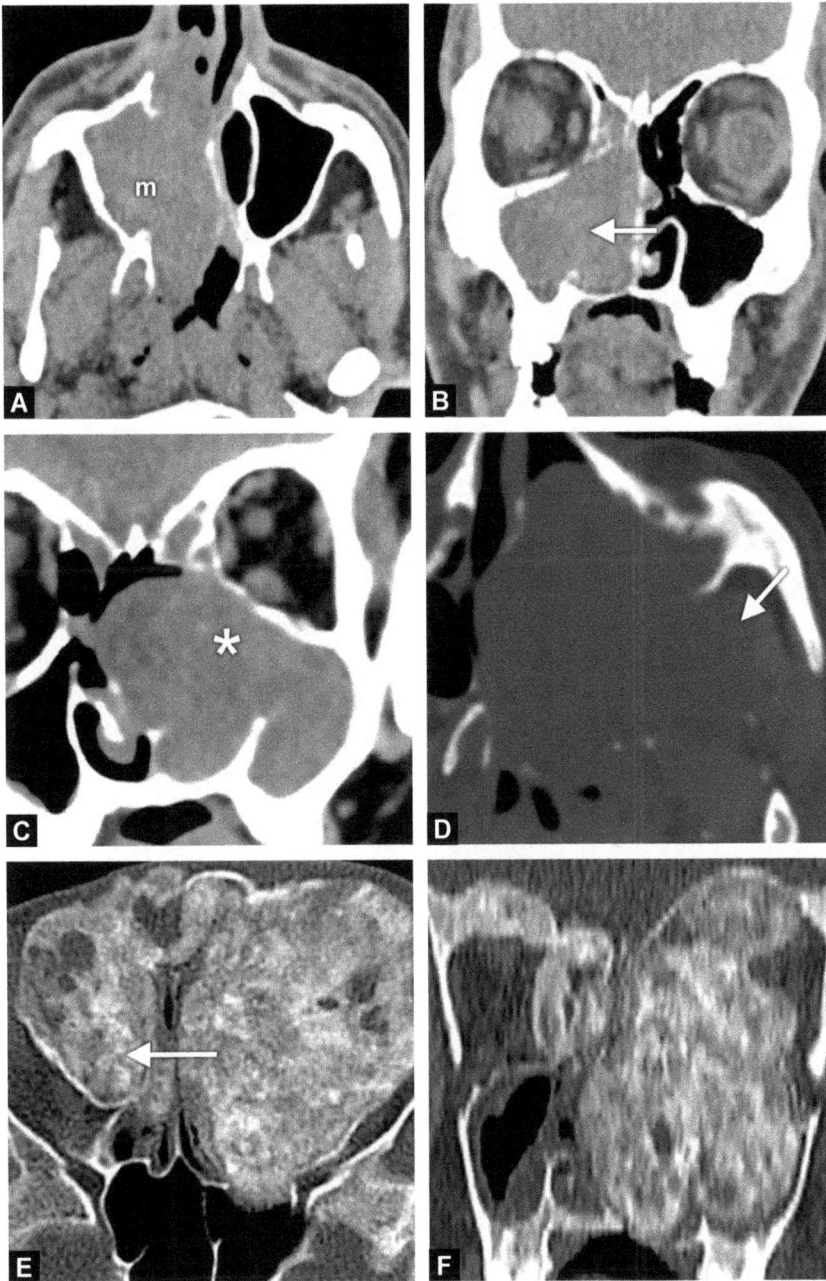

Figs. 26.5A to F: Nasal cavity lesions causing obstruction. (A) Inverted papilloma. Expansile mass lesion (m) involving right maxillary sinus and right nasal cavity; (B) Widening of maxillary ostium (arrow); (C) Neurofibroma. Large expansile soft tissue density mass (asterisk), left maxillary sinus, nasal cavity, and sphenoid sinus; (D) Widening of pterygomaxillary fissure and extension into pterygopalatine fossa and infratemporal fossa (arrow); (E and F) Ossifying fibroma. Large expansile mixed density masses in bilateral frontal and ethmoidal cells with mass effect over the globes bilaterally; and nodular sclerotic component (arrow in E).

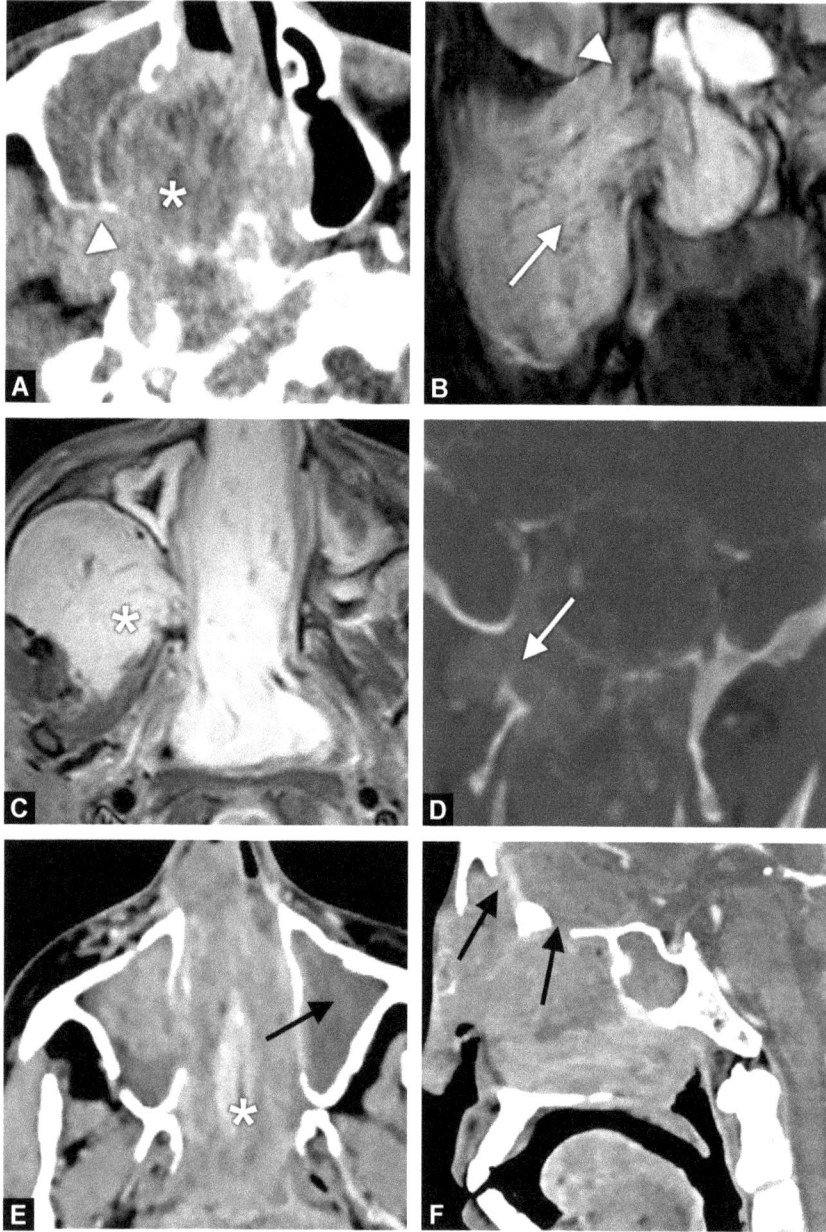

Figs. 26.6A to F: Nasal cavity masses causing obstruction. (A to D) **Juvenile nasopharyngeal angiofibroma.** Intensely enhancing heterogeneous mass lesion centered near right sphenopalatine foramen extending into, bilateral ethmoids, posterior choana, and nasopharynx (asterisk). Laterally extension into the pterygomaxillary fissure (arrowhead in A). Intermediate signal intensity with prominent flow voids on T2WI (arrow in B). Intense postcontrast enhancement (asterisk in C). Erosion of pterygoid base and widening of inferior orbital fissure (arrow in D). (E and F) **Nasopharyngeal carcinoma.** Large enhancing mass in nasopharynx, involving posterior wall of nasopharynx (asterisk in E). *Note:* Retained secretion in sinuses (arrow). Destruction of frontal bone (arrows in F).

Table 26.4: Clinical and imaging findings of nasal cavity/lateral nasal wall lesions causing obstruction.

Disease	Salient clinical/imaging findings
Rhinosinusitis (Figs. 26.4A to F)	Discussed in Chapter 4
Rhinolith (Figs. 26.4A to F)	• Rare, calcareous concretions which form in the nose due to deposition of salts around a foreign body • Result in foul smell and discharge • Exogenous foreign bodies usually located near the floor; may be endogenous (blood clots/tooth fragments) • Local inflammatory reaction leads to deposition of calcium, iron, magnesium salts, and organic substances • CT displays size and site of the rhinolith preoperatively. Appears as a well-defined, dense, and nearly osseous lesion within the nasal cavity. Mostly, no associated soft tissue lesion seen.
Inverted papilloma (Figs. 26.5A to F)	Numerous staging system used, Krause's system being most commonly followed • *Stage 1:* Confined to nasal cavity • *Stage 2:* Ethmoid sinuses, maxillary sinus (medial and superior region involved) • *Stage 3:* All paranasal sinuses but confined to nose/sinuses • *Stage 4:* Not confined to sinuses/malignant
Juvenile nasopharyngeal angiofibromas (JNAs)	• Mass with center in sphenopalatine foramen • Extension into the pterygopalatine fossa and bowing of posterior maxillary wall • Intense enhancement after contrast administration on CT/MRI
Nasopharyngeal carcinoma	• Mass in posterior nasopharyngeal wall • Older age, short duration of symptoms • Soft tissue mass with bone destruction • No calcification
Rhinoscleroma	Middle and inferior turbinate earliest site
Rhinosporidiosis	Inferior turbinate, inferior meatus, floor; spread to NLD and lacrimal sac

(CT: Computed tomography; MRI: Magnetic resonance imaging; NLD: Nasolacrimal duct).

Nasal Septal Lesions (Figs. 26.7 and 26.8)

The list of nasal septal lesions is exhaustive (Table 26.5), and imaging is indicated in the lesions associated with soft tissue. The diagnostic algorithm towards erosive nasal lesions is described in Flowchart 26.1. Most of the entities have been covered elsewhere in the book.

Table 26.5: Nasal septal lesions (Figs. 26.7 and 26.8).			
Causes			Key imaging points
Congenital			
Acquired	Traumatic	• Surgical • Iatrogenic • Self-inflicted	• No associated mass • More frequently iatrogenic • Occasionally self-inflicted (rhinotillexomania) consequent to chronic nose picking, e.g. in severe obsessive-compulsive disorders • Anterior and inferior part of septum involved first
	Infective	• Fungal • Tuberculosis • Syphilis • Leprosy • Rhinoscleroma • Actinomycosis	Collection of pus between the nasal septum and the mucoperiosteum or mucoperichondrium, depending on the part of the septum involved. • Following trauma or in immunosuppressed individuals • Adjoining sinusitis • Dental infection • Infection in underlying dermoid cyst
	Toxic	• Cocaine use • Other inhalants (chromium salts) • Nasal steroids	
	Inflammatory	• Granulomatosis with polyangiitis (GPA) • Sarcoidosis • LSS	
	Tumors	• Midline lethal granuloma (now recognized as a form of NHL) • Metastasis • Melanoma	• Midline lesion • May be associated with mass

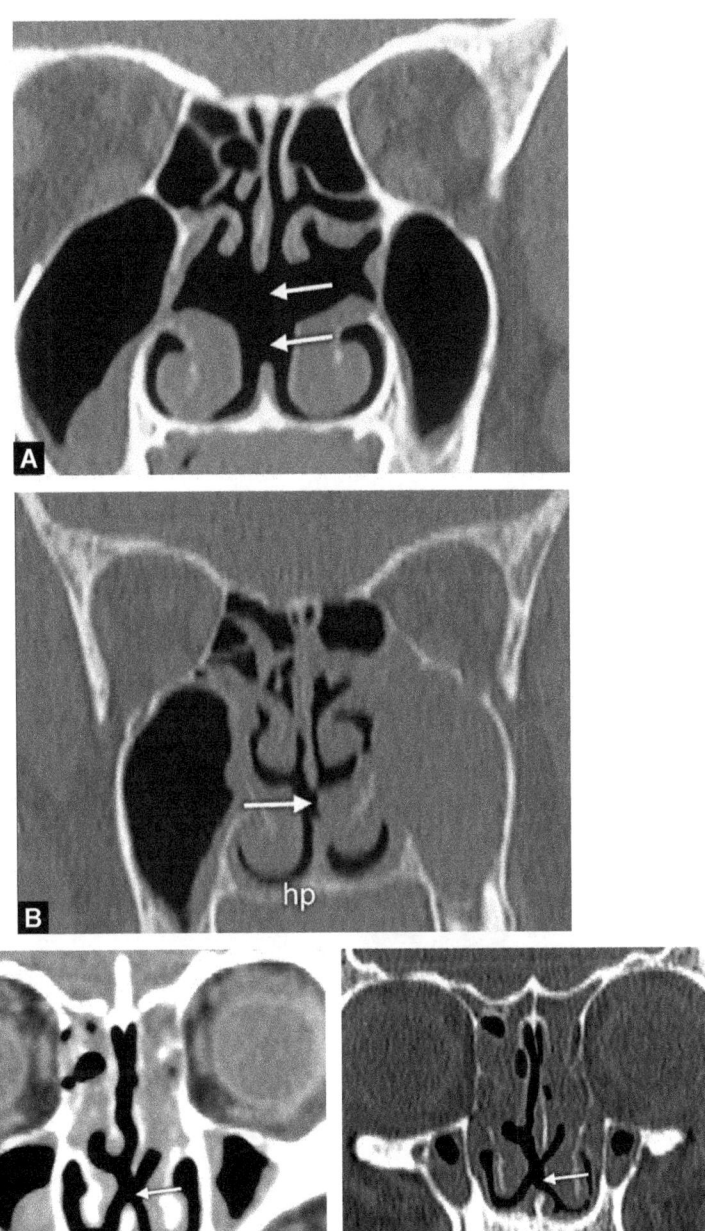

Figs. 26.7A to D: Nasal septal perforation without mass lesions (mucosal thickening may be present). (A) Septal perforation after fungal rhinosinusitis. Mucoperiosteal thickening of the turbinates and right maxillary sinus. Large septal perforation (arrows) at the bony part; (B) Nasal septal perforation in granulomatosis with polyangiitis (GPA). Left maxillary sinusitis. Perforation of the inferior nasal septum (arrow) but hard palate (hp) spared; and (C and D) Nasal septal perforation after functional endoscopic sinus surgery (FESS). Residual mucosal thickening in nasal cavity, ethmoid, and maxillary sinuses. Bony septal perforation at the inferior part (arrows).

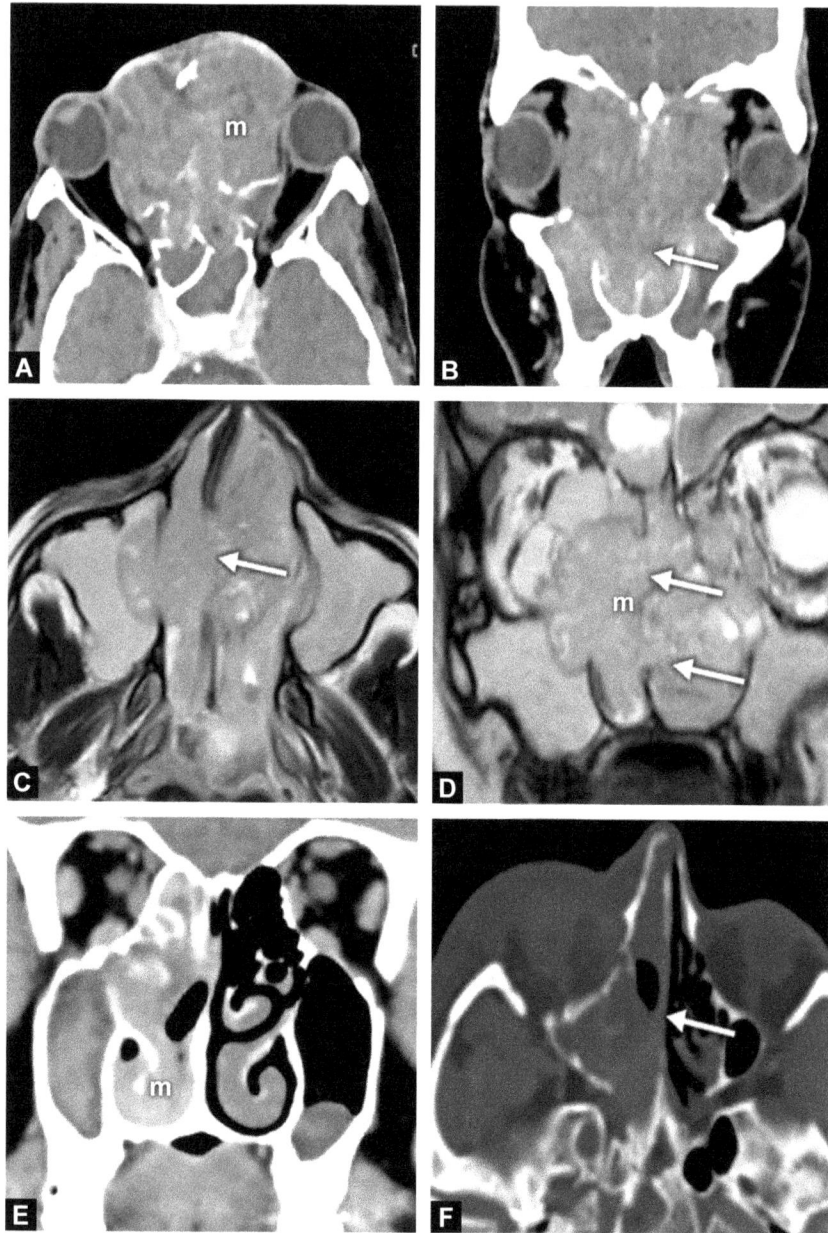

Figs. 26.8A to F: Nasal septal destruction associated with mass lesions. (A) Septal destruction in sinonasal PNET. Homogeneously enhancing mass lesion in the nasal cavity and ethmoids (m); (B) Destruction of the nasal septum (arrow) at the bony part; (C and D) Nasal septal destruction in esthesioneuroblastoma. Large mass (m) with epicenter at superior nasal cavity. Isointense signal on T2WI. Nasal septal destruction (arrows); and (E and F) Septal erosion in NK/T-cell lymphoma. Homogeneous mass (m) with erosion of bony nasal septum erosion (arrow).
(NK: Natural killer; PNET: Primitive neuroectodermal tumor; T2WI: T2-weighted image).

Flowchart 26.1: Differential diagnosis of common erosive nasal lesions based on distribution.

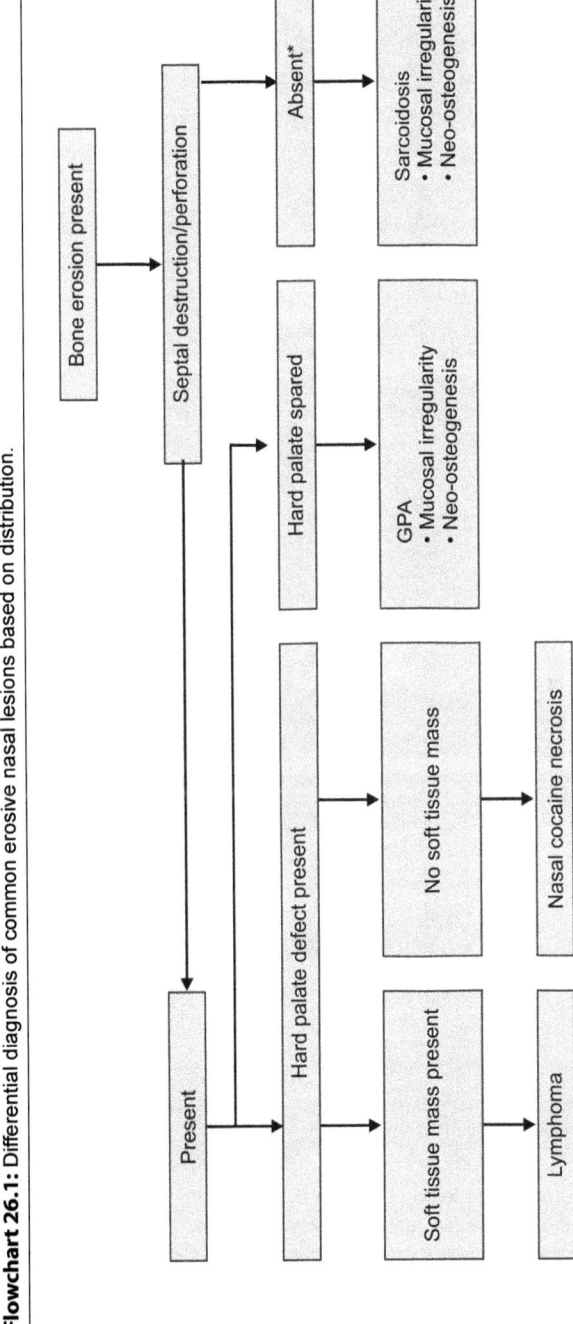

*Can occur, although rare.
(GPA: Granulomatosis with polyangiitis).

External Nose and Vestibular Lesion (Figs. 26.9 and 26.10)

The external nose and vestibular lesions are described in Table 26.6.

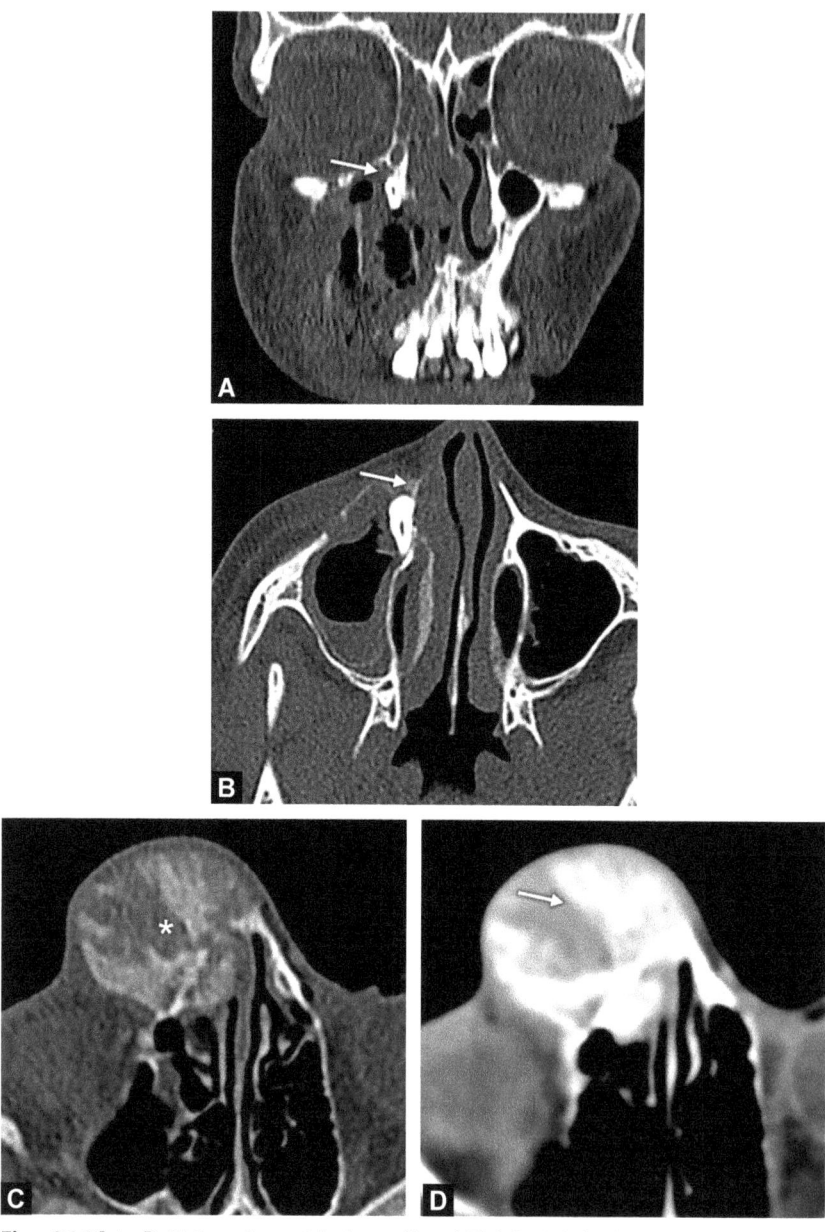

Figs. 26.9A to D: External nasal lesions. (A and B) Infected dentigerous cyst. Extensive inflammatory change in right maxilla and premaxillary spaces. Unerupted tooth in right maxilla (arrows); (C) Nasal bone hemangioma. Expansile lytic sclerotic lesion of right nasal bone with sun-burst appearance (asterisk); and (D) Heterogeneous contrast enhancement (arrow).

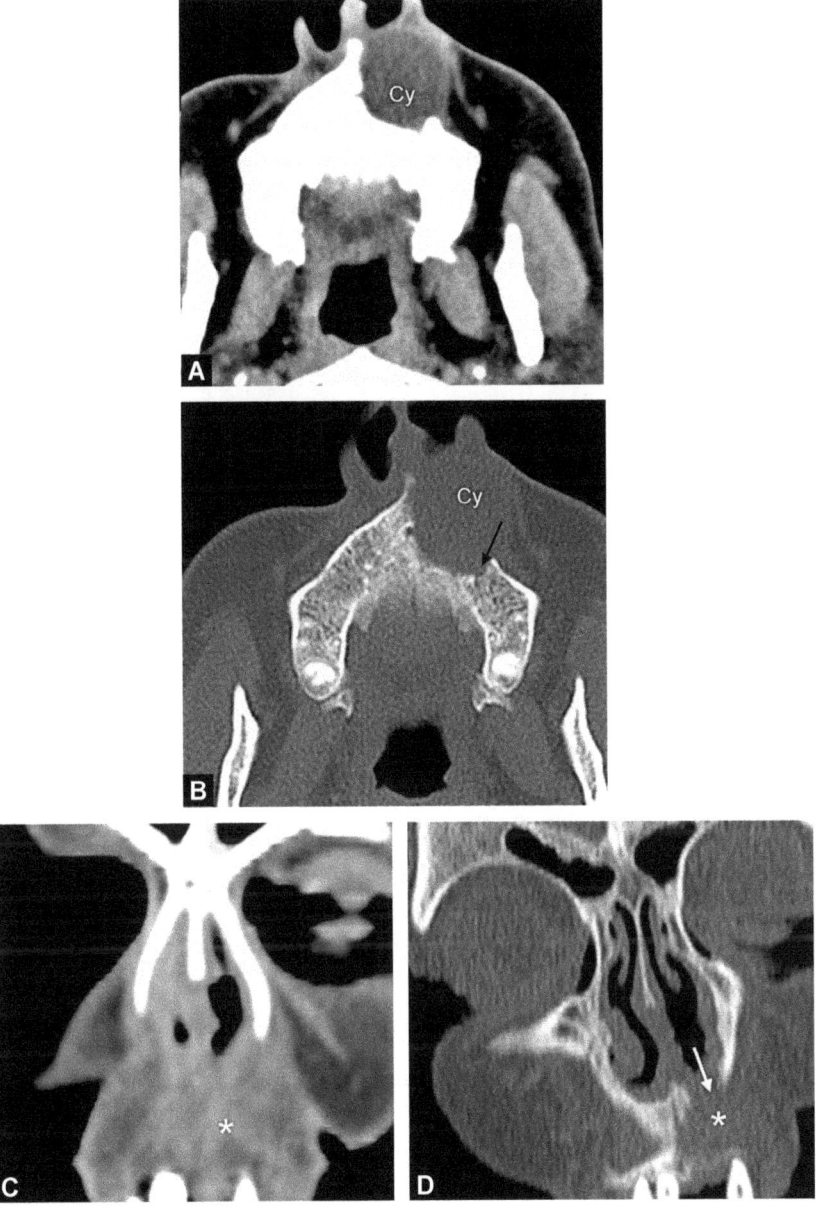

Figs. 26.10A to D: Lesions of nasal vestibule. (A) Nasoalveolar cyst. Hypodense cystic lesion (Cy) in left nasal vestibule; (B) Bony scalloping of the maxillary alveolus (arrow); (C) Basal cell carcinoma. Mass lesion in left side of columella (asterisks in C and D) Bone erosion of left maxillary alveolus (arrow).

Table 26.6: External nose and vestibular lesions (see Figs. 26.9 and 26.10).	
External nose lesions	Vestibular lesions
Most diseases do not require imaging and include cellulitis or deformities	Most commonly infective: Vestibulitis, furuncle
Deformities often result from abnormalities of the cartilage • *Saddle nose:* Depression of the dorsum due to involvement of bony/cartilaginous part or both • Following trauma or surgery or septal hematoma, abscess or midline lesions destroying the septum	• *Congenital:* Stenosis, atresia – Tumors/tumor-like condition: Nasoalveolar cyst/squamous cell carcinoma

• Masses:
 – *In the region of glabella:*
  - *Congenital lesions:* Dermoid cyst, encephalocele, glioma, hemangioma, and neurofibroma
 – *In the region of vestibule:*
  - *Malignant lesions:* Basal cell carcinoma, squamous cell carcinoma, and melanoma
	• *Nasoalveolar cyst:*
	 – Seen as a smooth swelling in nasal vestibule/lateral wall/floor
	 – Smooth, well-defined cystic lesion at the nasolabial fold with no deep extension
	• *Squamous cell carcinoma:*
	 – Irregular, ill-defined soft tissue mass with extension to floor of nasal cavity/collumella and upper lip

MANAGEMENT

Management in nasal obstruction depends on the cause of obstruction. It can be medical/conservative, endoscopic, or surgical.

DIAGNOSTIC ALGORITHM

- Flowchart 26.2 summarizes the approach to unilateral nasal obstruction associated with soft tissue/ 'mass lesion'
- Bilateral lesions are mostly infective or inflammatory in nature.
- However large masses which are initially unilateral become/appear bilateral due to erosion/ displacement of the nasal septum.

SUGGESTED READING

1. Borges A, Fink J, Villablanca P, et al. Midline destructive lesions of the sinonasal tract: simplified terminology based on histopathologic criteria. AJNR Am J Neuroradiol. 2000;21:331-6.
2. Gupta A, Hawrych A, Wilson WR. Cocaine-induced sinonasal destruction. Otolaryngol Head Neck Surg. 2001;124:480.
3. Provenzale JM, Allen NB. Wegener granulomatosis: CT and MR findings. AJNR Am J Neuroradiol. 1996;17:785-92.
4. Valencia MP, Castillo M. Congenital and Acquired Lesions of the Nasal Septum: A Practical Guide for Differential Diagnosis. RadioGraphics. 2008;28:205-23.

Flowchart 26.2: Diagnostic algorithm of unilateral soft tissue masses causing nasal obstruction.

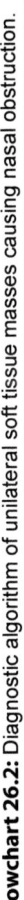

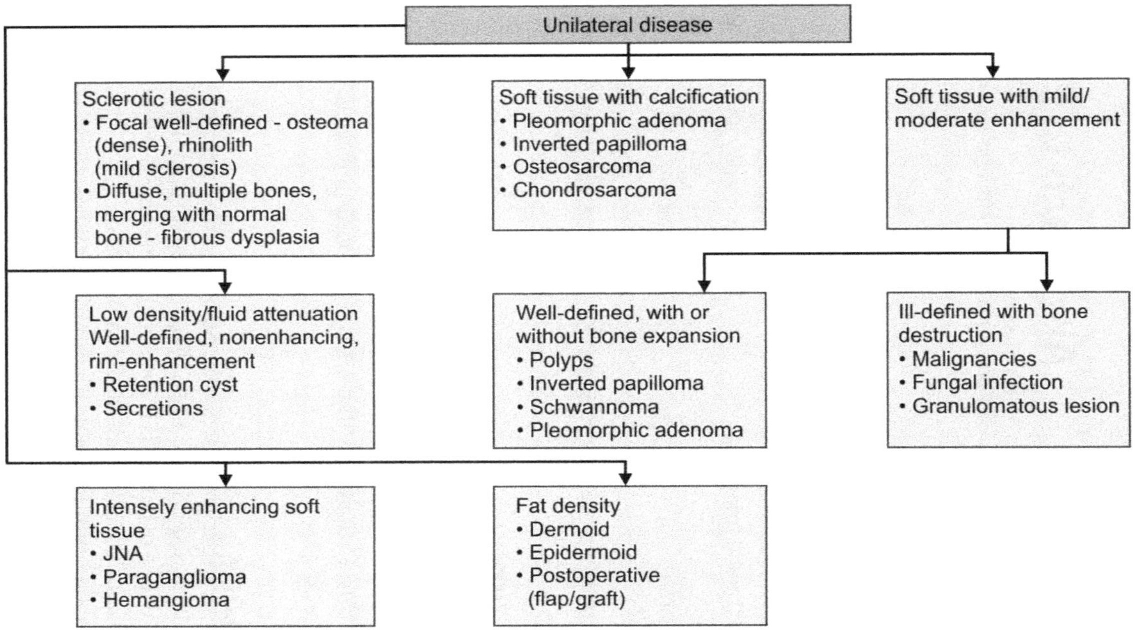

(JNA: Juvenile Nasopharyngeal angiofibroma).

CHAPTER 27

Approach to Epistaxis

David Victor Kumar Irugu, Manisha Jana, Ashu Seith Bhalla

- Introduction
- Epidemiology
- Relevant Anatomy
  - External Carotid Artery
  - Internal Carotid Artery
- Etiology
- Investigations
- Imaging
- Management
  - Cauterization
  - Nasal Packing
  - Surgical Management
  - Angiography and Embolization
  - Others
- Prevention

INTRODUCTION

- Epistaxis is defined as bleeding from nose or nasopharynx. The word epistaxis originated from Greek word "epistazein" which means to flow drop by drop.
- In 1784 Vogel suggested that the term should be used specifically for nasal bleeding.[1,2]

EPIDEMIOLOGY

- Many people experience nose bleeding at some point in their life and the prevalence of epistaxis is estimated to be about 108/100,000 per year.
- Of these about 6% need medical management.
- Epistaxis has bimodal age distribution and is most commonly seen under the age of 10 years and over 40 years. There is no race or gender predilection.[1-3]

RELEVANT ANATOMY

Blood supply to nose comes from both external and internal carotid arteries (Fig. 27.1A), through the following branches.

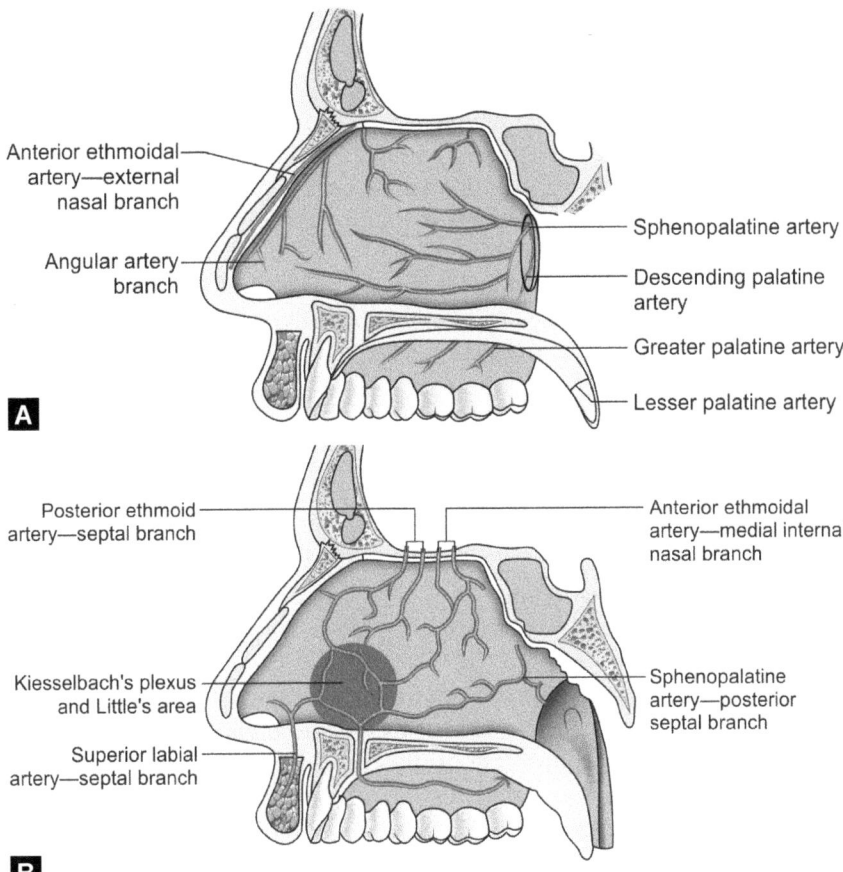

Figs. 27.1A and B: (A) **Blood supply of nasal septum** from external and internal carotid artery systems; and (B) **Little's area and Kiesselbach's plexus.**

External Carotid Artery

- *Internal maxillary artery:* It supplies blood to nose through its branches.
  - Greater palatine artery
  - Pharyngeal artery
  - Posterior nasal artery
  - Sphenopalatine artery (SPA) is the major supply to nasal cavity and to superior and medial turbinates.
- Superior labial artery branch of facial artery supplies to nasal vestibule.

Internal Carotid Artery

Ophthalmic artery, a branch of internal carotid artery (ICA) provides blood supply through:
- Anterior ethmoidal artery gives branch to superior turbinate.
- Posterior ethmoidal artery supplies to sphenoethmoidal recess area.

Both anterior and posterior ethmoidal arteries give medial and lateral branches. The medial branches supplies the superior septum and Little's area.

Anatomically important structures which are involved in epistaxis are (Fig. 27.1B):
- *Little's area:* Situated in the anteroinferior part of septum, described by James Little in 1879.[2] It contains *Kiesselbach's plexus,* a vascular network formed by branches from septal branches of SPA, greater palatine artery, and septal branch of superior labial artery, anterior, and posterior ethmoidal arteries. The vascular anatomy of this plexus was described by Wilhelm Kiesselbach in 1884.[2]
- *Woodruff plexus:* Situated at inferoposterior end of inferior turbinate; and formed by branches from ascending pharyngeal artery, posterior nasal branch of sphenopalatine and SPA.

ETIOLOGY

Epistaxis can be classified depending on anatomical location, onset, severity, causing/risk factors, and age as:
- Anterior or posterior
- Primary or secondary
- Traumatic or nontraumatic
- Acute or chronic
- Pediatric or adult.

About 90% of nose bleeding originates from Little's area.
- The most common cause of epistaxis in children is digital trauma and hypertension in people over 40 years of age. Most often primary epistaxis is idiopathic and the various causes of bleeding are documented in Table 27.1 and Figures 27.2 to 27.5.
- It is frequently seen in dry season and in less humid environments. These factors increase excoriation and cracking of nasal mucosa, loss

Table 27.1: Causes of epistaxis.	
Traumatic	Nontraumatic
• Nose picking • Facial injury • Impacted foreign body • *Surgery:* Ear-nose-throat (ENT)/maxillofacial/ophthalmic • Nasal intubation	• Septal spur/septal deviation/septal perforation • Allergic rhinosinusitis - Nasal polyps • Rhinosporidiosis • Benign tumors (e.g. inverted papilloma, juvenile angiofibroma) (Figs. 27.2 and 27.3) • Malignant tumors (e.g. squamous cell carcinoma) • Hereditary hemorrhagic telangiectasia • Vascular malformations (Figs. 27.4 and 27.5) • Granulomatosis with polyangiitis • Hypertension • *Coagulopathies:* Hemophilia, thrombocytopenia • Liver disease • *Drugs:* Nasal sprays, drug abusing, anticoagulants (heparin, warfarin) • Antiplatelet (e.g. aspirin, clopidogrel)

of mucosal integrity causing exposure of underlying vessels to trauma leading to nose bleeding.[1,2]

INVESTIGATIONS

The following investigations should be performed after stabilizing the patient (detailed later):
- Endoscopic examination to locate the site of bleed
- Complete blood picture to determine amount of blood loss
- Renal function tests to assess the renal damage in severe epistaxis
- Liver function tests for coagulation factors

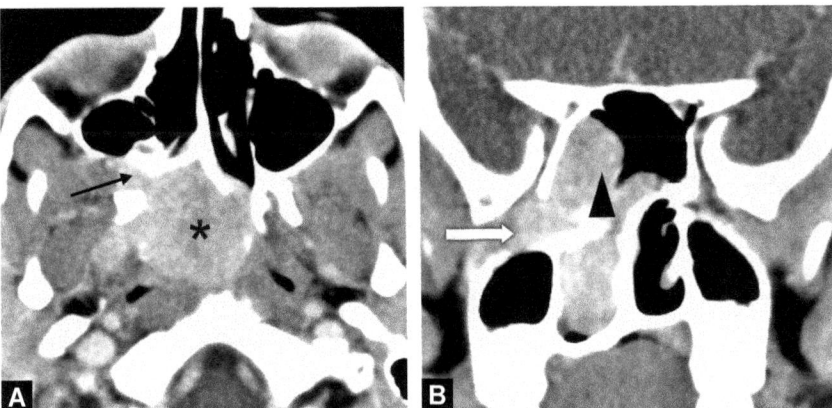

Figs. 27.2A and B: Juvenile nasopharyngeal angiofibroma. (A) Enhancing mass in the nasopharynx (asterisk). Widening of pterygomaxillary fissure (arrow); and (B) Extension into pterygopalatine fossa (block arrow) and sphenoid (arrowhead).

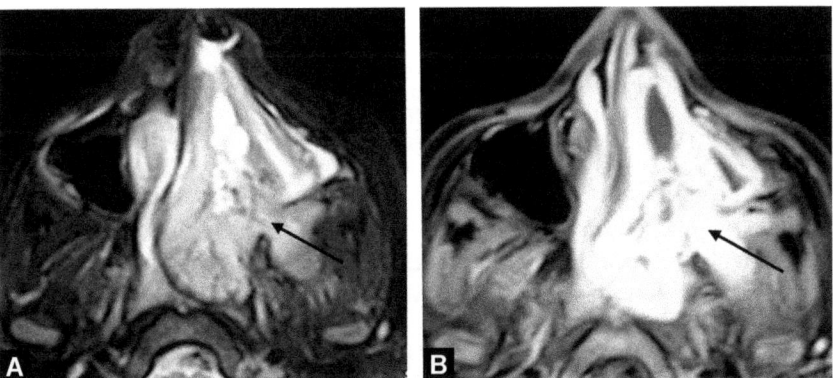

Figs. 27.3A and B: Magnetic resonance imaging (MRI) of juvenile nasopharyngeal angiofibroma. (A) T2W hyperintense mass lesion located in left nasopharynx. Widening of pterygomaxillary fissure (arrow); and (B) Intense enhancement after contrast administration (arrow).

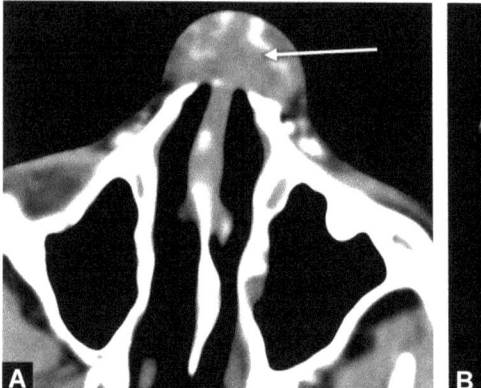
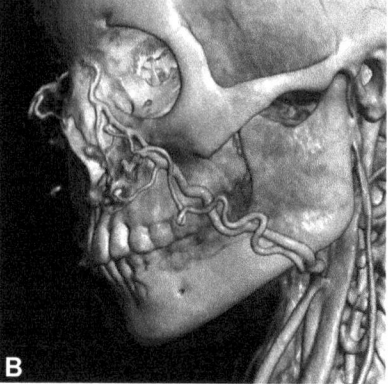

Figs. 27.4A and B: (A) High flow arteriovenous malformation (arrow) of nose causing epistaxis; and (B) Computed tomography (CT) angiogram showing large feeder from left linguofacial trunk.

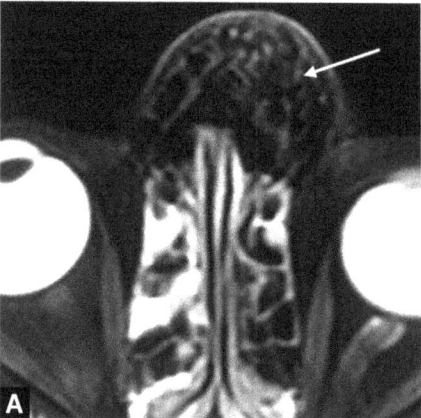
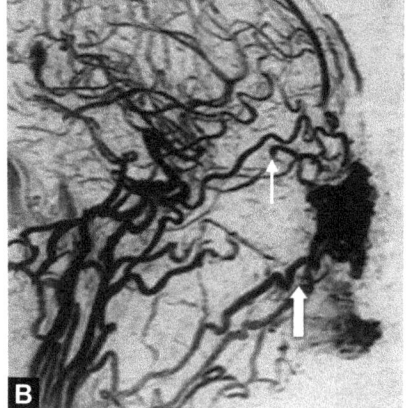

Figs. 27.5A and B: Arteriovenous malformation of nose causing epistaxis. (A) Multiple tortuous flow voids over root of nose on T2W fat suppressed MRI (arrow); and (B) MR angiography: Feeding artery from ICA (arrow) and ECA (block arrow).
(ECA: External carotid artery; ICA: Internal carotid artery; MRI: Magnetic resonance imaging).

- Prothrombin time (PT), activated partial thromboplastin time (APTT), and platelet counts
- Coagulation profile such as serum fibrinogen, plasminogen, fibrin breakdown products (FBPs), von Willebrand factor (VWF) antigen, etc.
- Imaging (vide infra)
- Diagnostic angiography if planning to embolize the patient.

IMAGING

- Cross-sectional imaging protocol for epistaxis depends on the severity of epistaxis and suspected cause based on clinical evaluation

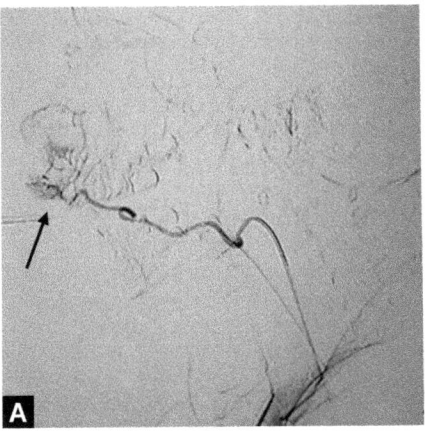 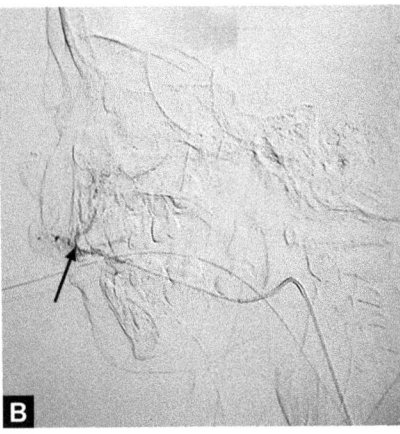

Figs. 27.6A and B: Idiopathic epistaxis. Left facial artery run showing abnormal blush (arrows) at anterior nasal cavity. Postembolization angiogram showing successful embolization.

- For suspected inflammatory disease noncontrast computed tomography (NCCT) would suffice for extent
- For suspected tumors it is essential to perform a contrast-enhanced CT (CECT)
- *Idiopathic epistaxis:* When no local or idiopathic cause is identified. If the bleeding is severe patients are taken up directly for angiography and embolization (Figs. 27.6A and B)
- In nose with milder bleeds being treated on outpatient basis, CT angiography should be performed to exclude vascular lesions, mainly arteriovenous malformations (AVMs).

MANAGEMENT

Stabilize the patient by universal airway, breathing, and circulation (ABC) method.

Careful history taking is important to know:[1,2]
- The frequency, severity, and side of the nasal bleed
- Aggravating and relieving factors
- Drug history like nonsteroidal anti-inflammatory drugs (NSAIDs), etc.
- Systemic disorders such as hypertension and diabetes mellitus
- Any surgical history or trauma.
- The amount and severity of blood loss can be estimated by clinical history, pulse rate, and blood pressure (BP).
- In case of moderate to severe blood loss secure intravenous (IV) access and start fluids immediately to avoid the circulatory failure.
- After stabilization of vitals, bleeding must be stopped and then proceed for evaluation to establish the cause.[1]
- Application of external pressure to anterior nares or pinching the nose (Hippocratic technique) or cold water/ice application is the first line of management.

Table 27.2: Interventions for epistaxis according to site.	
Anterior epistaxis	*Posterior epistaxis*
• Digital pressure application over anterior nares • *Cauterization:* Electric (monopolar/bipolar)/chemical silver nitrate (AgNO$_3$) • Anterior nasal packing (e.g. merocel, vaseline gauze, or gel foam)	• Rigid endoscopy-assisted electrocautery under local anesthesia • Posterior nasal pack (e.g. dental roll, Foley catheter, or Epistat) • Hot water irrigation • Angiography and embolization • *Arterial ligation:* Internal maxillary artery/sphenopalatine artery ligation (transantral or endoscopic)/anterior or posterior ethmoidal artery ligation/carotid artery ligation

- Table 27.2 outlines the interventions for epistaxis in a site-directed fashion. Application of pressure to anterior nares is first line of management. If the bleed persists, topical decongestants consisting of 1:1,000 adrenalin, 0.5% phenylephrine hydrochloride, 4% cocaine, or 0.05% oxymetazoline solution with cotton or gauze strips can be used for local application.[1]

Cauterization

- If the bleeding recurs frequently or the amount of bleeding is high in every episode, cauterization should be recommended.
- Silver nitrate (AgNO$_3$) and electrocautery are generally used for cauterization, with the aim to destroy the mucosa of the nasal septum, which heals with scar tissue with decreased vascularity.
- Silver nitrate is an oxidizing agent, used in a concentration of 2–10% for cautery. Increased concentrations can cause complications in the form of septal perforations, local infections, or synechiae formation.
- The second option is electric cauterization with bipolar or suction monopolar cautery, which produces thermal energy to destroy the selected area in a more controlled fashion, but it may not be easily available.
- In the follow-up period, local ointment with saline gel must be applied to prevent crusting and rebleeding. Complete recovery is generally achieved in 1 or 2 weeks.[1,2]

Nasal Packing

- If the bleeding is not controlled by earlier initial methods, nasal packing with traditional ribbon gauze (Fig. 27.7) or commercially available nasal dressings like merocel, spongostan with or without surgicel can be used.
- Spongostan is an absorbable hemostatic gelatin sponge which is biodegradable and can be used to stop bleeding. Nasopore foam provides strong initial compressive mechanical properties, whereas hydrophilic component takes up the water or blood and is gradually fragmented.[3]

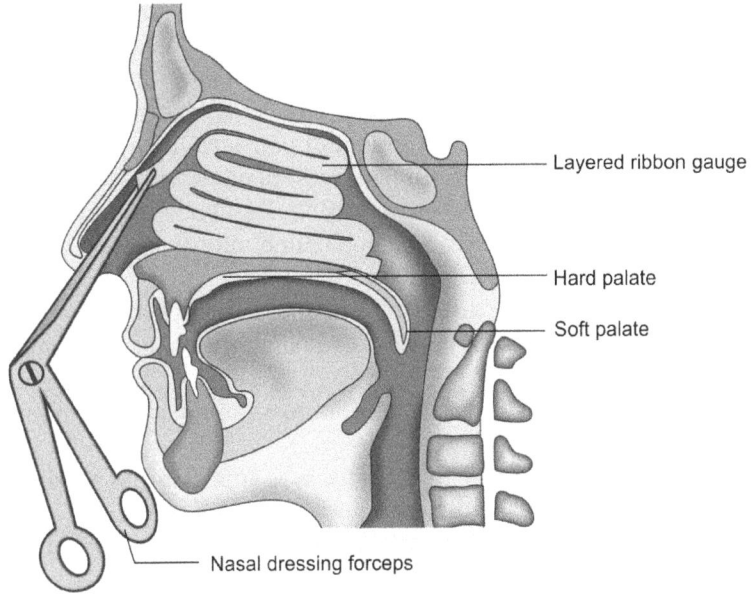

Fig. 27.7: Traditional ribbon gauze layered anterior nasal packing done in hypertensive epistaxis.

- If the anterior packing cannot stop bleeding, posterior packing with conventional gauze pack or catheters like Pope nasal packing Epistat or Postpac can be used (vide infra).
- Anterior packing is removed after 2 days, but posterior packing may stay up to 5 days according to the patient's general conditions.
- Antibiotic treatment should be used until the removal of nasal packaging for preventing toxic shock syndrome (related to staphylococcal toxins). Apart from nasal discomfort, nasal packing may also lead to other rarer complications like cardiorespiratory compromise, pneumocephalus, etc.[2]
- The usage of hemostatic compounds has increased in the recent years, such as Floseal which has bovine gelatin granules matrix which swell to produce a tamponade effect and also has high concentration of human thrombin which converts fibrinogen into fibrin monomers which accelerates clot formation.

Surgical Management

- Posterior nasal packing is a complicated procedure in which pack is kept in nasopharynx to maintain pressure effect in the posterior part of the septum as well as posterior choana. This is done with traditional dental roll nasopharyngeal packs, Foley catheters, or balloon tamponade products.
- Complications of anterior and posterior nasal packs include ulcerations, septal perforation, sinusitis, synechiae formation, hypoxemia, and

arrhythmias. Posterior packing can cause alar, columellar or palatal necrosis, apnea, and hypoxia which need oxygen supplementation.
- *Ligation techniques:* Ethmoidal artery, SPA or internal maxillary artery (IMA), and external carotid artery (ECA) can be ligated in any uncontrolled epistaxis by conventional/open or endoscopic approaches. SPA is the end artery which supplies most of nasal cavity and its ligation is frequent to control the bleeding. Various ligation procedures include:
  - Transnasal endoscopic sphenopalatine artery ligation (TESPAL) introduced by Budrovich and Saetti in 1992.
  - Anterior ethmoidal artery by endonasal approach (described by Woolford and Jones) or transcaruncular approach (approach through lamina papyracea).
  - Internal maxillary artery by canine fossa approach (Chandler and Serrins in 1965).
  - External carotid artery by transcervical approach has small risk of injury to hypoglossal and vagus nerves.
- *Septal surgery:* Reserved for correction of anatomical abnormalities such as deviated septum or spur and bleeding polyposis.

Angiography and Embolization (Figs. 27.8 and 27.9)

- Complete diagnostic angiogram of the ICA and ECA are performed.
- Angiography occasionally reveals site of bleed in form of extravasation, pseudoaneurysm, vascular malformation, or rarely an ECA source. All dangerous anastomoses between ECA and ICA are also mapped.
- A complete discussion of angiography technique/procedure is beyond the scope of this book. Essentially even if the diagnostic angiograms are normal ipsilateral internal maxillary is embolized using polyvinyl alcohol (PVA) particles or Gelfoam.
- Embolization of ipsilateral facial and contralateral IMA may also be required.

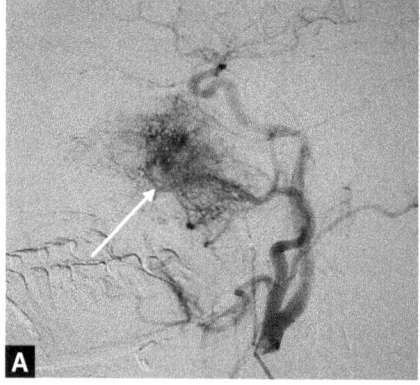
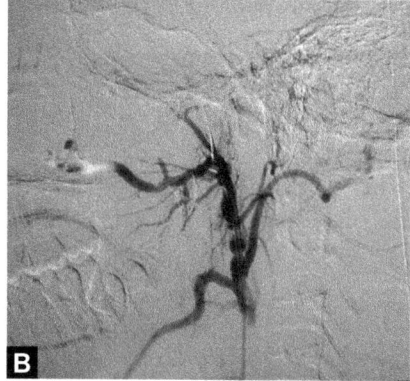

Figs. 27.8A and B: Juvenile nasopharyngeal angiofibroma causing epistaxis, treated successfully with angiographic embolization. (A) Internal maxillary artery run showing intense arterial blush (arrow); and (B) Postembolization angiogram showing absence of blush.

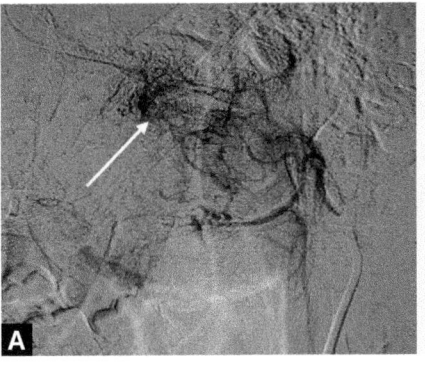 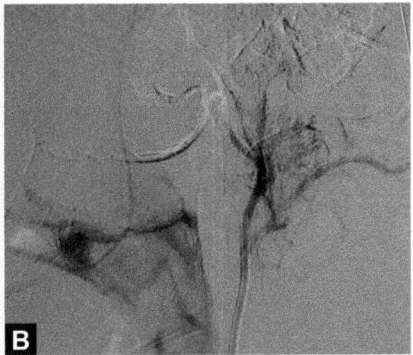

Figs. 27.9A and B: Juvenile nasopharyngeal angiofibroma causing epistaxis, treated successfully with angiographic embolization. (A) Ascending pharyngeal artery run showing intense arterial blush (arrow); and (B) Postembolization angiogram showing absence of blush.

- Coils are used in cases with contrast extravasation; platinum coils are used.
- Pseudoaneurysms arising from ICA are treated depending on the vessel involved by surgical ligation/coiling or detachable balloons or covered stents.
- High flow AVMs are treated with glue-lipiodol mixture or Onyx.

Others

- Sclerotherapy, septodermoplasty, and hormonal therapy are recommended in chronic epistaxis (especially in cases of hematological diseases and hereditary hemorrhagic telangiectasia).
- Sodium tetradecyl sulfate is used for sclerotherapy in chronic epistaxis.

PREVENTION

Preventive measures which can be taken include:
- Avoid nasal picking and manipulation.
- Home humidification.
- To preserve the mucosal integrity and to avoid intranasal excoriations apply petroleum jelly, saline spray, or saline nasal gels.
- Stop anticoagulants like aspirin and NSAIDs. These drugs do not initiate nose bleeding but may prolong bleeding.

REFERENCES

1. Bhadouriya SS, Raghuvanshi S. Aetiology and management of epistaxis—a prospective clinical study. Int J Clin Exp Otolaryngol. 2016;2(3):25-30.
2. Dubel GJ, Ahn SH, Soares GM. Transcatheter embolization in the management of epistaxis. Semin Intervent Radiol. 2013;30:249-62.
3. Pandey A, Gupta S, Rahul, et al. Clinical profile of patients of epistaxis: an experience from a tertiary level hospital in Jabalpur. IAIM. 2016;3(11):83-7.

CHAPTER 28

Imaging Approach to Sinus Lesions

Smita Manchanda, Ashu Seith Bhalla

- Introduction
- Laterality
- Size of Sinus
- Status of Bony Walls
- Density of Lesion
- MRI Signal
- Enhancement Patterns
- Diffusion-Weighted Imaging
- Pattern of Extrasinus Extension/ Involvement
- Location within the Sinonasal cavity:
  - Nasal Cavity
  - Frontonasal (Congenital lesions)
  - Specific sinus (Maxillary, Frontal, Sphenoethmoid)
- Important Differentials with Illustrative case

INTRODUCTION

Several diverse causes can lead to symptoms attributable to sinonasal cavity with/without opacification of sinuses on plain radiographs. Further diagnosis rests on clinical considerations and cross-sectional imaging, with computed tomography (CT) being the mainstay, and magnetic resonance imaging (MRI) being used in specific situations. The various considerations in formulating the approach to sinonasal disorders are enlisted in *Boxes 28.1 and 28.2*.[1] The clinical aspects are covered in Chapters 26 and 27. Imaging factors are discussed sequentially below.

Box 28.1: Clinical factors in approach.
- Age
- Clinical symptoms
- Duration
- History of surgery
- History of recent dental procedure
- History of trauma
- Immune status

Box 28.2: Factors on cross-sectional imaging for approach to differential diagnosis.
- *Laterality:* Bilateral/unilateral
- *Size of the sinus:* Small/ Expanded/ Normal
- *Status of Bony walls:* Bone expansion/ Bone destruction/ Sclerosis
- *Density on NCCT:* Hyperdense/osseous/mixed/calcification/cystic
- *MRI signal intensity:* T1WI and T2WI
- *Enhancement:* Mild/moderate/intense/specific pattern
- *Diffusion:* DWI/ADC
- *Extrasinus involvement:* Pattern/extent
- *Location within the sinonasal cavity:*
  - Nasal cavity
  - Frontonasal (congenital lesions)
  - Specific sinus (maxillary, frontal, and sphenoethmoid)

(ADC: apparent diffusion coefficient; DWI: diffusion-weighted imaging; MRI: magnetic resonance imaging; NCCT: noncontrast computed tomography)

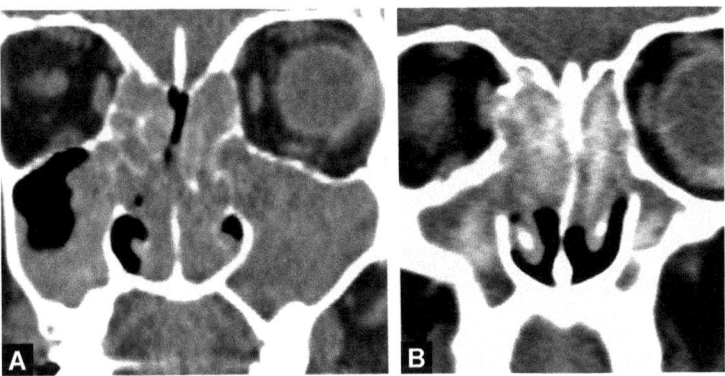

Figs. 28.1A and B: Bilateral disease. (A) Chronic rhinosinusitis with widening of OMU (polyposis pattern); and (B) Allergic fungal sinusitis.

LATERALITY

- *Bilateral disease (Figs. 28.1A and B):*
  - Bilateral disease is usually inflammatory.
  - Bilateral maxillary sinusitis may be seen in chronic rhinosinusitis (sinonasal polyposis pattern) and also in allergic fungal sinusitis.[2]
  - In bilateral rhinosinusitis, concurrent polyposis is suspected if osseous erosions and osteomeatal complex (OMC) widening is seen.
- *Unilateral disease (Figs. 28.2A and B):*
  - In unilateral disease tumors and tumor-like conditions are an important differential.
  - Unilateral inflammatory disease is usually due to obstruction of specific drainage pathways.
  - Unilateral maxillary sinusitis may also be in combination with anterior ethmoid and frontal sinusitis. This is because anterior ethmoid sinusitis secondarily causes obstruction of the frontal recess and osteomeatal unit.

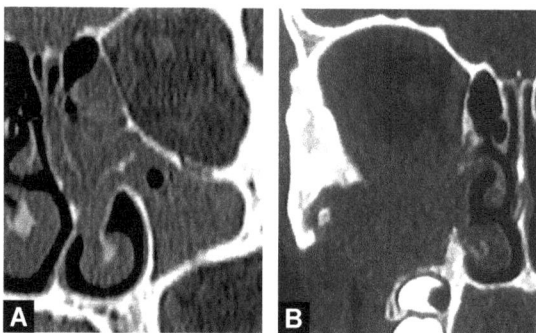

Figs. 28.2A and B: Unilateral disease. (A) Left osteomeatal pattern of chronic rhinosinusitis (CRS); and (B) Chronic invasive fungal sinusitis.

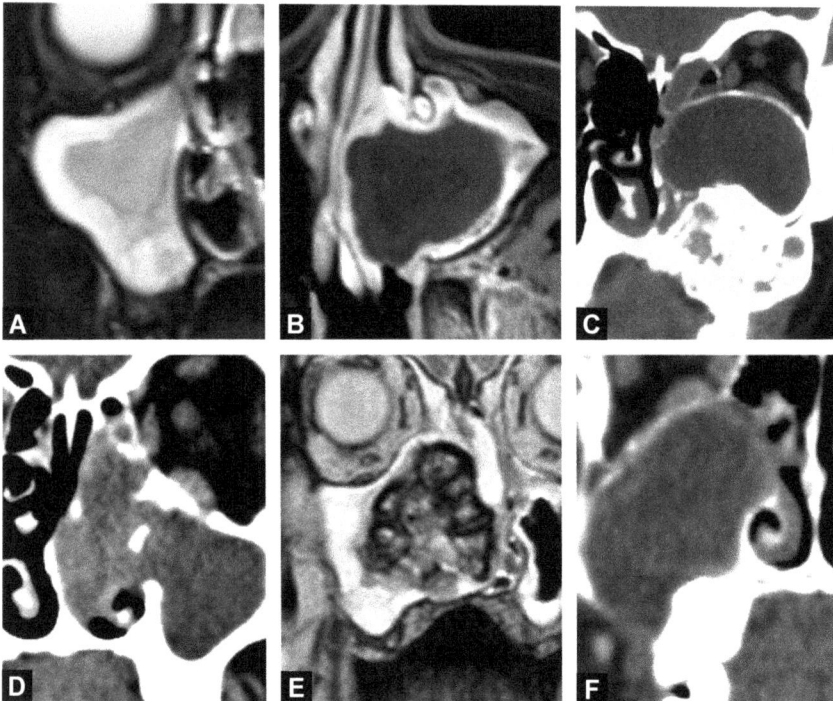

Figs. 28.3A to F: Expanded sinus with thin walls. (A) Retained secretions; (B) Mycetoma; (C) Mucocele with giant cell reparative granuloma; (D) Antrochoanal polyp; (E) Sinonasal angiomatous polyp; and (F) Odontogenic: Keratocytic odontogenic tumor.

SIZE OF SINUS

- There may be reduction in size of the sinus, expansion, or even normal size sinus.[2,3]
- Lesions which cause expansion will initially show normal-sized sinuses.
- Lesions which cause expansion of the sinus will result in thinning of its walls with decortication and focal erosions. However, these are not primarily destructive processes which are seen in more aggressive lesions (e.g. malignancies and osteomyelitis) (Figs. 28.3 and 28.4).

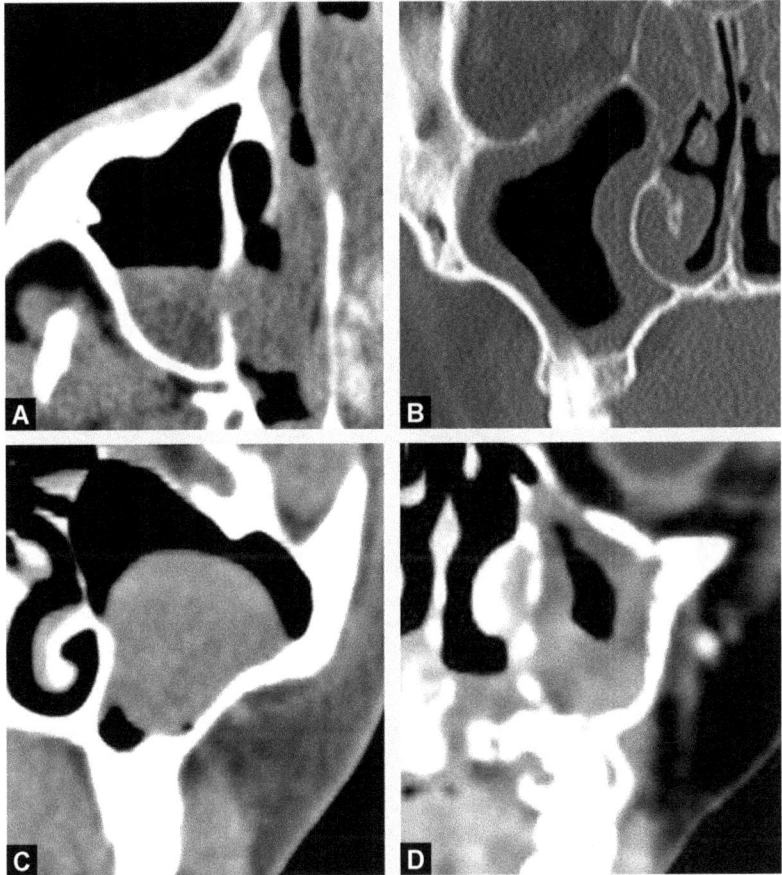

Figs. 28.4A to D: Normal size sinus. (A) Acute sinusitis; (B) Chronic sinusitis; (C) Retention cyst; and (D) Squamous cell carcinoma.

- Approach based on size of sinus is illustrated in Flowchart 28.1.

Flowchart 28.1: Differentials of lesions based on size of sinus.

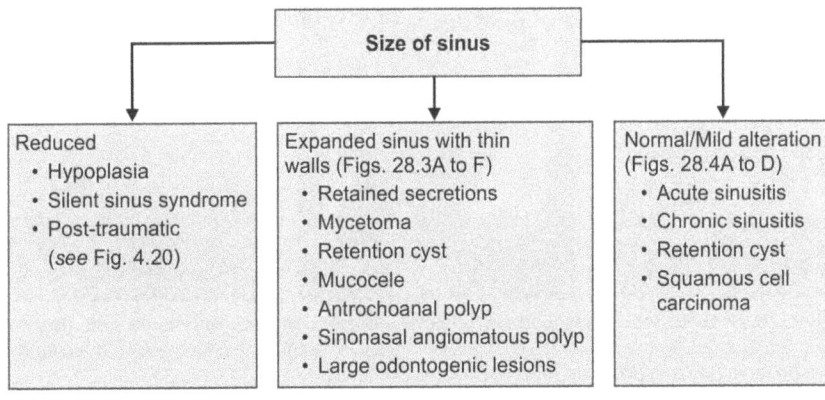

STATUS OF BONY WALLS

- The bony walls of the sinus can be thinned out, sclerosed, or eroded.[3,4]
- Lesions which cause expansion of the sinus will result in thinning of its walls with decortication and focal erosions. However, these are not primarily destructive processes which are seen in more aggressive lesions (e.g. malignancies and osteomyelitis) (Figs. 28.5 to 28.7).

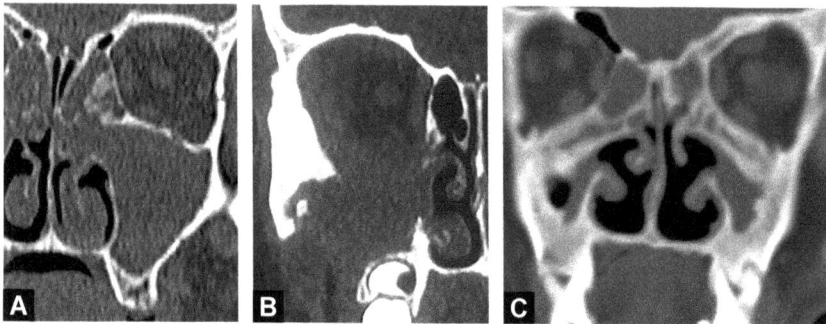

Figs. 28.5A to C: Bone sclerosis. (A) Neoosteogenesis: Chronic rhinosinusitis (polyposis pattern); (B) Chronic invasive fungal sinusitis; and (C) Granulomatosis with polyangiitis (GPA).

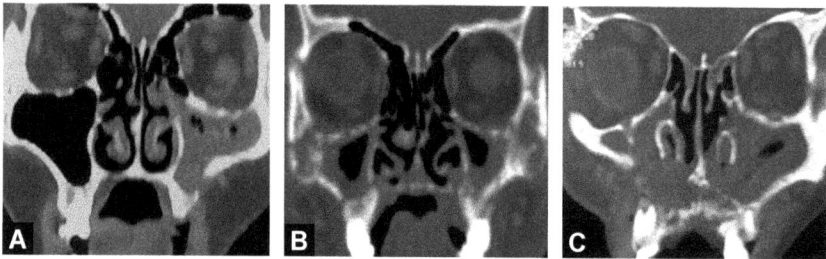

Figs. 28.6A to C: Infiltrative pattern of bone destruction with mild soft tissue. (A) Osteomyelitis (bacterial sinusitis); (B) Granulomatosis with polyangiitis (GPA); and (C) Osteoradionecrosis.

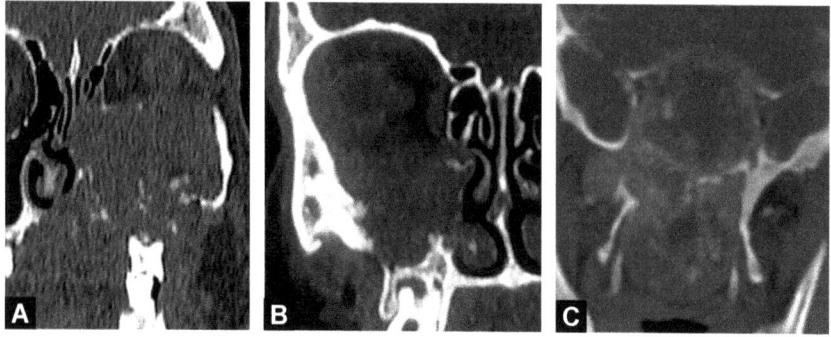

Figs. 28.7A to C: Infiltrative pattern of bone destruction with extensive soft tissue. (A) Squamous cell carcinoma; (B) Chronic invasive fungal sinusitis; and (C) Juvenile nasopharyngeal angiofibroma (atypical aggressive form).

- The differentials of lesions based on evaluation of the status of bony walls are detailed in Flowcharts 28.2 and 28.3.
- In general, malignant masses show erosive bone changes which have an ill-defined permeative pattern. Benign mass lesions such as

Flowchart 28.2: Differentials of lesions based on status of bony walls.

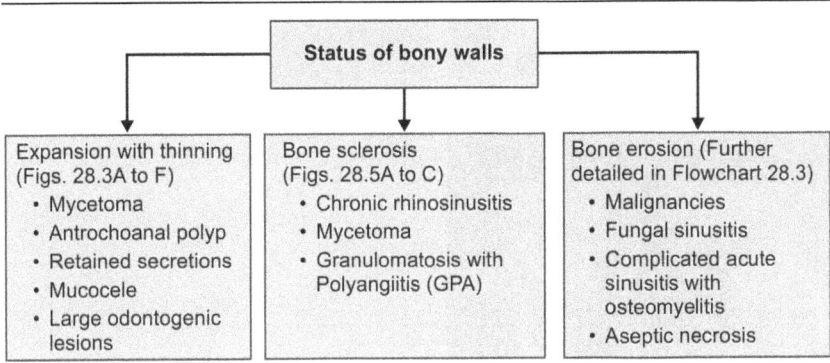

Flowchart 28.3: Differentials of lesions based on bone erosion.

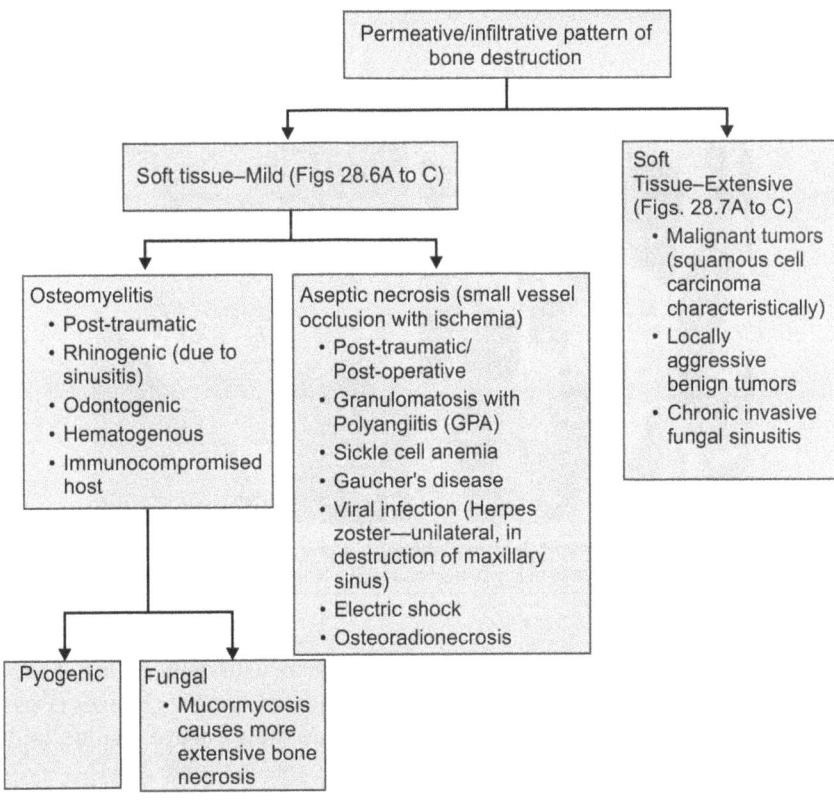

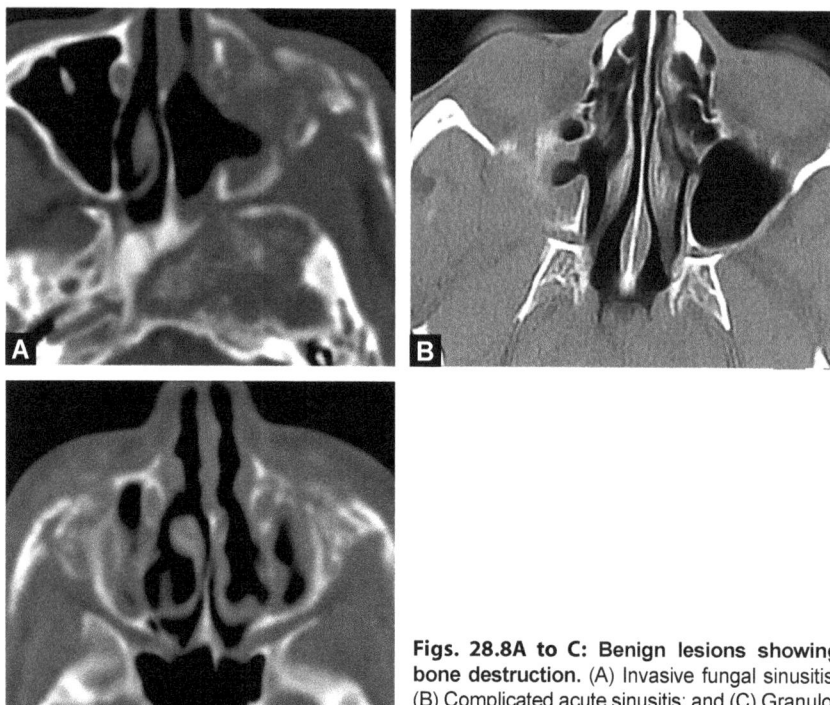

Figs. 28.8A to C: Benign lesions showing bone destruction. (A) Invasive fungal sinusitis; (B) Complicated acute sinusitis; and (C) Granulomatosis with polyangiitis (GPA).

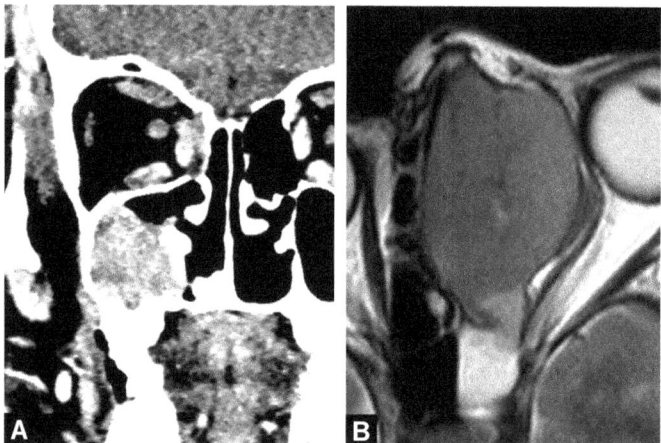

Figs. 28.9A and B: Malignant lesions showing bone expansion and remodeling: Lymphoma. (A) Diffuse large B-cell lymphoma; and (B) Non-Hodgkin's lymphoma.

inflammatory polyps display bone expansion with remodeling. Bone in these cases shows thinning but not ill-defined erosive changes (Figs. 28.8 and 28.9). However, benign lesions may show erosive change, and conversely malignant lesion may display expansion (Table 28.1).

Table 28.1: Atypical pattern of bony changes in benign and malignant lesions.	
Benign lesions showing bone destruction (Figs. 28.8A to C)	Malignant lesions showing bone expansion and remodeling (Figs. 28.9A and B)
• Invasive fungal sinusitis • Complicated acute sinusitis • Granulomatosis with polyangiitis (GPA) • Giant cell reparative granuloma	• Minor salivary gland tumors • Lymphoma

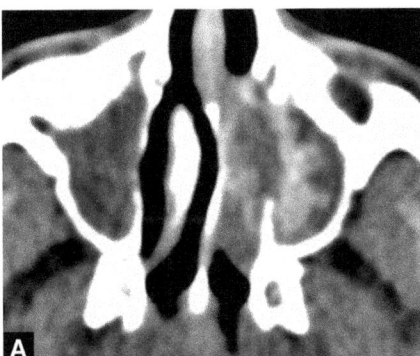
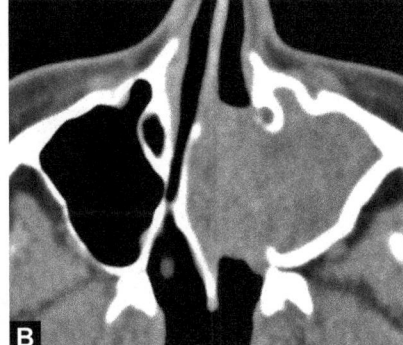
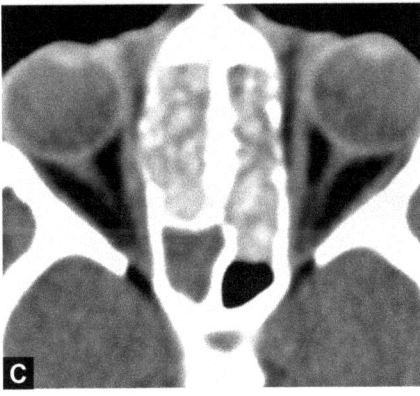

Figs. 28.10A to C: Hyperdense sinonasal lesions. (A) Chronic sinusitis (retained secretions); (B) Mycetoma; and (C) Allergic fungal sinusitis (AFS).

DENSITY OF LESION

- Lesions may be primarily hyperdense of osseous density, heterogeneous density, or cystic. The pattern of calcification can also give a clue to the etiology of the lesion.[1,4,5]
- The differentials of lesions according to the density are the following:
  - *Hyperdense (Figs. 28.10A to C):*
    ▶ Chronic sinusitis (retained secretions)
    ▶ Mycetoma
    ▶ Allergic fungal sinusitis (AFS).

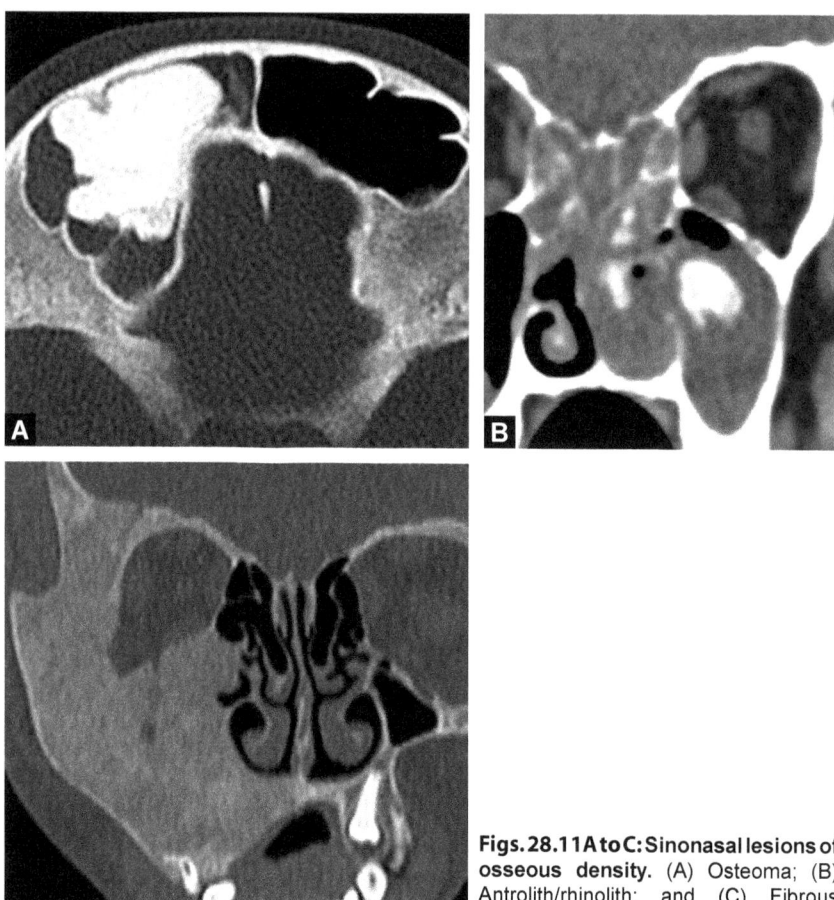

Figs. 28.11A to C: Sinonasal lesions of osseous density. (A) Osteoma; (B) Antrolith/rhinolith; and (C) Fibrous dysplasia (ground glass).

- *Osseous density (Figs. 28.11A to C):*
    - Osteoma
    - Rhinolith
    - Fibrous dysplasia (ground glass).
- *Heterogeneous density (Figs. 28.12A and B):*
    - Ossifying fibroma
    - Tumors.
- *Cystic lesions (Figs. 28.13 to 28.16):*
    - Detailed in Table 28.2.
- Specific pattern of *calcifications* (Figs. 28.17A and B) is seen in the following entities:
    - Inverted papilloma
    - Chondrosarcoma (arc like)
    - Osteosarcoma (dense, scattered).

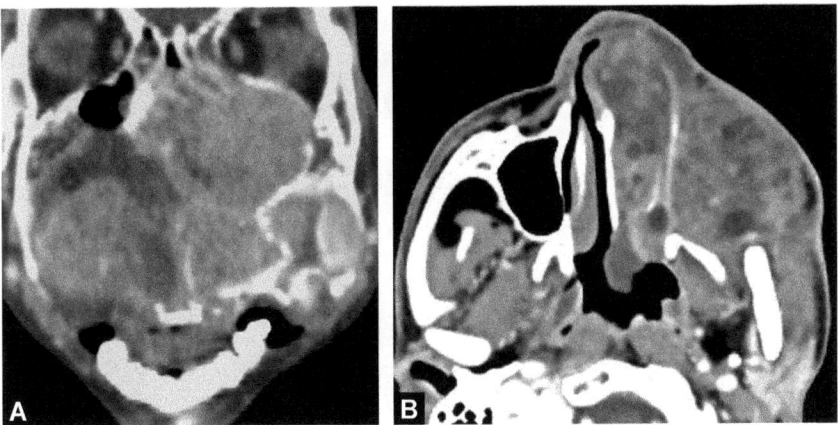

Figs. 28.12A and B: Sinonasal lesions of heterogeneous density. (A) Juvenile ossifying fibroma; and (B) Tumors: Maxillary nonseminomatous germ cell tumor.

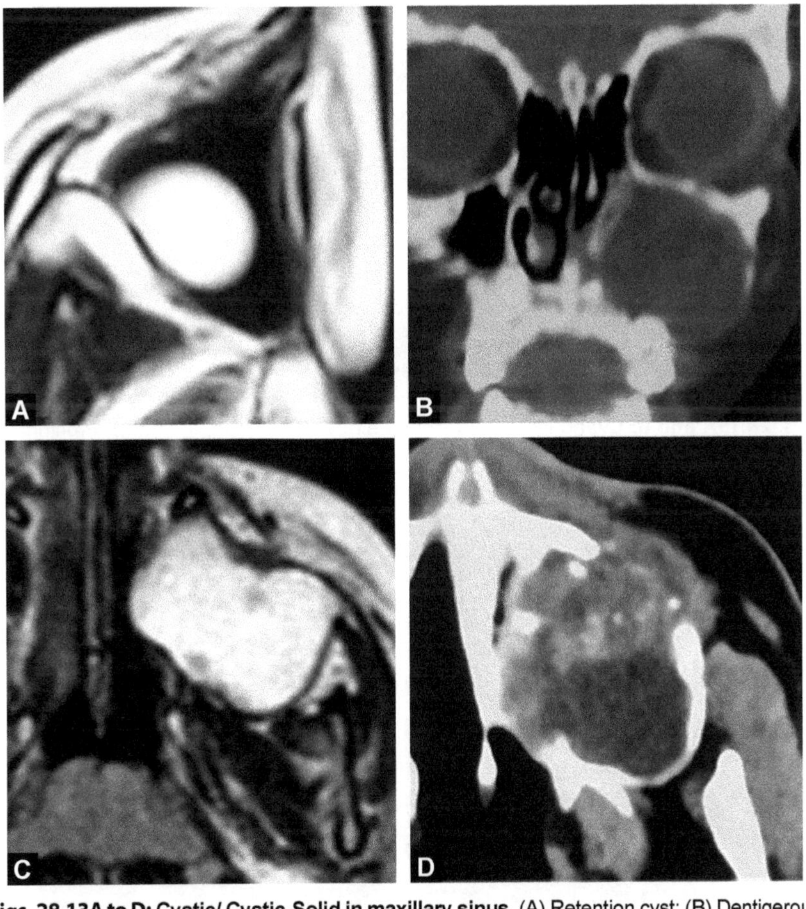

Figs. 28.13A to D: Cystic/ Cystic-Solid in maxillary sinus. (A) Retention cyst; (B) Dentigerous cyst; (C) Keratocystic odontogenic tumor (KOT); and (D) Ameloblastoma.

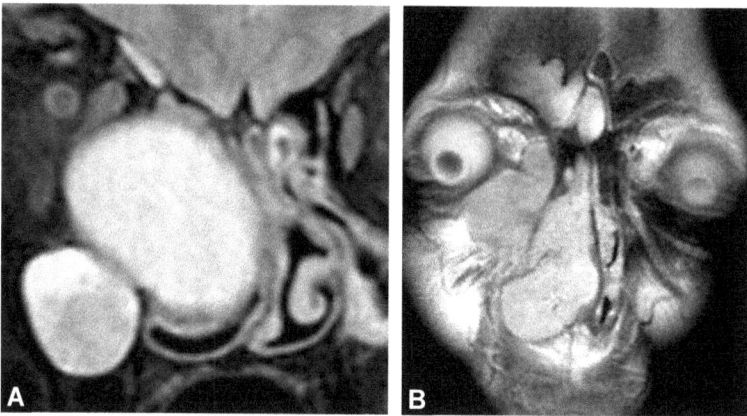

Figs. 28.14A and B: Cystic lesions in ethmoid sinus. (A) Mucocele; and (B) Esthesioneuroblastoma (solid cystic).

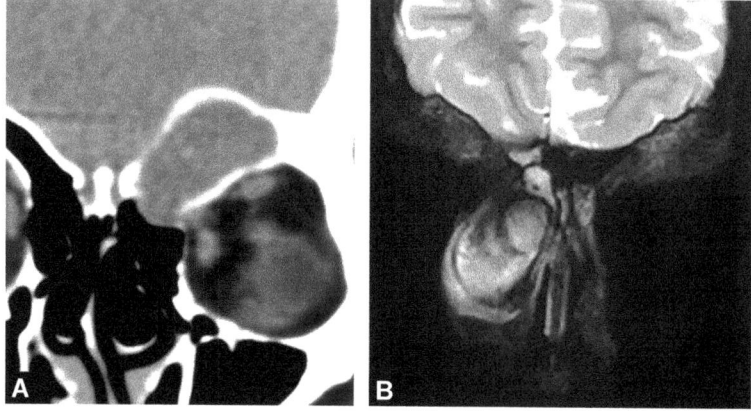

Figs. 28.15A and B: Cystic lesions in frontal sinus. (A) Mucocele; and (B) Frontonasal meningoencephalocele.

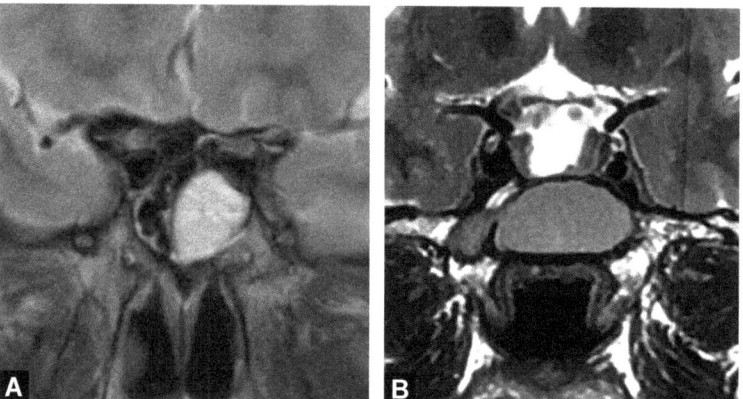

Figs. 28.16A and B: Cystic lesions in sphenoid sinus. (A) Mucocele; and (B) Retention cyst.

Table 28.2: Differential diagnosis of cystic lesions.

Location (sinus involved)	Cyst	Cyst with solid component
Maxillary sinus (Figs. 28.13A to D)	• Retention cyst • Dentigerous cyst • Ameloblastoma • Keratocystic odontogenic tumor (KOT)	• Ameloblastoma • KOT • Central giant cell reparative granuloma • Ossifying fibroma
Ethmoid (Figs. 28.14A and B)	• Cephalocele • Mucocele • Dermoid • Epidermoid	• Giant cell lesions • OF • Esthesioneuroblastoma
Frontal (Figs. 28.15A and B)	• Mucocele • Cephalocele	• OF
Sphenoid (Figs. 28.16A and B)	• Mucocele • Cephalocele • Dermoid • Epidermoid	• Craniopharyngioma • Chordoma

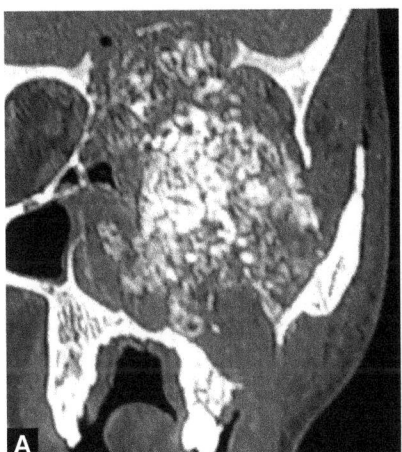 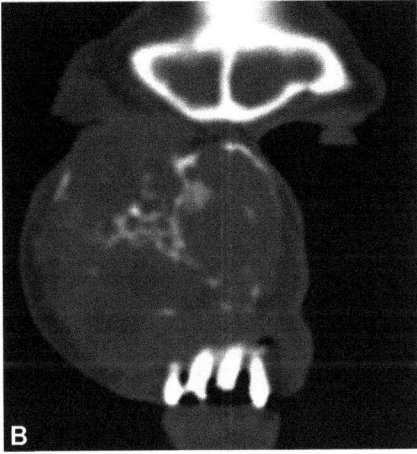

Figs. 28.17A and B: Specific patterns of calcification. (A) Chondrosarcoma: Dense, popcorn type; and (B) Chondrosarcoma: Ring and arc like.

MAGNETIC RESONANCE IMAGING SIGNAL

- Normal aerated sinus is hypointense on T1-weighted image (T1WI) and T2WI (Figs. 28.18A and B).
- Hence the lesions hypointense on T2WI simulate normal sinus and may thus underestimate the extent of disease (Figs. 28.19 to 28.21).
- Lesions can have hypointense or hyperintense signal on T1WI (Table 28.3) and hypointense, intermediate, or hyperintense signal on T2WI (Table 28.4).[5,6]

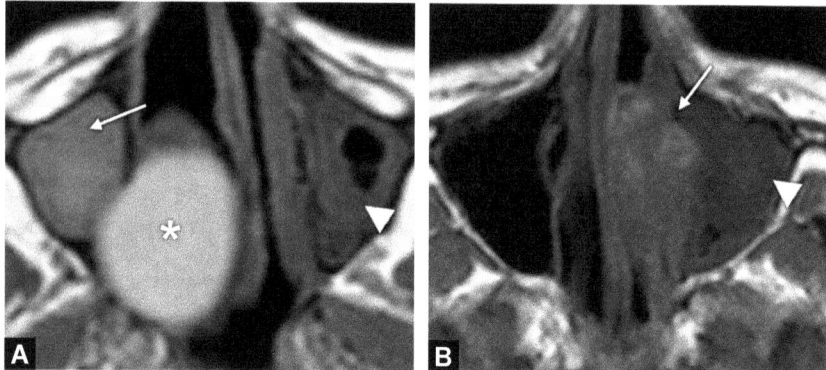

Figs. 28.18A and B: Signal intensity on T1WI (A and B)
Hyperintense: Inspissated secretions (arrow in A), Mucocoele (asterisk in A), Melanoma (arrow in B)
Hypointense: Mucosal thickening and secretions (arrowhead in A and B).

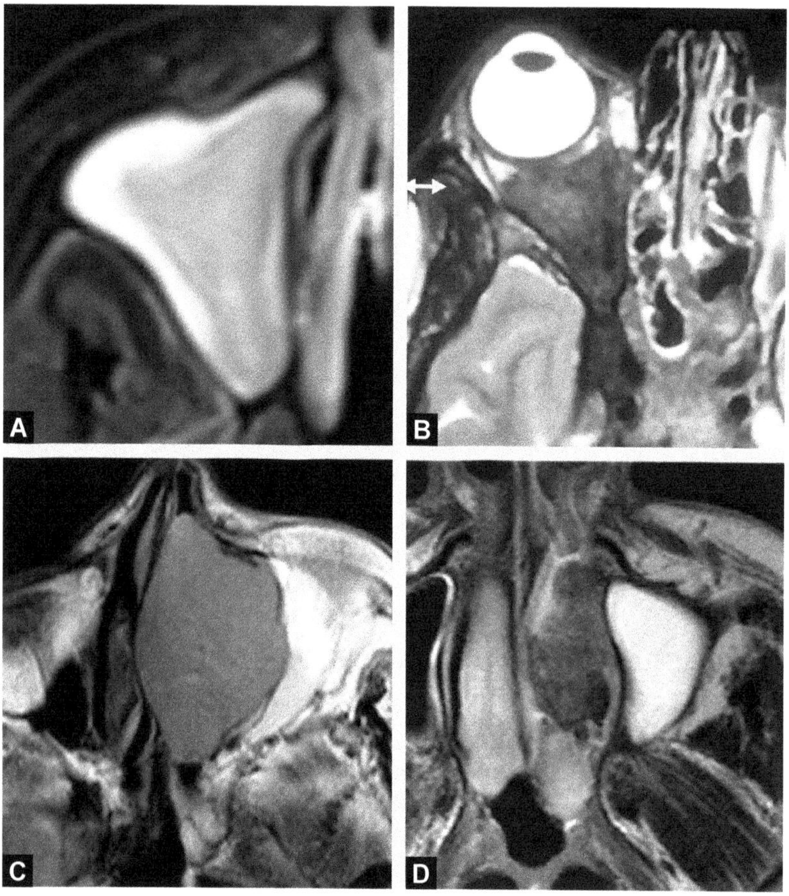

Figs. 28.19A to D: Hypointense SI on T2-weighted image (T2WI). (A) Inspissated secretions with high proteinaceous content; (B) Fungal sinusitis; (C) Lymphoma; and (D) Melanoma.

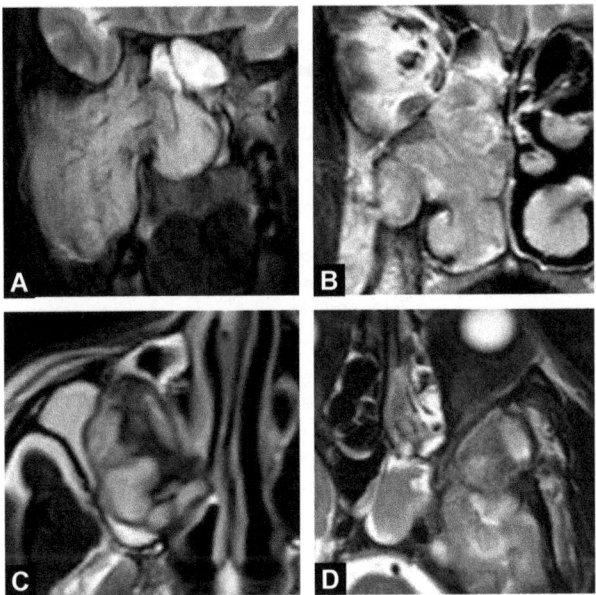

Figs. 28.20A to D: Intermediate SI on T2-weighted image (T2WI). (A) Juvenile nasopharyngeal angiofibroma; (B) Inverted papilloma; (C) Sinonasal angiomatous polyp; and (D) Fungal sinusitis.

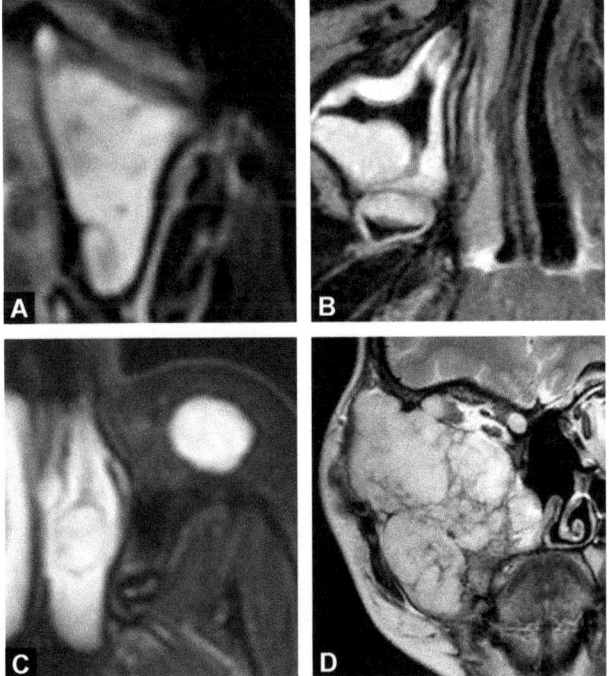

Figs. 28.21A to D: Hyperintense SI on T2-weighted image (T2WI). (A) Secretions; (B) Inflammatory polyps; (C) Pleomorphic adenoma; and (D) Chondrosarcoma.

Table 28.3: Differentials according to signal intensity on T1WI (Figs. 28.18A and B).

Hyperintense	Hypointense
• Inspissated secretions • Retention cysts • Melanoma	• Mucosal thickening with inspissated secretions

Table 28.4: Differentials according to signal intensity on T2WI.

Hypointense (Figs. 28.19A to D)	Intermediate (Figs. 28.20A to D)	High (Figs. 28.21A to D)
• Inspissated secretions with high proteinaceous content • Fungal sinusitis • Lymphoma • Melanoma	• Majority of tumors • Inverted papilloma • Fungal sinusitis • Lymphoma • Pseudotumor	• Secretions • Inflammatory polyps • Adenoid cystic carcinoma (low grade) • Pleomorphic adenoma (hypointense capsule) • Hemangioma • Chondrosarcoma • Nerve sheath tumors • Few inverted papillomas

ENHANCEMENT PATTERNS

- Lesions can be nonenhancing or show variable enhancement (ranging from mild/moderate to intense enhancement) (Figs. 28.22 to 28.25). These are detailed in Table 28.5.
- Certain lesions have a specific pattern of enhancement[7] which can give a clue to its etiology (Table 28.5).

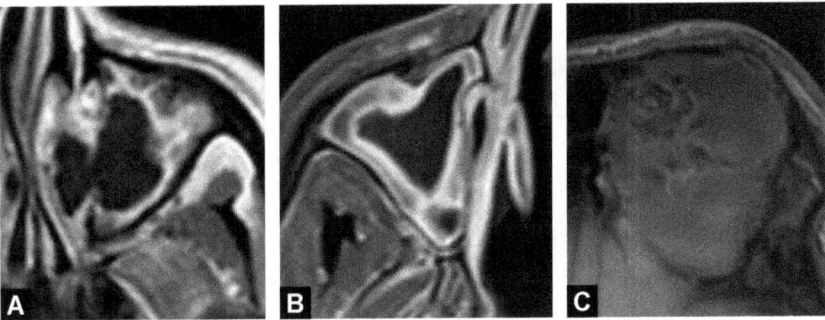

Figs. 28.22A to C: Nonenhancing masses. (A) Mycetoma; (B) Retained secretions; and (C) Frontal mucocele (with ossifying fibroma).

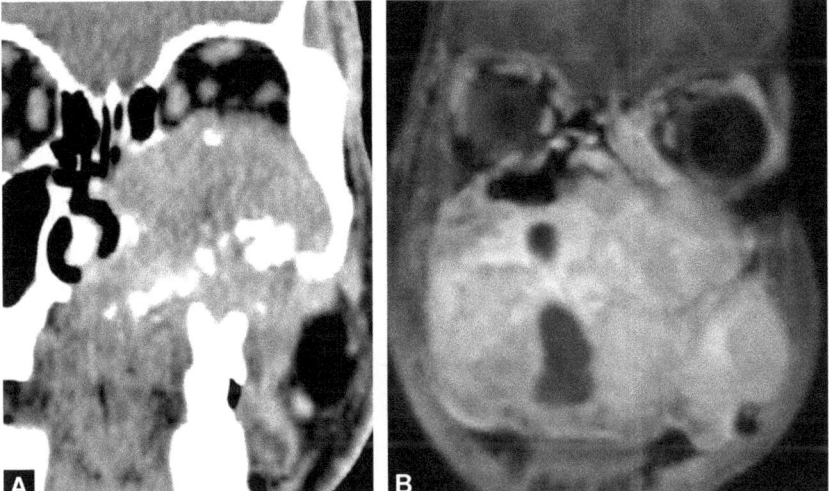

Figs. 28.23A and B: Masses with mild-moderate enhancement. (A) Malignancies: Squamous cell carcinoma (SCC); and (B) Large odontogenic lesions: Juvenile ossifying fibroma.

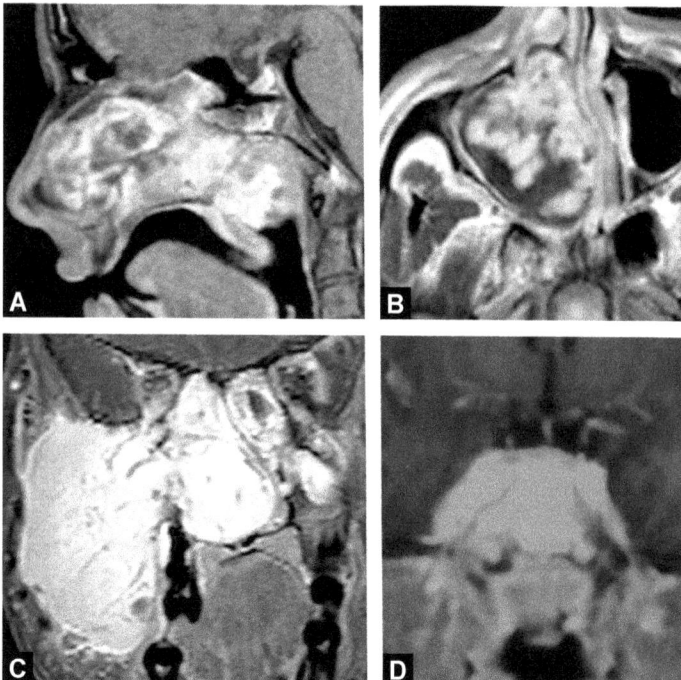

Figs. 28.24A to D: Masses with intense enhancement. (A) Antrochoanal polyp; (B) Sinonasal angiomatous polyp; (C) Juvenile nasopharyngeal angiofibroma; and (D) Hemangioma.

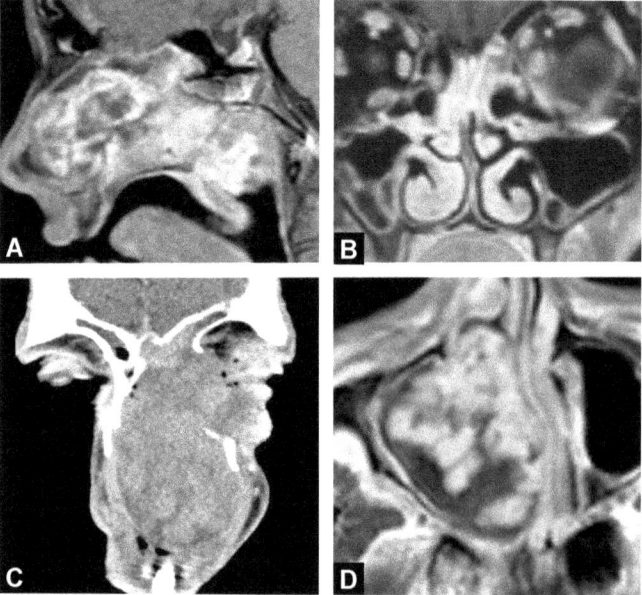

Figs. 28.25A to D: Specific patterns of enhancement. (A) Internal septal (linear) enhancement: Antrochoanal polyp; (B) Smooth rim/mural enhancement: Sinusitis; (C) Cerebriform pattern: Inverted papilloma; and (D) Lobular: Sinonasal angiomatous polyp.

Table 28.5: Differentials according to degree and pattern of enhancement on CECT/CEMRI.			
Nonenhancing (Figs. 28.22A to C)	Mild-Moderate (Figs. 28.23A and B)	Intense (Figs. 28.24A to D)	Specific pattern (Figs. 28.25A to D)
• Mycetoma • Retained secretions • Retention cyst • Mucocele	• Malignancies • Large odontogenic lesions	• Antrochoanal polyp • Sinonasal angiomatous polyp • Hemangioma • Juvenile nasopharyngeal angiofibroma.	• *Internal septal (linear) enhancement:* Polyps • *Smooth rim/mural enhancement:* Sinusitis, retention cysts, and mucocele • *Cerebriform pattern:* Inverted papilloma • *Heterogeneous enhancement with necrosis:* Tumors • *Lobular:* Sinonasal angiomatous polyp.

(CECT: Contrast-enhanced computed tomography; CEMRI: Contrast-enhanced magnetic resonance imaging).

DIFFUSION-WEIGHTED IMAGING

- In general, benign lesions show free diffusion and malignant lesions show restriction. Threshold apparent diffusion coefficient (ADC) value of 1.791×10^{-3} mm^2/s has been suggested for differentiation between benign and malignant lesions.[8]
- Juvenile nasopharyngeal angiofibromas (Fig. 28.26A) show high mean ADC values ($> 2.168 \pm 0.270 \times 10^{-3}$ mm^2/s).[8]
- However, certain lesions may show discordant behavior:[9]
  - *Benign lesions which can show restricted diffusion (Fig. 28.26B):*
    ▸ Meningioma
    ▸ Hemangiopericytoma
    ▸ Solitary fibrous tumor.
  - *Malignant lesions which can show facilitated diffusion (Figs. 28.27A and B):*
    ▸ Chondrosarcoma
    ▸ Fibromyxoid sarcoma
    ▸ Adenocarcinoma
    ▸ Adenoid cystic carcinoma.

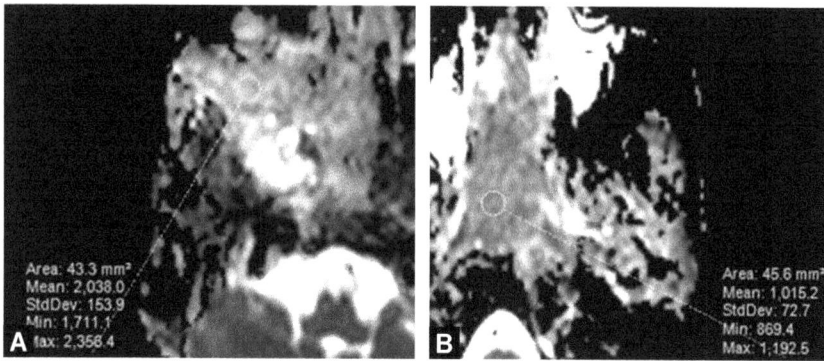

Figs. 28.26A and B: Benign lesions (DWI). (A) Facilitated diffusion with high ADC value (mean >2.168 ± 0.270 × 10^{-3} mm^2/s): Juvenile nasopharyngeal angiofibroma; and (B) Restricted diffusion: Meningioma. (ADC: Apparent diffusion coefficient; DWI: Diffusion-weighted imaging)

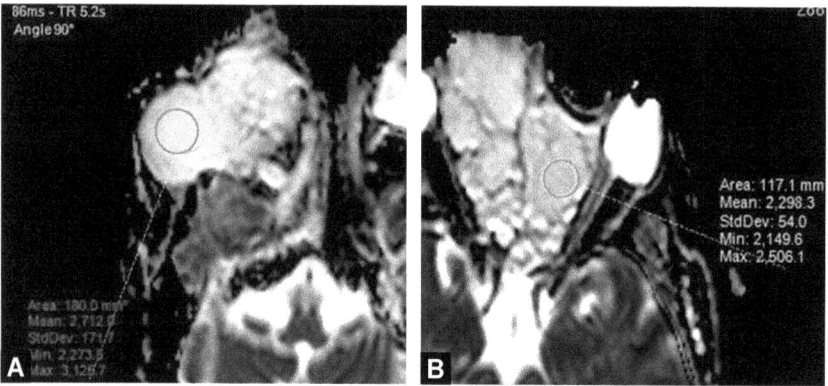

Figs. 28.27A and B: Malignant lesions which can show facilitated diffusion. (A) Chondrosarcoma; and (B) Adenocarcinoma.

LOCATION-WISE RADIOLOGICAL APPROACH

- Location within the sinonasal cavity is useful for suggesting possible etiology.
- The approach to lesions in the Nasal Cavity (Chapter 26) and Frontonasal: Congenital lesions (Chapter 20) have been described elsewhere.
- Specific sinuses (maxillary, frontal, sphenoethmoid) have certain disease processes limited to the respective sinus.

Radiological Approach to Maxillary Sinus

- Isolated involvement of unilateral maxillary sinus results from two mechanisms.
- This can be due to either ostium block or extension/complication of dental lesion.

Flowchart 28.4: Unilateral maxillary sinus disease.

```
         Isolated involvement of unilateral maxillary sinus
                    │                              │
                    ▼                              ▼
```

Ostium block (Figs. 28.28A to F)	Extension/Complication of Dental Lesion (Figs. 28.29A to C)
• Chronic rhinosinusitis • Fungal sinusitis • Tumors (inverted papilloma) • Antrochoanal polyp • *Expansion of ostium*: AC polyp, inverted papilloma, angiomatous polyp, Squamous cellcarcinoma (SCC) and rhinoscleroma	• Odontogenic cysts • Odontogenic tumours • Reactive mucosal hyperplasia • Infection following maxillary floor disruption • Results in displacement of sinus floor which forms superior margin of the lesion

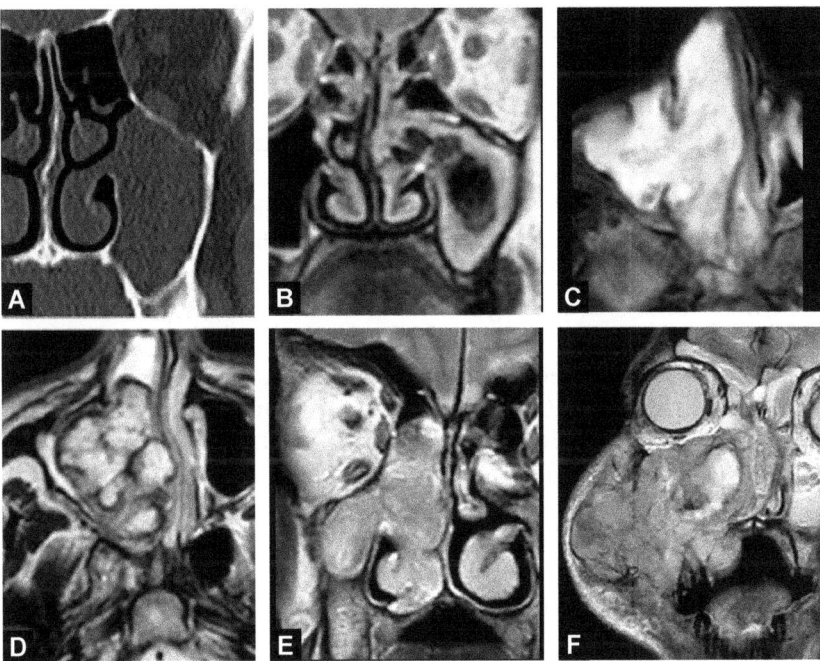

Figs. 28.28A to F: Unilateral maxillary sinus involvement (ostium block). (A) Chronic rhinosinusitis; (B) Mycetoma; (C) Antrochoanal polyp; (D) Angiomatous polyp; (E) Inverted papilloma; and (F) Squamous cell carcinoma.

- This is illustrated in Flowchart 28.4.
- Lesions which expand the infundibulum with unilateral maxillary sinus involvement include antrochoanal polyp, sinonasal angiomatous polyp, inverted papilloma, mycetoma, rhinoscleroma, and squamous cell carcinoma (Figs. 28.28 and 28.29).[4]

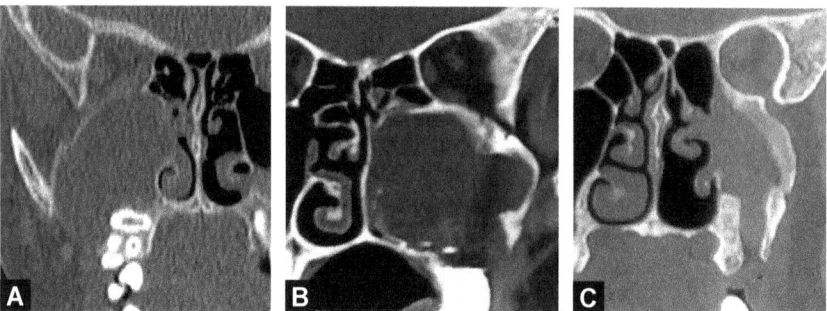

Figs. 28.29A to C: Unilateral maxillary sinus involvement (extension/complication of dental lesion). (A) Keratocystic odontogenic tumor (KOT); (B) Ameloblastoma; and (C) Infection following maxillary floor disruption.

Radiological Approach to Frontal Sinus Based on Various Considerations

- Acute bacterial rhinosinusitis: Although less common than maxillary or ethmoid sinusitis, intracranial and orbital complications are more frequent from this site. Erosion of its anterior table results in subperiosteal swellings called "Pott's puffy tumor".
- Frontal sinus is also least common site of involvement with acute invasive fungal rhinosinusitis (AIFRS), and is generally involved in combination with other paranasal sinuses.
- On the other hand, in allergic frontal sinusitis, the frontal sinus is involved in more than two-thirds of cases.
- Frontal sinus is the most common site of a mucocele.
- Cerebrospinal fluid (CSF) rhinorrhea may occur when fractures involve the posterior table, or with involvement of frontal sinus drainage pathway.
- Frontal sinus can also be site for encephalocele.
- Frontal sinus is a common site for osteoma, ossifying fibroma, and fibrous dysplasia.
- Inverted papilloma can also occur in frontal sinus, through far less frequently than the lateral nasal wall.
- Rare in frontal sinus with squamous cell carcinoma still being the most common (Figs. 28.30A to F).

Sphenoethmoidal Region (Figs. 28.31A to C)

- The sphenoid sinus (SS) and posterior ethmoidal cells are in close proximity, and their roof contributes to central skull base (CSB); these are hence often considered together.
- Lesions in this region may originate from within the sinonasal cavity or from adjoining structures. Pituitary gland lesions may extend into the SS inferiorly. Similarly, aggressive nasopharyngeal nasal masses may involve SS, while cavernous sinus lesions can enter from lateral walls. Posteriorly SS is bordered by the basisphenoid (joining upper part of

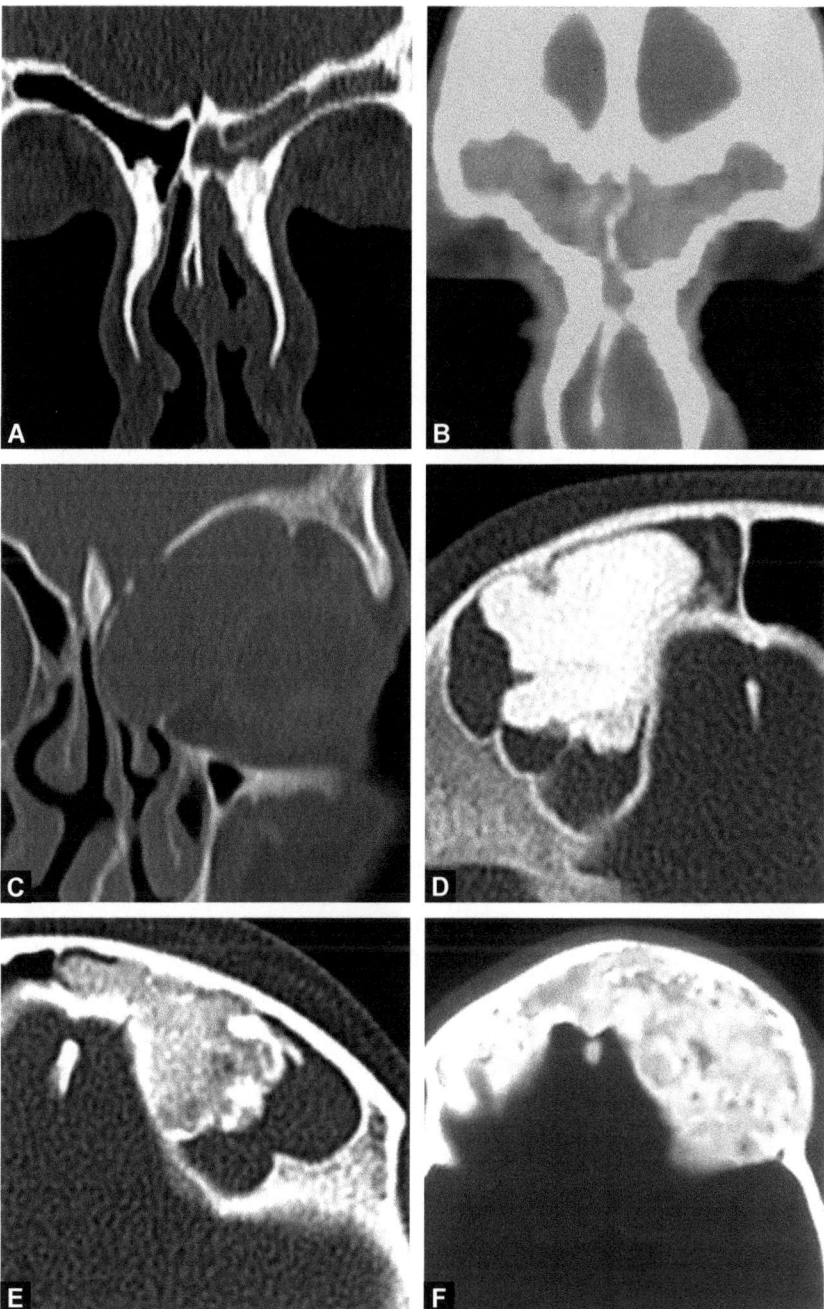

Figs. 28.30A to F: Major disease entities of the frontal sinus. (A) Chronic sinusitis; (B) Allergic fungal sinusitis; (C) Mucocele; (D) Osteoma; (E) Ossifying fibroma; and (F) Fibrous dysplasia.

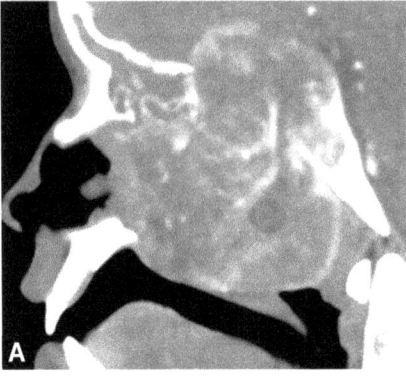
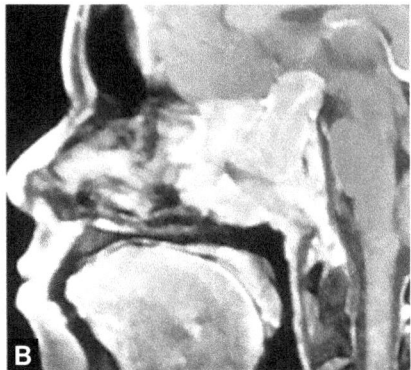
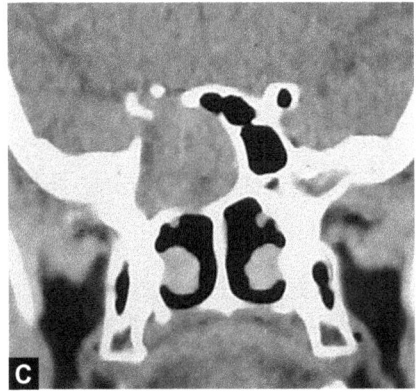

Figs. 28.31A to C: Disease entities of the sphenoethmoidal region. (A) Extension of juvenile nasopharyngeal angiofibroma; (B) Extension of pituitary macroadenoma; and (C) Mucocele.

clivus) and posterolaterally by the petro-occipital structures. Hence, osseous pathologies of these sites may also invade the sinus.[6]

- There are several routes of spread from this region to cranium – superiorly through planum ethmoidale and planum sphenoidale; laterally to cavernous sinus and to superior orbital fissure and posteriorly to clivus and even posterior fossa.
- Critical inferior and inferolateral relations are the vidian canal [vidian artery—internal carotid artery (ICA) branch] and foramen rotundum (maxillary nerve) and inferolaterally the pterygoid plexus.
- Anatomic variants of SS pose significant surgical risk due to proximity to critical structures particularly ICA and optic nerve.
- Variable pneumatization of sphenoid can appear as pseudolesions on both CT and MRI, as can the variable MR signal of basisphenoid.
- Sphenoid bone mostly contains medullary bone predisposing it to hematogenous spread of diseases.

IMPORTANT DIFFERENTIALS WITH ILLUSTRATIVE CASE (FIGS. 28.32A TO F)

The differentiating features between sinusitis and malignancy[2,5] are detailed in Table 28.6.

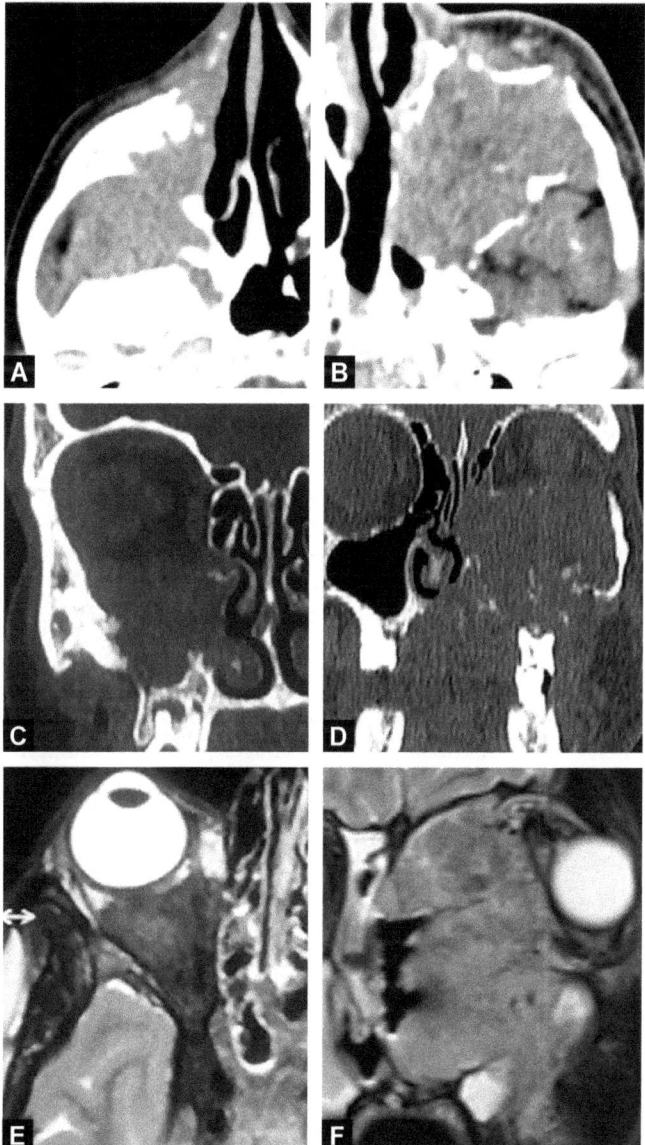

Figs. 28.32A to F: Differentiating features of chronic invasive fungal sinusitis and malignancy. (A) Mildly hyperdense, less extensive soft tissue in sinusitis; (B) Heterogeneously enhancing, extensive soft tissue in malignancy; (C) Focal erosions with bone sclerosis in sinusitis; (D) Extensive bone erosions in malignancy; (E) Hypointense signal on T2-weighted image (T2WI) in sinusitis; and (F) Intermediate T2 signal in malignancy.

Table 28.6: Differentiating features of sinusitis and malignancy.

	Sinusitis (chronic invasive fungal sinusitis)	Malignancy
CT		
Soft tissue	• Less extensive • May be hyperdense	• Extensive • Isodense to muscle
Bony changes	• Sclerosis present • Erosions in invasive forms • Short, irregular usually seen in region of normal dehiscence	• Sclerosis absent • Erosive changes more extensive • Certain areas, e.g. infratemporal surface in case of maxillary sinus eroded in malignancy, but not in sinusitis
MRI	*Chronic secretions:* • *T1WI:* Intermediate/hypointense • *T2WI:* Hypointense *Acute mucoid secretions* • *T1WI:* Hypointense • *T2WI:* Hyperintense.	• *T1WI:* Hypointense • *T2WI:* Intermediate (higher than T1WI)
	CEMR: Peripheral rim enhancement/mucosal enhancement	*CEMR:* Solid enhancement ± necrosis
Distribution	More diffuse	Mostly unilateral
Ancillary findings	–	Lymphadenopathy

(CT: computed tomography; MRI: magnetic resonance imaging; T1WI: T1-weighted image; T2WI: T2-weighted image; CEMR: Contrast enhanced MRI)

REFERENCES

1. Broderick DF. The opacified paranasal sinus: Approach and differential. Appl Radiol. 2015;44:9-17.
2. Mafee MF, Tran BH, Chapa AR. Imaging of rhinosinusitis and its complications: plain film, CT, and MRI. Clin Rev Allergy Immunol. 2006;30:165-85.
3. Sen S, Chandra A, Mukhopadhyay S, et al. Sinonasal tumors: Computed tomography and MR imaging features. Neuroimaging Clin N Am. 2015;25:595-618.
4. Whyte A, Chapeikin G. Opaque maxillary antrum: A pictorial review. Australas Radiol. 2005;49:203-13.
5. Sen S, Chandra A, Mukhopadhyay S, et al. Imaging approach to sinonasal neoplasms. Neuroimaging Clin N Am. 2015;25:577-93.
6. Connor SE. The Skull Base in the Evaluation of Sinonasal Disease: Role of Computed Tomography and MR Imaging. Neuroimaging Clin N Am. 2015;25:619-51.
7. Hur J, Kim JK, Byun JS, et al. Imaging characteristics of sinonasal organized hematoma. Acta Radiol. 2015;56(8):955-9.
8. Das A, Bhalla AS, Sharma R, et al. Can diffusion weighted imaging aid in differentiating benign from malignant sinonasal masses?: A Useful Adjunct. Pol J Radiol. 2017;82:345-55.
9. Das A, Bhalla AS, Sharma R, et al. Benign neck masses showing restricted diffusion: Is there a histological basis for discordant behavior? World J Radiol. 2016;8(2):17482.

Index

Page numbers followed by *f* refer to figure *fc* refer to flowchart, and *t* refer to table.

A

Accidental trauma 242
Acquired immunodeficiency syndrome 302
Adenocarcinoma 148, 192, 201, 207, 209, 362, 409, 410*f*
    intestinal 145, 145*f*
    non-intestinal type 145
Adenoid 296
    cystic carcinoma 142, 143*f*, 192, 193*f*, 194*f*, 207, 210, 354, 354*f*, 362, 409
    hypertrophy 361
        chronic 276, 296
Advanced trauma life support 249
AFRS *See* Allergic fungal rhinosinusitis
AFS *See* Allergic fungal sinusitis
Agger nasi 44
    cell 20, 21*f*, 42, 52, 70
AIFRS *See* Acute invasive fungal rhinosinusitis
Air cell 361
Allergic aspergillus sinusitis 308*f*
Allergic bronchopulmonary aspergillosis 101, 307
Allergic fungal
    rhinosinusitis 113-115, 115*f*, 116
    sinusitis 79, 100, 100*f*, 102*f*, 108, 108*t*, 109*f*, 139, 297, 393, 393*f*, 399, 399*f*, 413*f*
Allergic inflammatory sinusitis 141*f*
Allergic rhinitis 237
Allergic rhinosinusitis 94, 95
    diagnosis 94
    prevalence of 94
    treatment 95
Allergic sinusitis 140
    gross pathology 140
    histopathology 140
Allergy 363
    testing 94
Ameloblastoma 150, 338, 339*f*, 340*f*, 401*f*, 403, 412*f*
American Academy of Otolaryngology-Head and Neck Surgery 3
American College of Radiology 4
American Joint Committee on Cancer Staging System 202
Amino acid metabolism 100
Amyloidosis 309
Aneurysmal bone cyst 150, 156, 156*f*, 170, 171*f*, 286
    histopathology 156
Angiography 390
Angioinvasive fungal sinusitis 106
Angioma 363
Angiomatous polyp 411*f*
Anosmia 183
Anterior skull base 36
    arachnoid cyst 93
    fractures 317
    lesions 316
    meningioma 93
Antibiotics 96
Antihistaminics 95
Antral lavage examination 73
Apert's syndrome 332, 333
Aplasias 264
Aplastic anomalies 293
Arch 235
Arhinia 293
Arteriovenous malformation 386*f*, 387
    high flow 386*f*

Aspergillosis 106, 111f, 363
Aspergillus 99, 110, 116, 139, 140
   flavus 107
   fumigatus 103, 107, 307
   sinusitis 307
Aspirin 384
Asthma 308
ATLS *See* Advanced trauma life support
Atresia 266
Atretic anomalies 294
Atrophic rhinitis 71, 73f, 370f
Atypical retention cyst 362
Autosomal recessive
   disorder 306
   inheritance 306
AVMS *See* Arteriovenous malformations

B

Bacteria, gram-negative 310
Bacterial infection
   chronic 296
   secondary 95
Bacterial rhinosinusitis, chronic 296
Barotrauma 60
Basal cavity 16
Basal cell carcinoma 200f, 379f
Basal encephaloceles 319
   characteristics of 291t
Basal lamella 15, 48
Beam radiotherapy, external 212
Behcet disease 309
Benzodiazepines 362
Bicoronal incision 251
Biopsy 258
Bisphosphonate 186, 345
Black turbinate sign 106
Bone 235
   benign tumors of 168
   destruction 398f
   erosion 72, 122
      lesions based on 397fc
   expansion 122
   marrow transplant recipients 307
   sclerosis 122, 396f
   tumors of 160, 198
   windows 8

Bowel disease, inflammatory 308
Brachytherapy 212
Brain
   herniation 245f
   parenchyma 122, 245f
Broad aseptate fungal hyphae 139f
Bronchiectasis, extensive 307f
Brown tumors 168
Bulla ethmoidalis 21f, 35f, 44, 48, 52
Burkitt's lymphoma 197

C

Caldwell-Luc procedures 186
Candida 140
Canine fossa 76
Canthal tendon, medial 231t
Canthus masses, medial 284
Carcinoma 137, 138, 143
   alveolus infiltrating maxillary sinus 189f
   in situ 203
   palate eroding into maxillary sinus 344f
Carotid artery
   external 383, 390
   internal 122, 383, 414
   systems
      external 383f
      internal 383f
Carotid canal 46
Cartilage
   benign tumors of 168
   tumors of 160, 198
Cartilaginous sinonasal tumors, pathology of 150
Catarrhal stage 311
Cavernous hemangioma 142
Cavernous sinus 101
   thrombosis 271
Cells
   frontoethmoidal 20
   inflammatory 142f
   layer, epithelial 142f
   lymphomas 146
Cellular stroma 142f, 143f
Cellulitis 61f
Cemento-ossifying fibroma 152

Cephalocele 91, 403
    classification, anterior 319
Cerebellar tonsils, low-lying 246
Cerebral abscess 61*f*, 62, 231
Cerebrospinal fluid 236, 245*f*, 319, 321, 366, 412
    leak 118, 236, 238, 246
    rhinorrhea 4, 129, 231, 231*f*, 247*fc*, 249, 251
        causes of 242, 251
        investigations 252
        management 252
        signs 252
        symptoms 252
        traumatic 243*f*, 244*f*
Cervical lymphadenopathy 196
CGCGs *See* Central giant cell granulomas
Chemoradiotherapy, concurrent 211
Chemotherapy 202, 209, 213
Chloroma 198, 286
Choanal atresia 259, 266, 295
Choanal polyps 80
    types of 82*t*
Cholesterol crystals 85
Cholesterol granuloma 85
Chondroblastoma 150
Chondroma 150
Chondromyxoid fibroma 150
Chondrosarcoma 150, 157, 157*f*, 158, 189, 199, 200*f*, 369, 403*f*, 405*f*, 409, 410*f*
    histological features 157
    primary 199
    secondary 199
Chordoma 150, 362, 369
Churg-Strauss syndrome 306, 309
CIFS *See* Chronic invasive fungal sinusitis
Ciliary dyskinesia, primary 295, 306, 307*f*
Clopidogrel 384
Cocaine abuse 72
COF *See* Cemento-ossifying fibroma
Computed tomography 59, 228
    axial image 267*f*
    cisternography 238
    techniques 8*t*

Concha bullosa 11*f*, 17*f*, 70, 361
Conchal sphenoid sinus 37
Cone-beam computed tomography 11*f*
    advantages of 11*t*
    disadvantages of 11*t*
Contrast enhanced
    computed tomography 202, 273*f*, 409
    magnetic resonance imaging 65, 202, 409
Contrast magnetic resonance cisternography 240, 241*f*
Coronal computed tomography image 307*f*, 308*f*
Coronal contrast enhanced computed tomography 269*f*
Coronal soft tissue window 8
Cosmetic recontouring surgery 186
Cranial nerve palsy 271
Craniofacial clefts 294
Craniofacial resection 206
Craniopharyngeal wall, lateral 37
Cribriform plate 44, 235, 242, 321
    anatomy 122
    defects of 366
    disruption 231
    superior 15*f*
Crista galli 32*f*, 34*f*, 44, 48, 366
Crouzon's syndrome 92*f*, 332, 333
Cryptococcus 140
CSB *See* Central skull base
CSF *See* Cerebrospinal fluid
Cushing's syndrome 207
Cyst
    dentigerous 336*f*, 401*f*, 403, 403
    dermoid 261, 270*f*, 291, 292, 316, 321, 321*t*, 362, 403
    epidermoid 261, 284, 316, 362, 403
    glial-lined 319
Cystic lesion
    hypodense 379*f*
    mixed solid 340*f*

D

Dacryocystitis 231, 268*f*, 284
Dacryocystocele 270*f*, 284
    congenital 268, 270*t*
    infected bilateral 269*f*

Dental
  caries 333
  etiology 332
  infection 73, 333, 334f
  lesions, imaging of 332
Dermoid cyst, intranasal 278
Diabetes mellitus 387
Diagnostic provocative tests 94
Diethylenetriaminepentaacetic acid 241
Diffusion weighted imaging 12, 192
Digital subtraction angiography 130
Diplopia 202
DNS *See* Deviated nasal septum
Drainage pathways, obstruction of 66
DSA *See* Digital subtraction angiography
Duct, frontonasal 235
Dutcher body 159
Dysphagia 213

E

ECA *See* External carotid artery
Empty nose syndrome 132
Encephalocele 284, 291, 292, 321, 321t
  congenital frontoethmoidal 245f
  intranasal 280
Endophthalmitis 351
Endoscopic sinus surgery 118, 127, 130t, 185
  imaging, pre-functional 118, 119
  post-functional 107f, 118, 126127t
Enophthalmos 231
Epidural abscess 231
Epiphora 231
Epistaxis 390f, 391f
  anterior 388
  causes of 384t
  epidemiology 382
  etiology 384
  hypertensive 389f
  idiopathic 387f
  investigations 385
  management 387
  posterior 388
  prevention 391

  recurrent 86
  relevant anatomy 382
Epithelial tumors, benign 161, 172
Epstein-Barr virus 143
ESS *See* Endoscopic sinus surgery
Esthesioneuroblastoma 362, 369, 366f, 402f
Ethmoid
  bony margins, left posterior 79f
  cells, posterior 35f, 36
  roof of 238f
  sinuses
    malignancy 204t
    right 351f
  skull base height, posterior 35f
  trabeculae
    deossification of 70f
    sclerosis of 66f
    thinning of 79f
Ethmoidal air cell, anterior 21f, 23
Ethmoidal artery
  anterior 231
  canal, anterior 31f
  posterior 231
Ethmoidal bulla, enlarged 70
Ethmoidal cells
  anterior 21f, 24f, 25f
  frontal 70
  infraorbital 122
  posterior 35f, 36f, 46, 50
  supaorbital 124
Ethmoidal sinuses, anterior 18
Ethmoidectomy
  anterior 119
  posterior 119
  procedures, external 186
Ewing sarcoma 189, 195, 286
Expansile cystic lesion, unilocular 336f
Expansile mass lesion 342, 371f
Expansile polypoidal soft tissue bilateral ethmoids 79
Eye
  congestion of 213
  proptosis, right 115f
Eyebrow, loss of 213
Eyelash, loss of 213

F

Face fractures
  middle third 251
  upper-third 251
Facial
  artery, left 387f
  deformity 186
  fractures 251, 356t
    complex 231t
    complications of 232t
  hair loss 213
  injuries, complex 221
  pain 202
  swelling 202
  trauma 249
FD *See* Fibrous dysplasia
FESS *See* Functional endoscopic sinus surgery
Fibroma 364
Fibrosis, cystic 271, 295, 306, 362
Fibrous capsule, development of 85
Fibrous dysplasia 93, 150, 155, 155f, 176, 177f, 179, 179t, 180f, 186, 286, 288, 289, 343, 343f, 364, 400f, 413f
  histologic features 155
  management of 186
Fibrovascular stroma 152
FLAIR *See* Fluid-attenuated inversion recovery
Fluid-attenuated inversion recovery 351fc
Foley catheters 389
Foramen rotundum 46
Fossa, infratemporal 106f, 191f
Fovea ethmoidalis 33, 34f, 235, 238f
Fracture
  anterior skull base 242f
  comminuted 225
  complex 225
  fragment 232f
  frontobasal 322, 322f
Frontal sinus 18, 18f, 42, 44, 48, 121, 185, 235, 242, 261, 402f, 403, 412, 413f
  drainage pathway 19, 20f, 21, 21f, 44
  fracture 227, 227f, 232
  hypoplastic 260f
  ostium 19
  posterior wall fracture, left 227f
Frontobasal fractures, classification of 322
Frontoethmoidal air cells, types of 22f
Frontoethmoidectomy 184
FSDP *See* Frontal sinus drainage pathway
Functional endoscopic sinus surgery 16, 97, 118, 119, 132t, 296
  basic principles 119
  complications of 129
  early complications 129
  immediate complications 129
  indications 119
  late complications 132
  orbital complications 129
  rare complications 132
  steps of surgery 119
Fundus 183
Fungal ball 102, 114
Fungal diseases 113
  classification 113
  diagnosis 116
  treatment 116
Fungal infection 79f, 362
  invasive 302
  superadded 79
Fungal rhinosinusitis 375f
  invasive 114, 412
Fungal sinusitis 74, 99, 111, 140, 351, 396f, 404f, 405f
  acute invasive 104, 104f, 105f, 116f
  chronic invasive 107, 107t, 108, 108t, 109f, 306f, 394f
  chronic nongranulomatous invasive 111, 111f
  classification of 99
  complicated 106f
  imaging modalities 100
  invasive 4, 99, 104, 107f, 115, 117, 139, 351, 351f, 398f
  noninvasive 99, 100
  symptoms 104
  types 100

Fungiform papilloma 162
Fungus balls 113
Furstenberg sign 320

G

Gastroesophageal reflux disease 272, 295
GC *See* Gigantiform cementoma
GCRG *See* Giant cell reparative granuloma
GCT *See* Giant cell tumors
GERD *See* Gastroesophageal reflux disease
Germ cell tumor 160, 286
Giant cell 156f
 granuloma 341
  central 150, 151, 151f, 158
 lesions 168
 reparative granuloma 168, 170f, 341, 342f, 394f
 tumor 168, 169, 170f
Gigantiform cementoma 152
Gillies incision 251
Glands, admixture of 142f
Glioceles 319
Glioma 291, 292, 362
 intranasal 280
Globe injury 231
Glomangiopericytoma 146f, 164, 165f
Glucocorticosteroids, topical 95
GnRH *See* Gonadotropin-releasing hormone
Gorlin-Goltz syndrome 338, 338f
Gossypiboma 130, 132
GPA *See* Granulomatosis with polyangiitis
Granulomas 363
Granulomatosis 140, 141, 302, 305, 313, 362, 377, 396f, 398f
Granulomatous disease 309, 311, 363
Granulomatous disorders 79, 309, 311
Granulomatous invasive fungal sinusitis, chronic 107, 110f
Grunwald, interlamellar cell of 70
Guitar-Pick sign 351

H

Haemophilus influenzae 95, 139
Haller cell 25f, 70f, 122
Halo sign 252
Hamartoma 273, 362
Hard palate 46, 50
Head and neck tumours, classification of 137
Headache 183, 186
Hemangioma 142, 165, 282, 362, 408f
 aggressive 286
 capillary 142, 273f
 intraosseous 166
 sphenoid sinus 166f
Hemangiopericytoma 326, 329
Hematolymphoid 138
 neoplasms 196
 tumors 146, 160, 189
Hematoma 86
Heminasal aplasia 292f, 293
Hemoglobinopathy 345
Hemophilia 384
 A 175
 B 175
Hemorrhage, intraorbital 130
High-resolution computed tomography, normal 238f
Holman-Miller sign 174
HPV *See* Human papilloma virus
Human papilloma virus 137, 148
Hyperostosis 120
Hyperparathyroidism 189
Hyperplasias 264
Hypersinus 91
Hypertension, intracranial idiopathic 246f
Hypertrophy 276, 306
Hypoplasia 74, 75f, 76t, 264
Hyposmia 183

I

ICA *See* Internal carotid artery
Idiopathic intracranial hypertension, radiological signs of 246t
IFS *See* Invasive fungal sinusitis

IMA *See* Internal maxillary artery
Immunodeficiency, severe combined 302
Immunotherapy 95
Inappropriate antidiuretic hormone secretion, syndrome of 207
Infantile frontonasal capillary hemangioma 272
Infection 302, 348
  intracranial 231
  severe 349
Infectious rhinosinusitis, recurrent acute 95
Inflammatory disorders 348, 352
  chronic 303
  gamut of 301
Influenza 139
Injuries, intracranial 130
Intracranial tumors, primary 329*t*
Intrasinus synechiae 271
Ipsilateral metastatic lymph node
  multiple 204
  single 204
Itraconazole 117

J

JPOF *See* Juvenile psammomatoid ossifying fibroma
JTOF *See* Juvenile trabecular ossifying fibroma
Juvenile nasopharyngeal angiofibroma 173, 173*fc*, 174*f*, 175*f*, 186, 263, 354*f*, 362, 372*f*, 373, 381, 385*f*, 390*f*, 391*f*, 396*f*, 405*f*, 408*f*, 410*f*
  extension of 414*f*
Juvenile ossifying fibroma 401*f*, 407*f*, 153
Juvenile psammomatoid ossifying fibroma 152, 154, 154*f*
Juvenile trabecular ossifying fibroma 152

K

Kallmann syndrome 321
Keratocystic odontogenic tumor 336, 337*f*, 394*f*, 401*f*, 403, 412*f*
  multiple 338*f*

Keros classification 31
Kiesselbach's plexus 384
Klebsiella ozaenae 72
Klebsiella rhinoscleromatis 310
KOT *See* Keratocystic odontogenic tumor

L

Lacrimal drainage system, disruption of 130
Lacrimal duct injury 231
Lacrimal sac injury 231
Lamella
  lateral 44, 46
  medial 44, 46
Lamina papyracea 15, 16*f*, 25*f*, 27, 30*f*, 35, 44, 46, 122, 129, 235
  bulging of 79*f*
Large B-cell lymphoma, diffuse 197*f*, 398*f*
Le Fort fractures 221, 223*f*
  types of 222*f*, 222*t*
Leprosy 140, 302, 303*f*
Lesions
  benign 398, 399*t*, 410*f*
  congenital 332
  cystic 400, 402*f*, 403*t*
  density of 399
  fibro-osseous 176, 179, 341
  inflammatory 139
  malignant 399*t*, 410*f*
Leukemia
  acute 198
    myelocytic 276*f*
  clinical background of 198*f*
Ligation techniques 390
Lipoblastoma 273
Lipodermoid 284
Lipogranuloma 132
Lobular capillary hemangioma 142
Lund-Mackay system, modified 65
Lupus vulgaris 363
Lymph node
  contralateral metastatic 204
  involvement 211
  regional 204
Lymphatic spread pathway 210, 210*t*

Lymphoepithelial carcinoma 143
Lymphoid tissue, mucosa-associated 158
Lymphoma 189, 196, 197f, 286, 362, 398f, 404f
  B-cell type 196
Lymphovascular invasion 211
Lynch incision 184, 185f

M

Macroadenomas 326
Magnetic resonance
  cisternography 239
  imaging 59, 192, 321, 337f
    of paranasal sinuses 12f
    planning 12t
Mandible, irregular lytic-sclerotic destruction of 214f
Mapping sinus involvement 120
Markowitz and Manson classification 225
Masses 335
  benign 286
  congenital 277fc
  differential diagnosis of 284
  frontonasal 282
  lesion, heterogeneous 191f, 193f, 195f
  malignant 286
  with intense enhancement 408f
  with mild-moderate enhancement 407f
Maxilla
  frontonasal process of 19
  osteonecrosis of 344, 345f, 346f
Maxillary alveolus, bony scalloping of 379f
Maxillary antrum
  infrastructure of 210
  suprastructure of 210
Maxillary artery, internal 390
Maxillary bone 39, 195f
Maxillary buttress
  lateral 220, 221f
  medial 220, 221f
  posterior 220, 221f
Maxillary cancer 209
Maxillary dentition, abnormal 266

Maxillary fracture, posterior 229f, 232
Maxillary mucosal disease, right 61f
Maxillary nonseminomatous germ cell tumor 401f
Maxillary ostium 21f, 27f, 30f, 44, 46, 371f
  abnormal 30f
  plane of 30f
Maxillary sinus 15, 25, 42, 63, 68f, 80f, 121, 174, 185, 201, 212, 235, 261, 304, 332, 401f, 403, 410
  anatomy of 24
  bilateral 12f, 64f, 260f
  cancers 209
  carcinoma 190f
  diseases, bilateral 346
  fractures 229, 229f
  granulocytic sarcoma, left 276f
  hypoplastic 70
  left 26f
  malignancy 202, 203t, 204t
  medial wall of 16f
  mucosa 203
  mucosal thickening, hyperintense bilateral 13f
  opacified left 68f
  ostium 69
  parts of 42
  right 371f
  roof fractures 232
  roof of 35f
  small 75f
  superior wall of 26f
Maxillary sinusitis 333, 334f
  bilateral 104f
  chronic left 74f
Maxillectomy 186
  infrastructural 206
  medial 184, 205, 205f
  posterior 206
  total 184, 206, 206f
Maxillofacial trauma 219
Meatal antrostomy, middle 119
Meatus
  inferior 44, 46
  middle 44, 46
Medial rectus muscle entrapment 230f

Melanoma 195, 404f
    malignant 362
Meningioma 329, 362, 410f
Meningitis 61f, 231
Meningoceles 246
Meningoencephalocele 290
    frontonasal 402f
Mesenchymal cells 151f
Mesenchymal tumors 362
Messerklinger technique 119
Metastasis 199, 286, 328, 362
Metastatic lymph node 204
    bilateral 204
Metastatic lymphadenopathy, low
    incidence of 192
Methyl green-pyronin 159
Midface
    anomalies 261
    hypoplasia 92f
Midnasal stenosis 294
Mikulicz cells 311
Moraxella catarrhalis 139
Mouth, dryness of 213
MRI *See* Magnetic resonance imaging
Mucocele 77, 87, 91f, 126, 186, 286, 394f,
    402f, 403, 413f, 414f
    causes of 90
    ethmoidal 90f
    frontal 88f, 89f, 407f
    secondary 91f
Mucociliary deficiency 271
Mucormycosis 104f, 106, 107f, 303f, 363
Mucosal atrophy 73f
Mucosal disease 349f
Mucosal lesions 344
Mucosal thickening 64
    inflammatory 90
Mucositis, esophageal 213
Mucous form 85
Multidetector computed tomography
    120t, 219, 265
Muscle injury, extraocular 130
Muscle, extraocular 351
Mycetoma 102, 103f, 113, 114, 116, 394f,
    399, 399f, 407f, 411, 411f
Myeloma, multiple 197

Myeloproliferative disorders, spectrum
    of 198
Myoepithelial cell layer 142f
Myofibroblastic tumor, inflammatory
    164, 165f

N

Nasal bone 42, 238f, 235
    comminuted fracture
        bilateral 228f
        right 228f
    fracture 227, 232
        left 228f
    hemangioma 167f
    hypoplastic 264f
Nasal cavity 14, 57, 79f, 80f, 191f, 209,
    210, 235, 274f, 311, 369, 373t
    anatomy of 15
    anomalies 265
    anterior 387f
    boundaries 15f
    lateral wall of 16f
    lesions 370f
        causing obstruction 371f
    masses 278, 280, 372f
    right 371f
    superior 366f
    tumors of 209
    vascular polyp of 312f
    walls of 259
Nasal conditions, inflammatory 55
Nasal cycle, physiological 361
Nasal decongestants 363
    topical 95
Nasal dermal sinus 261, 316
    tract 278
Nasal dermoid 292f
Nasal discharge 182
    causes of 237
Nasal duct pathway, frontal 122
Nasal encephalocele 261
Nasal endoscopy 96
Nasal glioma 261, 280, 317
Nasal hair loss 213
Nasal lesions
    common erosive 377fc
    external 378f

Nasal melanoma 213f
Nasal mucosal atrophy 306
Nasal obstruction 182, 201, 361
  causes of 362t
  clinical
    examination 363
    presentation 361
    diagnostic imaging 364
Nasal packs 388
  anterior 389
  posterior 389
Nasal polyps 77
  etiology 77
  imaging 78
  pathology 78
Nasal pyriform aperture stenosis 294
  congenital 265, 265f
Nasal septal
  destruction 376f
  deviation 17f
  lesions 374, 374t
  perforation 131f
    without mass lesions 375f
Nasal septum 16, 42, 44, 46, 122, 130, 185, 304, 365
  blood supply of 383f
  destruction of 309f, 311
  deviated 70, 122
  injury 227, 313
  parts 16f
Nasal sinus 318f
Nasal turbinates 17, 191f
  destruction of 197f
Nasal vestibule 210, 212
  left 379f
  lesions of 379f
Nasal wall
  lateral 185
  lesions, lateral 373t
Nasoalveolar cyst 379f
Nasobuccal membrane, developmental errors of 295
Nasociliary groove 228f
Nasoethmoidal cephalocele 319
Nasoethmoidal encephalocele 320f
Nasoethmoidal lesions 365
Nasoethmoidal masses 368f, 369t
  of bony origin 367f

Nasoethmoidal polyposis 79f
Nasofrontal cephalocele 319
Nasofrontal encephalocele 319f
Nasofrontal suture 220
Nasolacrimal apparatus anomalies 268
Nasolacrimal duct 42, 48, 50, 259, 263, 270, 311, 354, 354f, 362
  bilateral cystic dilatation of 269f
  block 72
  dilatation 269
  inflammation 350f
  melanoma 355f
  stenosis 268, 268f
Nasomaxillary suture 228f
Naso-orbital encephalocele 319
Naso-orbitoethmoid complex fractures 225, 225f, 231
Naso-orbitoethmoid fracture 221, 225f, 226f, 228f
Nasopharyngeal
  angiofibroma 138, 142, 143f
  carcinoma 191f, 373
  mucosal inflammation 306
  soft tissue, posterior 277f
  tumors, benign 173
Nasopharynx 122, 364
  angiofibroma 364
  carcinoma 364
Natural killer T-cell lymphoma 147f, 197f, 309f
NB See Neuroblastoma
NEC See Neuroendocrine carcinoma
Neck
  dissection 203
  nodes, regional 204t
  swelling 202
Necrosis, avascular 304
Neo-osteogenesis 396f
Neoplastic lesions
  benign 141
  malignant 143
Neovascularization, subsequent 85
Nerve
  canal, infraorbital 25, 76
  entrapment, infraorbital 230f
  sheath tumor, nasal benign 274f, 282
Neuroblastoma 148, 286

Neuroectodermal malignancies 195
Neuroectodermal tumor 160
　malignant 147
Neuroendocrine carcinoma 148
Neurofibroma 167, 169f, 371f
Neurofibromatosis 167
Neuropore errors, types of anterior 292t
Neutrophils 145f
Nodular mucosal thickening 304
Nonallergic rhinitis 363
Noncontrast computed tomography 59, 80, 80f, 275f, 346
Nonenhancing masses 407f
Nongranulomatous disease 107t
Non-Hodgkin's lymphoma 146, 147f, 398f
Non-intestinal adenocarcinoma 146f
Non-keratinizing squamous cell carcinoma 143, 144f
Non-neoplastic
　lesions 137, 139
　sinonasal lesions 138t
Nonodontogenic lesions 333, 341
Nonpneumatized frontal sinus 19f
Nonpneumatized sphenoid sinus 37
Nonsteroidal anti-inflammatory drugs 308, 387
Nontraumatic cerebrospinal fluid 317
　rhinorrhea 324
Nose 113, 204t, 363
　benign tumors of 160, 363
　causing epistaxis 386f
　congenital malformations of 290
　external 378, 380t
　lesions, external 380
NSAIDs *See* Nonsteroidal anti-inflammatory drugs

O

Obstructive right maxillary sinusitis 90f
Obstructive sinusitis 186
OCS *See* Orbital compartment syndrome
Odontogenic cysts 335
Odontogenic lesions 333
　large 407f

Odontogenic myxoma 340, 341f
Olfactory bulb 32f
Olfactory fossa 44, 46
　anatomy of 31
　bilateral deep 128f
　boundaries 32f
　types of 33f
Olfactory nerve injury 324
Olfactory neuroblastoma 147, 147f, 207
Olfactory neuroepithelium, basal cell of 207
Olfactory schwannoma 328f
OMU *See* Osteomeatal unit
Oncocytic papilloma 163
Onodi cells 36, 36f, 122, 124
Opaque maxillary sinus, small 71f
Opaque sinus 75f, 76
Ophthalmic injuries 130
Optic canal 46, 235
Optic nerve 355
　anatomy 122
　canal 38f
　injury 130, 231
Optic neuritis, infectious 271
Oral azole antifungals 117
Orbit 235, 348t
　boundaries of 39f
　enlargement of 71f, 75f
　granulocytic sarcoma of 198f
　ipsilateral 195f
Orbital abscess 349
Orbital apex 46
　syndrome 231
Orbital blowout fracture 229, 232
　right inferior 230f
Orbital cellulitis, right 350f
Orbital compartment syndrome 349
Orbital complication 60, 129
　evolution of 350, 350fc
Orbital extension 311
Orbital fissure
　inferior 61f, 235, 354, 354f
　syndrome 231, 235
　widening of inferior 168
Orbital nerve
　canal, inferior 26f, 44
　inferior 44

Orbital penetration, risk of 25
Orbital plane, mid 34*f*
Orbital pseudotumor 352
Orbital wall blowout fracture, left inferior 230*f*
Oroantral fistula 74*f*
    post-tooth extraction 334*f*
Oronasal fistula 333
Orthopantogram 335, 339
Ossifying fibroma 91*f*, 150, 152, 153*f*, 177, 179, 179*t*, 180*f*, 186, 286, 288, 289, 342, 343*f*, 364, 407, 413
Osteitis 79*f*
Osteoblastoma 150, 171
Osteochondroma 150
Osteoclastic multinucleated giant cells 151*f*
Osteoid osteoma 150
Osteoma 150, 152, 152*f*, 171, 286, 362, 364, 400*f*, 413*f*
    frontoethmoidal 172*f*
Osteomeatal complex 27*f*, 78*f*, 119
    widening of 79*f*
Osteomeatal unit 127
    anatomy of 26
    components of 44
    pattern 68*f*
    widening of 64*f*, 70*f*
Osteomyelitis 271, 394, 396, 396*f*
Osteonecrosis 189
Osteoradionecrosis 213, 214*f*, 396*f*
Osteosarcoma 150, 189, 199
Ostium block 411*f*
Otolaryngological procedures 244
Otolaryngology 96
Otorrhea 236

P

Pain, severe 186
Palatine bone 39
Palliative radiotherapy 211
Pamidronate 186
Panoramic radiography 346
Papilloma 362, 363
    antrochoanal 82*t*
    inverted 82*t*, 142*f*, 161, 162*f*, 185, 363, 371*f*, 373, 405*f*, 408*f*, 411*f*
    recurrent inverted 163*f*
    squamous 363
Paradoxical middle turbinate 70
Parainfluenza viruses 139
Paranasal sinuses 3, 5*t*, 7*f*, 15, 113, 146, 160, 191*f*, 201, 307*f*, 364
    computed tomography of 8
    development of 259
    maturation of 260*t*
    radiograph of 6*f*, 7*f*
    radiographic development of 259*f*, 260*f*
    tumors of 209
Parathormone 168
Pediatric chronic sinusitis 271
Pediatric sinonasal disorders 257
    classification of 261, 262*t*
    congenital 261
    inflammatory 270
    masses 263*fc*
Perineural invasion 211
Periodic acid-Schiff stains 139*f*
Periodontitis 333
Periorbital lipogranuloma 130
Periostitis 61*f*
Peripheral hypodensity 102*f*
Peripheral nerve sheath tumors 167
Persistent sinonasal disease 332
Pharynx 57
Pituitary macroadenoma 92*f*, 326, 329
    extension of 414*f*
Plain magnetic resonance cisternography, normal 241*f*
Planum sphenoidale 321
    meningioma 325*f*
Plasma cell
    mature 158
    neoplasm 189, 197
Plasmacytoma 150, 158, 158*f*
    differential diagnosis 159
    histopathology 158
    of nasal bone 158*f*
Pleomorphic adenoma 141, 142*f*, 163, 164*f*, 362, 405*f*

PNET *See* Primitive neuroectodermal tumor
Pneumatized basal lamella 124
Pneumocele 92
Pneumocephalus 244f
Pneumosinus 91
  dilatans 91, 92f
Polyangiitis 140, 141, 302, 303, 305, 313, 362, 377, 396f, 398f
Polyarteritis nodosa 306
Polychondritis 305
Polycyclic hydrocarbons 201
Polyp
  antrochoanal 82, 286, 297, 394f, 408f, 411, 411f
  basis of imaging appearance of 81t
  ethmoidochoanal 83f, 84
Polypoid mucosal disease 64f
Polypoidal mass 81f, 83f
Polypoidal soft tissue 313
Polyposis 79f, 97, 286, 370f
  diagnosis 97
  treatment 97
Polyps 77
  inflammatory 405f
Polyrhinia 264
Positron emission tomography 4, 192
Postcontrast slight enhancement 269
Postembolization angiogram 387f
Posterolateral wall 235
Posteromedial wall 235
Post-FESS
  appearance 128f
  complications 131f
  contralateral disease 129f
  polyp recurrence 128f
Postviral infection 345
Pott's puffy tumor 62, 271, 412
Premaxillary soft tissue, left 104f
Primitive neuroectodermal tumor 195, 196f, 353f, 376
Proboscis lateralis 264, 264f, 294
Proptosis 202
Psammomatoid bodies 154
Pseudoaneurysm 130
Pseudotumor 352f
  hemophilic 175, 176f, 275, 275f
  inflammatory 165f

Pterygoid plate 46, 220, 224f, 229f, 235
  medial 46
Pterygoid tubercle 229f
Pterygomaxillary fissure 385f
  widening of 385f
Pterygopalatine fossa 235, 385f
Purulent nasal discharge 363
Pyogenic granuloma 142
Pyomyositis 271
Pyriform aperture 259

R

Radiation 209, 213
  dermatitis 213
  dose, lower 11
Radioallergosorbent test 94
Radiofrequency ablation 127
Radionuclide cisternography 241
Radiotherapy 202, 211
  adjuvant 211
  intensity-modulated 212
  management, site-specific 212t
  treatment, modes of 212t
Radkowski staging 186, 187t
Rectus muscle, inferior 356f
Red nasal mucosa 363
Respiratory
  disease, aspirin-exacerbated 308
  tract infection, recurrent upper 271
Restricted diffusion 410f
Retention cyst 84, 85f, 395f, 401f, 402f, 403
RFA *See* Radiofrequency ablation
Rhabdomyosarcoma 189, 198, 263, 286
Rhinitis 306, 362
  medicamentosa 362
Rhinolith 364, 373
Rhino-orbito-cerebral mucormycosis 101f
Rhinorrhea 130, 236, 246f, 317
Rhinoscleroma 138, 309, 310, 373, 411
Rhinosinusitis 57, 138, 270, 295, 362, 363, 373
  acute 296
  infectious 95
  invasive 116

bacterial 296, 412
chronic 62, 65, 66f, 67t, 78, 94, 95, 97, 98t, 370f, 393, 393f, 394f, 396f, 411f
    infectious 95
    invasive 115
    forms of 100
    infectious 95, 96t
    infective 139
    treatment, chronic infectious 96
Rhinosporidiosis 138, 139, 140f, 311, 312f, 364, 373
Rhinosporidium 140
    seeberi 139, 311
Rhinotomy
    incision, lateral 184, 185f
    lateral 186
Rhinovirus 139
Rhizopus 116
Root of nose, region of 277fc
Russell bodies 311

S

Salivary gland
    tumors 138, 141
    type adenomas 163
Samter's triad 308
Sarcoid 363
Sarcoidosis 304
Sarcoma
    fibromyxoid 409
    granulocytic 189, 198
Sarcomatoid 143
SCC *See* Squamous cell carcinoma
Schwannoma 167, 362
Scleroma, histopathology of 310
Sclerosis 66f, 305f
    bony 368f
Sclerotic bone, hypointense 305f
Sellar sphenoid sinus 37
Septal cartilage 232
Septal deviation 16
Septal pneumatization 17
    posterior 17f
Septal spurs 17

Septum
    bony 26f
    cartilaginous 42
    fibroangioma of 363
Shock, electric 345
SIADH *See* Syndrome of inappropriate antidiuretic hormone secretion
Sickle cell anemia 345
Silent sinus syndrome 68, 71f, 75f, 76t
Silver methenamine stains 139f
Silver nitrate 388
Sincipital encephaloceles, characteristics of 291t
Sinonasal
    anatomy
        section-wise 41
        structure-wise 14
    angiomatous polyp 85, 87f, 394f, 405f, 408f, 411
    cancers 209t
    carcinoma 195f
    cavity 14, 93, 236, 301, 302, 302fc, 332, 333t, 341, 348t
        bilateral 70f
    chloroma 275
    complications 130
    diseases 4
    epithelium and cysts 142f
    fractures 221
    glomangiopericytoma 145
    infections, diagnosis of 140t
    inflammation, chronic 311
    inflammatory pathology 3
    injuries, bony 250
    lesions
        classification of 138
        congenital 366
        hyperdense 399f
        of heterogeneous density 401f
        of osseous density 400f
        pathology of 137
    malignancy 188, 210t, 211, 211t
    malignant tumors 148fc
    nerve sheath tumors 274
    neuroendocrine carcinoma 194
    organized hematoma 85
    origin, epithelial tumors of 202

papillomas 138, 141, 161
polyposis 60, 66, 70f, 77, 78f, 393
polyps 79, 140
sarcoma, biphenotypic 137, 145
schwannoma 282
tract 137, 196
trauma 219, 249
tuberculosis 73
tumors 160, 189, 207, 214
   benign 180, 182
   cartilaginous 150t
   classification of 150
   malignant 201, 202, 209
   of epithelial tumors, malignant 202
undifferentiated carcinoma 144
Sinus 195f
   angioma of 363
   drainage of 25
      pathways 70t
   drains 15
   ethmoid 23, 63f, 92f, 102f, 121, 185, 193f, 196f, 203t, 210, 235, 243f, 244f, 245f, 261, 308f, 309-311, 402f, 403
   expansion 235
   floor 235
   hypoplasia 25
   large air filled 91, 92f
   lesions 392
      laterality 393
   masses 286, 288
   normal size 395f
   opacification of 63f, 65, 235
   parts of frontal 42
   pneumatization of 121
   septae 235
      cell, interfrontal 22f, 70
   sets of 15
   size of 394
   walls, status of 120
   window 8, 102f
Sinusitis 12f, 13f, 73, 306, 408f, 416t
   acute 59, 60, 62t, 271, 395
   bacterial 396f
   chronic 4, 58f, 60, 72, 271, 395f, 399, 399f, 413f

   complicated acute 59, 348, 398f
   complication of 4, 61f
   ethmoid 307f
   intracranial complications of 61f
   orbital complication of 349f
   recurrent 4
      chronic 140
Sjögren's syndrome 306
Skull base
   complications 130
   foramina, widening of 246
   intact of 239f
   lesions
      anterior 317t
      congenital anterior 316
      median anterior 31, 36
Smell function 366
Soft palate 46
Soft tissue
   density 80f, 351f
      mass 164f
   edema 105
   injuries of face 250
   mass 200f
      expansile 78f, 79f
      hyperdense 276f
      mild 396f
      opacification 370f
      premaxillary 335f
   thickening 303
   tumors of 160, 198
      benign 138, 165
      low malignant potential 164
      malignant 138, 145
      nasopharynx 138
   windows 8
Solitary fibrous tumor 326, 329
Sphenochoanal polyp 84
Sphenoethmoidal recess 37, 37f, 69f, 122
   obliteration of 69f
Sphenoethmoidal region 412
   disease entities of 414f
Sphenoid 127
   bone, small 92f
   cells 50
   mucocele 89f
   mucosal enhancement 61f

ostium 50, 52
sinus 35f-37f, 38f, 46, 52, 83f, 107f,
    121, 185, 209, 210, 235, 242,
    245f, 261, 349f, 402f, 412
  anatomy of 36
  presellar 37
  types of 37f
Sphenoidotomy 127
  posterior 119
Sphenopalatine artery 383
Spindle cell 143
Spindle-shaped cells 154
Spontaneous cerebrospinal fluid 246f
  rhinorrhea 324
Spontaneous leaks 242, 246
Sprengel's deformity 338
Squamous cell carcinoma 143, 148, 189,
    201, 209, 353f, 362, 395f, 396f,
    407f, 411, 411f
  keratinizing 143, 144f
  of maxillary sinus 191f
  staging system 202
Stenosis 266
Streptococcus pneumoniae 95, 139
Stroma, edematous 140
Structured reporting format 121t
Subdural empyema 271
Subepithelial large sporangia 140f
Subfrontal schwannoma 327, 329
Subperiosteal abscess 61f, 271, 349f
Supernumerary nostril 264, 294
Supraorbital cells 24f
Surgery 184, 202
Symphysis menti 235
Synechiae 72
Syphilis 363
  infection 303
Systemic corticosteroids 95
Systemic disorders 299
  chronic 272
  classification of 302fc
Systemic lupus erythematosus 302, 306

T

T cells, nuclear factor of activated 151
Teeth, loosening of 202

Tegmen tympani 242
Telecanthus 231
Temporal fossa 193f
Temporal hairline 251
Temporalis muscle 106f
Tennis racket 340
Teratocarcinosarcoma 146
Teratoma 272
  mature 172
TESPAL *See* Transnasal endoscopic
    sphenopalatine artery ligation
Tetrapod fracture 226f, 231
Trabecular juvenile ossifying fibroma
    153
Transnasal endoscopic sphenopalatine
    artery ligation 390
Transsphenoidal encephalocele 320f
Transverse mandibular buttress, lower
    220, 220f
Transverse maxillary buttress, lower
    220, 220f
Transverse sinuses, stenosis of 246
Trauma 321, 355, 317
  complications 324
Treponema pallidum infection 303
Tuberculosis 140, 302, 363
Tumor 91f, 158, 204, 324, 348, 352, 401f
  benign 150, 151
  cartilaginous 158t
  cells 143f, 145f
  contiguous perineural extension of
      194f
  direct extension 352
  epithelial 160
  evaluation 4
  extension, intracranial 190
  fibro-osseous 186
  head and neck 160
  high grade 211
  like lesions 150
  location 210
  malignant 157
  meningioma 324
  node and metastasis staging 202,
      203t, 204t
  of nose, malignant 201

of sinonasal cavities, malignant 188
  spillage 211
Turbinate, inferior 42, 44, 46

U

Unilateral disease 394f
Unilateral maxillary sinus 411f, 412f
  disease 411fc
Unilocular cystic lesions, multiple 337f
Upper transverse
  mandibular buttress 220, 220f
  maxillary buttress 220, 220f

V

Vascular injury 130
Vascular tumors, benign 165
Vasculitides 140
Vasoconstriction, severe 72
Vertebral anomalies 338
Vessel vasculitides, types of small 141
Vestibular lesions 380, 380t
Vidian canal 46
Vision
  field of 183
  loss 231

Visual acuity 183
Vital structures, compression of 186
Volume rendering technique 10
Voriconazole 117

W

Wait and watch policy 184
Weber-Ferguson incision 184, 185f
Wegener's granulomatosis 137, 141, 362, 363
Widal's triad 308
Wigand technique 119
World Health Organization classification of sinonasal tumors 138t

Z

Zygoma 224f, 305f
Zygomatic bone 39, 223f, 226, 235
  erosion of 61f
Zygomaticofrontal suture 220, 226f
Zygomaticomaxillary
  complex fracture 221, 226, 231
  suture 226f, 235
Zygomaticotemporal suture 226f
Zygomycosis 139f, 140

EU GSPR Authorised Reprsentative
Logos Europe, 9 rue Nicolas Poussin
1700, La Rochelle, France
Phone: +33 (0) 6 67 93 73 78
E-mail: contact@logoseurope.eu